OP

Burt Alperson
1969

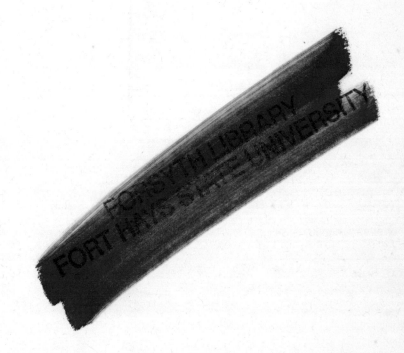

The Measurement of
Psychological States
Through the Content Analysis
of Verbal Behavior

The Measurement of Psychological States Through the Content Analysis of Verbal Behavior

by Louis A. Gottschalk, M.D.
and Goldine C. Gleser, Ph.D.

University of California Press
Berkeley and Los Angeles 1969

University of California Press
Berkeley and Los Angeles, California
University of California Press, Ltd.
London, England

FOREWORD

This book is a superb example of the application of diverse techniques to the understanding of human functioning and psychodynamics. The psychoanalytic techniques of skilled perception and empathic understanding of trends and hidden meanings, of seeing significant configurations and sequences, of understanding the intrapsychic and interpersonal forces at work, are used to develop categories of thematic content for the study of verbal productions. These categories, in turn, are treated by psychometric methods which translate the raw data of observation into sensitive quantitative scales. Furthermore, the data are collected using modern experimental design and are analyzed with the aid of statistical inference.

While a probabilistic approach is used in the quantification of content scales, it is used with imagination and appreciation for the subtleties of the psychodynamic concepts with which it deals. We have here, then, a significant development in the field of a scientific understanding of human behavior and psychodynamics, viz. a dialog (metaphorically speaking) between psychodynamic formulation and probability theory. Each contributes to the total understanding; each provides starting points for the other approach; each provides checks and corrects excesses in the other approach. Inherent in such a dialog, and perhaps the most important development in the field of psychodynamics, has been the increasing sophistication of both approaches.

In this and in other ways, this book represents work of the highest quality: original and creative. The book itself is a well-integrated report of an outstanding series of unique and significant investigations, and is, therefore, a major contribution.

The authors have different professional backgrounds and experience, but they have an extensive heritage in common. Their comment, using a lighthearted phrase to make an important point, is that both acquired a healthy skepticism from having been raised in the state of Missouri. Both are dedicated to empirical research, on direct observation, using a variety of techniques, as the "royal road" to increased knowledge.

In their approach, one central and productive emphasis is on the many potential uses of a meaningful content analysis in the systematic investigation of interindividual and intraindividual processes. It may even be possible with their method to make a quantitative and qualitative study of the sequential interplay of emotional states during an hour of psychotherapy.

In one phase of their work, they have used their content scales to explore several areas of possible relationship between immediate emotional states and biochemical and physiological functioning. These areas can be regarded as small samples of extraordinarily large areas which may be studied with comparable research techniques.

In brief, this book presents well-documented evidence that a systematic study of a five-minute verbal sample is highly productive. It serves also as convincing evidence that focused techniques can be devised which are applicable to many of the most important, most crucial questions in the field of psychiatry today.

Maurice Levine, M.D.
Professor and Chairman
Department of Psychiatry
College of Medicine
University of Cincinnati
Cincinnati, Ohio

PREFACE

History of the Development of
the Method of Content Analysis

The method of verbal content analysis presented in the following chapters had antecedents in earlier work of the authors.
Even prior to this collaborative endeavor, the senior author had
committed himself to the investigation of verbal behavior.

While a research associate at the Institute for Psychosomatic
and Psychiatric Research and Training of the Michael Reese Hospital in Chicago, Illinois (1948–1951), Dr. Gottschalk became
interested in exploring emotional factors that contribute to or trigger epileptic convulsions. It was during the process of these psychophysiological studies of epilepsy that he decided to pursue the
systematic and microscopic analysis of verbal behavior. Briefly,
the sequence of events that aroused his interest was the following.
He took three boys into psychotherapy; one, 17 years old, received psychoanalytic psychotherapy, and the other two, 4½ and
8 years old, received child psychoanalysis. The results of this
study (Gottschalk, 1953, 1956) provided strong evidence that
psychological factors played a causal role in the occurrence of
the epileptic seizures of these children. On moving to the National
Institute of Mental Health at Bethesda, Md., in June, 1951 to become a research psychiatrist there, Dr. Gottschalk decided to pursue further the psychophysiological factors in epilepsy. Dr. David
McK. Rioch, Director of the Division of Psychiatry and Neurology,
Post-Graduate School at the Walter Reed Army Institute of Research, made available to Dr. Gottschalk rich clinical material
and provided electroencephalographic laboratory facilities. Several longitudinal investigations were begun of military personnel
who had developed seizures during their tour of duty. Patients
were selected for study who had frequent discrete paroxysms
(about one every 2-3 minutes) of readily distinguishable high-

amplitude fast or slow waves in their electroencephalograms. The choice of subjects was based on the hope that it might be possible to relate the acute arousal of emotions and psychological conflicts to the abnormal, high-amplitude, paroxysmal brain waves. The experimental procedure that was used consisted of having patients free-associate while recording their electroencephalogram, electrocardiogram, electromyogram of gross muscular tension of upper and lower extremities, and galvanic skin response. The patients' free associations were tape-recorded and synchronized with the electrical findings. From these studies Dr. Gottschalk was able to make the observation that speaking as well as doing silent mental arithmetic tended to suppress the frequency of paroxysmal electroencephalographic activity and that the arousal of separation anxiety appeared to trigger many of the epileptic seizures of the patients (Gottschalk, 1955). He was dissatisfied, however, with the precision with which he could measure the intensity of separation anxiety or other affects of possible relevance to the abnormal, high-amplitude brain-wave activity from the patients' recorded free associations. It was, in fact, the problems encountered in measuring emotions and other psychological states from typescripts of speech obtained in the studies that led Dr. Gottschalk to resolve to pursue further the content analysis of speech.

At the National Institute of Mental Health he now teamed up with a long-time friend and fellow psychiatrist and psychoanalyst, Dr. Gove Hambidge, Jr., to pursue methods of analyzing and measuring communication processes. The two men explored a number of ways of eliciting and recording different channels for the communication of affects and other psychological states, for example, by lexical features in speech, by paralanguage features (vocalizations, voice quality, voice set), by linguistic features (junctures, stress, pitch), and by kinesic features (posture and gestures) of behavior. They studied tape recordings of speech obtained under different circumstances and also 16 mm. movies of action sequences. Although both of them were accustomed, as clinicians, to using cues from all possible channels of communication as to how a person was feeling and what he was thinking, they finally decided that it was impossible for them to analyze and note systematically all the elements in all these communication channels and to determine how quantitative as well as qualitative aspects of psychological states were communicated separately and conjointly through these different channels. They decided to narrow and focus their attention on characteristics of speech, especially lexical content features. They devised two standardized techniques of eliciting speech, both attempting to maximize the human tendency toward projection of intrapsychic qualities, response sets, and attitudes. The *verbal* method of eliciting speech used instructions which told subjects that this was a study of speaking and conversational habits and asked the subjects to talk for five minutes about any interesting or dramatic personal life experience they had ever had. The *visual* method of induction of speaking involved asking subjects to tell stories for five minutes about certain pictures from Murray's Thematic Apperception Test (1943). Two types of analysis of the speech were carried out: (1) *form analysis,* which involved such variables as rate of speech, frequency and duration of pauses, and frequency of "fills" (uhs, ahs, ers), of incomplete words, of sequential repetitions, of nonlexical vocalizations (laughs, coughs, sneezes, throat clearings, sniffles, etc.), and of aposiopeses (instances in which the speaker suddenly breaks off the expression of a thought and introduces another); and (2) *content analysis,* which involved a consideration of the meaning, relationships, objects, concepts, and processes symbolized by the verbal elements in speech. Content analysis was at the level of single words rather than groups of words or themes. Every word was categorized by a system of codification of language largely derived from psychodynamic principles, and this classification was labeled a "psychological" one. A second system of classification of the words was a grammatical one.

The "psychological" system of classification was as follows. One class of words included all those which referred to environmental *objects.* These in turn differentiated into self and nonself. Nonself was broken down into other human objects, animals, flora, and inanimate objects. A second class of words was *concepts* or *abstractions.* A third class included subgroups of words expressing *neuromuscular actions, motivation, perceptions,* and *thought,* all of which represented types of processes between objects or concepts. Other word classes included references to measure, qualification, gender, part-whole differentiations, and negations.

Measure references consisted of words indicating some relativity of time, space, or quantity regardless of part of speech or context in which used.

The *grammatical* classification included adjectives, adverbs, nouns, pronouns, verbs, prepositions, conjunctions, and interjections.

The first paper published from these early investigations (Gottschalk and Hambidge, 1955) indicated that the methods of eliciting speech (*verbal* and *visual*) evoked different percentages of these categories of words from the same individual and that certain patterns of words in five-minute verbal samples obtained after psychoanalytic sessions with two patients were associated with recurring focal conflicts occurring during the psychoanalytic sessions.

The next study involved an examination and comparison of the differences in the *form* and *content* of the speech patterns of a small group of psychotic and nonpsychotic individuals. Differences were found between the two groups in both form and content of five-minute verbal samples elicited by the so-called *verbal* method. Formwise, the psychotic subjects showed a decreasing word rate per minute as compared to the nonpsychotic subjects. Contentwise, the psychotic patients showed a greater number of references to the self and to negations; greater use of verbs; lesser use of "we" and "us," of words referring to inanimate objects, and of qualifying words; and a significantly smaller use of words which denote or connote location or spatial relationship (regardless of grammatical use) as compared to the nonpsychotic subjects (Gottschalk *et al.*, 1957).[1]

In another study carried out about this time (Hambidge and Gottschalk, 1958), 80 verbal samples were obtained from a single subject on a once-a-week basis over a period of a year while this individual underwent a psychoanalysis. The verbal samples were all obtained by the psychoanalyst (G. H.) at a regular time following one of the psychoanalytic sessions. Forty of the 80 verbal samples were elicited by the "visual" method, which simulates the projective test situation, and 40 were elicited by the "verbal"

---

[1] This data, although collected in 1952–1953 by Dr. Gottschalk while at the National Institute of Mental Health, Bethesda, Maryland, was not fully analyzed and prepared for publication until 1956, after Dr. Gottschalk had moved to Cincinnati; Dr. Gleser assisted in the structuring and statistical analysis of the data.

method, which simulates the psychiatric interview situation. Again evidence was obtained supporting the hypothesis that the choice and frequency of use of certain words in the verbal samples were related to the dynamic state of the patient both quantitatively and qualitatively, as observed in analytic treatment sessions. Consistent differences were found between verbal samples obtained in the projective test situation (*visual* induction of speech) and psychiatric interview situation (*verbal* induction of speech). Further evidence was obtained which indicated that the psychoanalytic experience and the state of therapeutic progress at the time of giving the verbal sample influence the way a patient expresses himself in terms of the choice and use of language variables in the visually induced and verbally induced verbal samples.

The last two studies terminated the collaboration of Louis Gottschalk and Gove Hambidge, Jr., for Dr. Gottschalk moved in September, 1953, to Cincinnati, Ohio, to become a faculty member of the Department of Psychiatry, University of Cincinnati, College of Medicine.

Gradually Dr. Gottschalk made further efforts to explore the use of content features in language as a possible tool for the quantitative analysis of psychological states; for the first time, an effort was made to examine thematic content categories, using the grammatical clause instead of a word as the unit of communication. It was found in a double-blind drug-placebo study that a psychoactive pharmacological agent, pipradrol—a medicament similar in action to dextro-amphetamine—significantly increased thematic references to achievement strivings (Gottschalk *et al.*, 1956). In another study, a very complex psychological position (a masochistic problem-solving approach to obtaining support and love) was found to be significantly associated with the percentage of streptococcal bacteria that could be cultured from the oropharynx of a woman with rheumatic heart disease (Kaplan, Gottschalk, and Fleming, 1957). A cross-validation study tended to confirm this hypothesis by finding a significant correlation (0.40, p < .05) between a frequency count of relevant themes in 20 five-minute verbal samples and the relative percentage of streptococcal bacterial colonies cultured from the patient's throat (Gottschalk and Kaplan, 1958*b*; Kaplan and Gottschalk, 1958).

In 1955, Dr. Gottschalk obtained a U.S. Public Health Service research project grant enabling him to pursue verbal behavior studies on a broader scale. At this point he met Dr. Goldine C. Gleser, a psychologist from St. Louis, Mo., with extensive experience in interdisciplinary research and mathematical statistics, and he invited her to collaborate with him. They decided to study speech at both the "atomistic" level (words) and "molecular" level (themes). A first step taken was to obtain five-minute verbal samples from 90 "normative" individuals, all medically healthy and capable of gainful employment. The group was stratified for sex and intelligence. From this investigation came a contribution to the "atomistic" approach to content analysis, giving in detail the relationship of sex and intelligence to the choice of words (Gleser, Gottschalk, and John, 1959). Data obtained from the study were also used in a number of reports featuring the thematic approach to content analysis (Gleser et al., 1961; Gottschalk et al., 1960a, 1963; Gottschalk and Gleser, 1964a).

The atomistic approach was applied to a set of false and genuine suicide notes collected by Shneidman and Farberow (1957) in an investigation to determine factors contributing to suicide. Analysis of the notes yielded a set of characteristics by which the genuine suicide notes could be distinguished from the pseudo-suicide ones. The criteria of differentiation were further substantiated by applying them to another set of genuine suicide notes obtained from the Cincinnati Police Department. The practical application of the distinctive features of the genuine suicide notes to the problem of ascertaining whether any suicide note was a genuine or false one was illustrated using a decision model. For example, it was observed that, if those notes were considered genuine in which the percentage of auxiliary words minus the percentage of references to others (second and third person) is less than 14 percent plus those remaining notes in which the percentage of references to inanimate objects is greater than 1 percent (Gottschalk and Gleser, 1960a), it would be possible to identify successfully 94 percent of the genuine suicide notes while misidentifying only 15 percent of the false ones.

The suicide note study marked the last of the published reports using the atomistic approach to content analysis. The ensuing period of research marked the beginning of the systematic development of verbal behavior measures of transient affects, such as anxiety and hostility, at the level of thematic content. Dr.

Gottschalk and Dr. Gleser worked toward evolving principles whereby the specification and quantification of psychological states could be derived from brief samples of a subject's speech. Reliability and construct validation studies were carried out with different samples of subjects under different treatment situations over a period of many years. The Public Health Service Research Project Grant to pursue these verbal behavior studies was renewed in 1957, and financial support has continued to the present time from one or another division of the National Institute of Mental Health. Other sources of research funds (Public Health Service, M-1055, M-6005, MH-08282, K3-MH-14,665; Foundations Fund for Research in Psychiatry, T57-74; National Association for Mental Health; Veterans Administration; Schweppe Research and Education Foundation; Defense Atomic Support Agency Contract #Da-49-146-xz-315; Robert D. Stern Fund) were obtained to help support continuing investigation and development of this content analysis method. An exposition and elaboration of these studies and the method constitute the subject matter of this book. The theoretical underpinnings, reliability studies, construct validation studies, "normative" and demographic data for various scales, applications (and further construct validation studies) in the areas of research in psychotherapy, psychoanalysis, psychophysiology, psychosomatic medicine, psychopharmacology, psychology of affects, prediction of outcome with various treatments, and so forth, are covered in considerable detail. Finally, a glimpse is provided into future directions and possible applications of the content analysis method.

CONTENTS

CHAPTER I
Problems and Goals in Content Analysis

One of the basic problems in psychology and psychiatry is that of obtaining precise measurements of the kind and intensity of psychological experiences. Almost everyone believes that he knows and can speak authoritatively about the presence or absence of his own psychological states. In fact, most of us assert we can distinguish quite accurately between subtle differences in the intensity of our emotional states, and we usually deny an inability to differentiate one of our feeling states or attitudes from another. Nonetheless, the science of psychology, challenged first by the solipsistic school of philosophy and spurred on by the discoveries and contributions of psychoanalysis, has wavered in its assumption that reporting of subjective experiences is a reliable or valid guide to what is going on inside the individual.

The solipsistic position, that one's own experience is knowable only by oneself and that there is no way of discerning whether one's experience corresponds to that of anyone else or to the inanimate world, threatened to destroy a science of psychology, for no community of experience, no consensual validation, would be possible if this view told the whole story. Indeed, no valid appraisals or predictions of events outside oneself would be possible. Though solipsism is not accepted as an important model in modern psychology and psychiatry, in attenuated form it has attracted more than mild attention from most behavioral scientists and clinical psychiatrists. It is evidenced among those who emphasize the limits of the reliability of human perception, learning, cognition, and memory and even more so among those who emphasize individual differences in behavior and personality.

Clinical psychoanalysis has empirically determined that we are strongly influenced by unconscious motives and that, because of factors of which we are largely unaware, we are all capable of distorting our perception, memory, and thinking. These dis-

1

tortions are said to be based on the programming into our mind of taboos and inhibitions during childhood. The psychoanalytic procedure has shown that reports of subjective experience may be imperfect and that our appraisals of others may be subject to as many distortions as our self-appraisals. Methods of correcting these distortions have been evolved, and these include therapeutic psychoanalysis or self-analysis and self-scrutiny, using decoding procedures that have been found by psychoanalysis to be pertinent and corrective.

There have been adverse criticisms of psychoanalysis and its solutions to the problem of what individuals are really thinking and feeling. One type of criticism hinges on the matter of theoretical preference and a reservation about the scientific usefulness of a psychology of drives and motivations of the kind represented by psychoanalysis, and a preference for a theoretical model of the mind which makes few if any inferences about the inner psychological state of man. The behavior and learning theory model, for example, focuses on behavior and action, frequency of response, and so forth, and it avoids consideration of psychological constructs of inner, subjective states. This model may approach such constructs through what is called "response class," but the focus remains on observing and recording behavior that is manifest and easily recognizable, broken down into units that are relatively simple and countable. The principal advantage claimed by psychologists of this theoretical persuasion is that their data of observation is quantifiable, is accessible to mathematization, and can be relatively easily organized for predictive purposes.

The claim may be granted that the behavior and learning model provides a perspective and method that promotes quantification and minimizes the need for inference and guesswork in what one is measuring. On the other hand, one of the primary weaknesses of this model is that it has been obliged to take manifest behavior literally as a sign of what the human being is thinking or feeling. For example, an assertion by a man that he is or is not angry is taken as a valid appraisal of how he feels. If the man says he is not angry and behaves nonverbally in an angry fashion, the contradictoriness is likely to be noted, but if the verbal and nonverbal data regarding feelings of "no anger" are congruent, this is likely to be evaluated as the presence of "no anger." Statements by the speaker that other individuals are angry would not likely be counted as indicating in any way how the speaker himself is feeling.

Psychoanalytic psychology, on the other hand, takes the position that a man is often not able to report accurately how he feels because of the influence of wishful (primary process) thinking and various mechanisms of defense. In fact, psychoanalytic observers have offered an excellent empirically derived set of guidelines for decoding from the individual's speech the probable state of feeling of the man. A shortcoming of psychoanalytic psychology, according to some psychoanalysts (Grinker *et al.*, 1961; Seitz, 1966), has been low interobserver consensus or reliability, although other psychoanalytically oriented observers have reported adequate reliability when the research design and clinical procedures are carefully planned (Bellak and Smith, 1956; Bellak and Small, 1965; Knapp *et al.*, 1966; Strupp *et al.*, 1966; Gottschalk and Auerbach, 1966).

PURPOSE

It is our aim to demonstrate how the respective strengths of the psychoanalytic model, the learning theory model, and the linguistic theory model can be utilized in the evaluation of certain important personality dimensions by the systematic analysis of verbal behavior. We will try to show how directly observable and recordable speech behavior, especially its lexical content features, when processed and analyzed per communication unit from the perspective of scales derived from an empirical psychodynamic frame of reference, provides a numerical approximation (assessable in terms of probabilities) of complex psychological states.

USES

The underlying principles of this method have been applied to and tested with respect to only a few of the immense number of feeling, motivational, and cognitive states communicated by language. It is likely that these underlying principles are applicable to many other facets of possible theoretical and practical interest in both the content and form of speech behavior. For example, we will describe in detail how measures of anxiety and hostility, of social alienation and personal disorganization, and of other complex psychological states and psychiatric conditions can be derived from verbal content and can be applied to many heretofore technically unapproachable problems in the behavioral, social, and medical sciences (see Chapter X). The development of this system has not, in our experience, been rapidly achievable because of the necessity of empirical testing and retesting and revision along the way. The development of new scales to the level of pertinence and proficiency of the anxiety, hostility, and schizophrenic scales, therefore, may require considerable time and work. But many of the details of this method of assessing intensity as well as quality of a psychological state are generalizable to the assessment of other complex psychological dimensions.

CHAPTER II

The Theoretical Bases for Qualifying and Quantifying Psychological States through the Content Analysis of Speech

A SUMMARY OF THE VARIOUS CURRENT THEORETICAL APPROACHES

The analysis of content and form of speech as a means of evaluating the emotional status, the psychosocial position, or the cognitive functioning of an individual has beeen approached from a number of points of view and theoretical positions. Scientists and scholars from many different disciplines have interested themselves in language, its origins, its structure, its meaning, and its function as a means of communication. Philologists, philosophers, linguists, sociologists, anthropologists, economists, psychologists, psychiatrists, neurologists, and psychoanalysts have all considered the language behavior of man as their rightful and sometimes their exclusive domain. When they have interested themselves in the aspects of language that convey a certain psychological dimension, such as emotion, they have naturally enough tackled these problems from a theoretical frame of reference stemming from their own scholarly specialty. It is enlightening to review some of the theoretical stances taken in the developing field of psycholinguistics.

Saporta (1961) has attempted to characterize some of these stances insofar as they involve linguists and psychologists. He states that a distinction must be made between language in its abstract aspect and language in its physical aspect. This distinction is implied in such pairs of terms as language and speech, metalanguage and object language, code and message, and system and process. The abstract aspect of language is a system of habits, described in terms of a set of signs and rules. The physical aspect of language consists of actual verbal statements. Psychological

5

analysis of language is primarily concerned with meanings; whereas, linguistic analysis is concerned with the properties of language as a code for the transmission of communication (Pool, 1959; Saporta and Sebeok, 1959). The type of question a linguist asks is "Can a speaker ever properly say this?" or "Is this a grammatical sentence?" or "Are these phonemes the same or different?" Although linguists have pursued a strategy of emphasizing structural considerations, linguistics is nonetheless eventually concerned with meaning (Carroll, 1955). Furthermore, linguistics is entering a period of development in which its methods are being applied to extralinguistic problems in cooperation with specialists in other disciplines. One result of this collaboration is a more immediate concern with the problem of meaning (Carroll et al., 1951; Hoijer, 1954; Firth, 1956; McQuown, 1957; Pittenger and Smith, 1957; Pittenger et al., 1960; Dittmann and Wynne, 1961; Scheflen, 1966; Trager, 1966).

The psychologist sees language, spoken or written, as a variety of learned human behavior, like maze-running and lever-pushing. There are sets of factors influencing the learning process, and, characteristically, the psychologist's question is: "What factors are operating to cause the speaker to say this at this time?" Psychologists have not succeeded in adequately formulating a psychology of grammar exclusively in terms of habit strength, generalization, frequency, reinforcement, and so forth (Saporta, 1961). Nor have psychologists, relying solely on learning theory models, been satisfactorily able to evolve a method of measuring emotions or attitudes or the more cognitive aspects of speech content.

Pool (1959) and Marsden (1965) have described how psychologists and others interested in the content analysis of speech have approached such issues as qualitative and quantitative analysis. Their reviews are recommended to the interested reader. One useful classification system of content analysis includes classical, pragmatic, and linguistic analysis.

Classical Content Analysis

The so-called classical model of content analysis does not necessarily limit content analysis to lexical content but may include investigation of the musical, pictorial, plastic, and gestural systems of communication (Berelson, 1952). "Manifest" content has been limited by Berelson to the semantic and syntactic aspects of communication and has not included the pragmatic aspect of communication, which has been thought of as the relationship between the communication symbol and its user.

Pragmatic Content Analysis

In the so-called pragmatic model (Marsden, 1965), content units are coded into categories descriptive of some condition of the communicator or of the relationship between him and his communication; whereas, in the classical model the units are coded to categories descriptive of the content itself. In the pragmatic model, inference is used at the time of coding and is the basis of coding pertinent semantic and syntactic content units to the categories of the content analysis system. For example, to code the statement "he is afraid" to signify that the speaker is himself afraid follows the pragmatic model. With the classical model, once the units are coded, further inferences may be made about the internal state of the communicator and these inferences are subject to validation only by other procedures. Following the classical model, the statement "he is afraid" could be coded to the category he (other) afraid, and only subsequently could one hypothesize that perhaps such a statement might indicate something about the internal state of the speaker.

According to Marsden (1965), "the classical model places a premium on objectivity and is designed so that workers with minimal special training can reliably perform the analysis. . . . The price paid for this precision is often a superficiality of results."

The pragmatic model attempts to realize psychological meaningfulness by working with complex clinical constructs, and it utilizes the skills and knowledge of the clinician while formalizing the conditions under which these skills are used to insure procedural rigor.

Nonquantitative Analysis: Linguistic Analysis

Whereas the pragmatic model promotes research with psychodynamic constructs for which behavioral cues cannot be easily specified, linguistic analysis has begun to try to make possible identification of these cues through a nonquantitative approach or through a combination with appropriate statistical techniques.

Pittenger, Hockett, and Danehy (1960) combined the tools of linguistics and paralinguistic analysis and clinical inference and applied them to the first five minutes of an initial psychiatric interview. These investigators showed that linguistic techniques applied to interview material might add understanding not otherwise obtainable. Eldred and Price (1958) have tried to explore the relationship between some dimensions of "vocalization" and the clinical impression of certain affect states in a patient. Dittmann and Wynne (1961) have explored the relationship between linguistic phenomena and the clinical impression of affect. They found that paralinguistic features could not meet statistical reliability standards and that linguistic features could be identified reliably but were not related to affect. Trager (1966) has expressed the hopeful view that, with further collaborative work between linguistics and clinicians, more fruitful applications of linguistic analysis to content analysis will come forth.

THE PROBLEM OF ASSESSING INTENSITY

The classical model and many pragmatic model systems measure intensity of feeling or behavior in terms of the frequency of occurrence of units in a speech category. Advocates and antagonists alike have asked, How much of the intensity variance might the frequency be expected to explain? The additional question has been asked: What factors other than frequency of occurrence of specific units are significant cues to degree of intensity?

Contingency analysis is another quantitative procedure that involves counting, but the form of the hypothesis and of the critical observations is different from that in a simple frequency analysis. Contingency analysis asks not simply how often a given symbolic form appears in the content of verbal behavior, but how often it appears in conjunction with other symbolic units. Contingency analysis seeks to determine the probability that a specified content category will occur, given that other specified categories are found in that or related units. The difference between frequency and contingency analysis can be expressed most clearly as the difference between a simple probability statement and a conditional probability statement.

Many content analysts have considered inadequate the assumption that frequency of response is the sole indicator of intensity. Some have turned to linguistic theory for aid, looking for an enumeration of the nonlexical and structural forms of language through which intensity is conveyed. Some leads have been turned up by this approach (Starkweather, 1956a, 1956b; Mahl, 1959; Boomer and Goodrich, 1961; Ostwald, 1963), but the results to date are meager.

GENERAL FEATURES OF OUR THEORETICAL APPROACH

There are certain general features of our theoretical approach to the measurement of psychological states which might be clarified at this point. At least three major aspects of our method can be identified, each of which involves certain theoretical issues. A first consideration is that of the interrelationship between the procedure used in eliciting verbal material and the ensuing thematic content. A second consideration concerns the formulation of specific qualitative and quantitative relationships between thematic content and psychological states. The third set of issues involves the choice of appropriate procedures for scale development and validation. We shall consider each of these briefly in this section.

Theories Pertaining to the Method of Eliciting Verbal Behavior

The principal method we have used to evoke speech has been to ask subjects to talk for five minutes, in response to purposely ambiguous instructions, about any interesting or dramatic personal life experiences. This method of eliciting speech has been used in order to maximize the projective aspects of the human communication relationship so that the speaker will be more likely to present evidence of his internal psychological state rather than a reaction to cues from the interviewer. The procedure minimizes the effects of the personality of the interviewer, but subtle effects of the interviewer can be studied with appropriate research designs (see Chapter IX).

The measurement procedure has also been applied to language produced under a variety of circumstances other than that involved in our standard five-minute interview. Thus, the spoken language of dream reports, reactions to pictures (the Thematic Apperception Test), responses to interview questions, and even written material have been analyzed by this procedure. It is likely that there may be differences in the magnitude of psychological states as assessed from language obtained under one condition or another (see e.g., Gottschalk and Hambidge, 1955, and Chapter IX of this book). Such differences in language, however, are to some extent a reflection of the differential instructions and circumstances under which the verbal sample is obtained, which in turn produce differences in the psychological state of the subject. To the extent that differences occur in the communication messages of subjects as a consequence of the method used to elicit speech, we have assumed that only the mean and standard deviation but not the relative ordering of measures is affected.

Theories Relating to Our Approach to Content Analysis

Marsden (1965) has classified our theoretical approach to content analysis as one that follows the pragmatic model. In a number of respects, our system cannot be readily classified as being based on the pragmatic model as Marsden describes it. It does not fit this model very well for technical reasons, for although clinical inferences have been built into the categories to be coded, nonprofessional technicians can be trained to do the coding with approximately the same level of reliability as they could code "manifest" lexical content categories. Moreover, our system is unusual from a theoretical point of view in that it borrows from several different bodies of theory—learning theory, linguistic theory, and psychoanalytic theory are all involved. For these reasons, we think that our approach could be designated more correctly as an *eclectic* one.

Our approach to the problem of quantification has been to include both frequency and nonfrequency aspects of specific types of statements to assess intensity. This is accomplished by differentially weighting the specific content categories of a scale in proportion to the assumed intensity represented by statements classifiable in these content categories. The weights are initially assigned on the basis of clinical psychoanalytic theory and experience. They are later revised on the basis of further empirical studies where either comparisons of scores with other criteria or the results of predictive studies warrant a modification of the weights assigned to a content item within a category. Furthermore, linguistic lexical features (such as comparative adverbs—"very," "much") are included as indicators of the magnitude of the psychological state and are given additional weight. Also, the unit of speech that is analyzed is the grammatical clause in its lexical context, which again is a linguistic facet of speech.

Our approach requires repeated exposure to verbal phenomena, so that hypotheses can be derived about the ways in which information regarding psychological events and states is typically conveyed via verbal behavior. Also needed is a set of circumstances—natural or experimental—permitting testing and revision of tentative hypotheses. The clinical practice of psychiatry and psychoanalysis has been the source and testing grounds for the initial approach to content analysis to be described here. Many other avenues have been followed from this point to the eventual development and validation of this system of scoring written and spoken language to provide measures of various psychological states. The avenues have been selected from whatever disciplines or sciences appeared to be necessary to accomplish our goals. Included were such medical sciences as biochemistry, physiology, pharmacology, bacteriology, internal medicine, surgery, psychiatry, dermatology, gynecology, and radiology. Some of the behavioral sciences, such as clinical and experimental psychology, sociology, cultural anthropology, and measurement theory and statistics, have been utilized at every step of the way.

In the following sections, we will describe in more detail how we have formulated our theoretical and experimental approaches in different psychological areas.

Theoretical Approaches to Scale Development and Validation

There are those who will question why correlational approaches, such as factor analysis or multiple regression analysis, were not used in scale development, particularly in the determination of category weights. Such approaches did not seem appropriate to us, however, in most instances. The factor analytic model assumes that every subject obtains a score on each measure used, whereas this assumption is not made regarding verbal behavior. Different persons have different preferred modes of expression. Certainly, in any one five-minute verbal sample, the subject is likely to utilize only a limited number of categories. In fact, since a message unit is coded in only one scale category, and successive communication units tend to be somewhat redundant as to subject matter, negative correlation can be expected between categories of the same scale. Categories are assumed to be alternative ways of expressing the same psychological state at different times and in different situations, but they are not necessarily all used by a particular subject, regardless of the intensity of his affect. Thus the basic model of factor analysis is violated.

Whereas category intercorrelations and factor analyses are conceivable approaches to the problem of differential weighting from internal considerations, multiple regression is a method of determining weights in order to maximize the correlation of the total scale with a suitable criterion. The difficulty in this approach lies in the problem of obtaining suitable criteria. While many indicators of a specified psychological state are available, no one measure can be taken as a criterion. Rather, we have sought to determine those category weights that maximize the correlation of the verbal measure with all the reasonably valid indicators of the same state. This technique has involved waiting until enough examples could be found for the use of a particular category to enable us to determine its contribution to several different validity indicators. Only on the basis of such multiple evidence has the decision been made to modify the weight or even in some cases to reduce the weight to zero.

SPECIFIC ASPECTS OF OUR THEORETICAL APPROACH

The Quantification of Affects [1]

One of the general problems involved in the quantification of affect is the formulation of a satisfactory working definition of affect. Theoreticians and experimentalists have approached this problem in different ways, and these differences, as we have mentioned, have led to varying conclusions.

We have chosen to define affect from an intrapsychic frame of reference, and we have based our assessment of immediate affect on two types of verbal communications. One type is the direct verbal report of a subjective affective experience, such as "I am anxious." The other type of verbal communication provides indirect evidence of the occurrence of affect, for example, the

[1] This section has been excerpted in part from L. A. Gottschalk et al., "The measurement of emotional changes during a psychiatric interview: A working model towards quantifying the psychoanalytic concept of affect," in Methods of Research in Psychotherapy, ed. L. A. Gottschalk and A. H. Auerbach (New York: Appleton-Century-Crofts, 1966)—with permission of the publishers.

spontaneous remark "I am not anxious." Only by inference can the latter type of verbal statement be taken to signalize the presence of affect. Such an affect might be one which the individual is aware of but does not care to acknowledge or which he does not recognize as a specifiable emotional feeling but experiences as a feeling tone which is capable of influencing the quality and intensity of the individual's general feeling state, ideation, and behavior.

Many kinds of behavioral and psychological manifestations other than verbal communications have been used by investigators to determine the presence of affects (see, e.g., Darwin, 1955; Knapp, 1963). The signs used have been external behavior, including facial expression, criteria frequently used by investigators experimenting with subhuman animals (Massermann, 1943; Seitz, 1954, 1959; Mirsky, 1958); physiological measures (Darrow, 1929; Cannon, 1936; Ax, 1953; Lacey, 1959); biochemical indicators (Funkenstein, 1952, 1956; Persky et al., 1958; Hamburg, 1962; Gottschalk et al., 1965b; Mason et al., 1966a); the report of subjective experience alone, as in the Taylor Anxiety Scale (1953) and Cattell Scale (1957) and in various adjective checklists (Nowlis and Nowlis, 1956; Zuckerman, 1960; Lubin, 1966); kinesics (Birdwhistell, 1963); and so forth.

It is our opinion that the essential feature of affects is that they are qualitative feelings of varying intensity about which the individual has various degrees of verbal articulateness or discriminatory capacity, these depending on the relative amounts of awareness he has about these feelings and drive states. We do not intend to differentiate here between affects, emotions, and feeling states.

We presume that, at a neurophysiological level, the qualitative and quantitative differences typifying emotional states are associated with the activation of different configurational patterns of the cerebral cortex and the visceral brain (see, for example, Gellhorn and Loofbourrow, 1963; MacLean, 1955; Brady, 1962). Although the nature of the neurophysiological concomitants of affects are of serious interest to our working concept of affect and affect quality and intensity, an integration of neurophysiological and psychological theories and facts related to affects is not our aim at this time. Neurophysiological bases of affects require even more research than the psychodynamic features of affects, and it is premature and pretentious to attempt to invent a workable, unified psychophysiological theory of emotion. In our opinion, it is a wiser procedure at this time to sketch out only roughly the principles afforded by our overlapping knowledge of emotions at the psychological and neurophysiological levels and to maintain a tentative position about the principles governing their psycho-physiological interrelationships.

The usual objection to using an intrapsychic frame of reference as a vantage point from which to determine the amount or intensity of an affect is that subjective and intrapsychic data have not generally been considered suitable for scientific investigation. There is sound evidence to support the viewpoint, however, that such data can be used as reliably and validly as any other phenomena subjected to scientific scrutiny provided adequate research designs and controls are used (Gottschalk et al., 1956; Beecher, 1959; Sargent, 1961; and others).

Our working definition of affect, in summary, is as follows. Affects are feeling states that have the attributes of quality and quantity. Affects and emotions have subjective, purely psychological components as well as physiological, biochemical, and behavioral concomitants. Continual mixtures of affects of relatively long duration occur, and these constitute what is ordinarily designated as mood. Upon the background of mood, feeling states of relatively high intensity and variability may play, and these are generally referred to as emotions. Relatively smaller fluctuations of feeling states which occur irregularly are sometimes referred to, in a narrower sense, as affects. Since we are attempting to develop an instrument to measure immediate affect rather than the more prolonged feeling states usually referred to as mood, we do want to point out that we are not here equating affect with mood.

To go from verbal behavior to an estimate of the relative intensity of certain affects experienced by an individual during brief units of time has required a series of assumptions that should be made explicit at this point. Some of these assumptions have been partially substantiated. Some have not and perhaps cannot be, for they may be more in the nature of representational models than testable hypotheses. It would require more space than is appropriate to take at this time to give here in detail the evidence that tends to favor one assumption or another; instead, reference will be made here and there to investigations providing supportive data for some of our working assumptions.

(*a*) The relative magnitude of an affect can be validly estimated from the typescript of the speech of an individual, using solely content variables and not including any paralanguage variables. In other words, the major part of the variance in the immediate affective state of an individual can be accounted for by variations in the content of the verbal communications (Gottschalk *et al.*, 1958*a*, 1958*b*, 1961*a*, 1961*b*, 1963, 1967*b*; Gleser *et al.*, 1961). (See also Chapter IX, pp. 250 ff.)

Features other than the content of verbal behavior, especially pitch, volume, tone of voice, accent, rhythm, cadence, stress, and so forth, constitute paralanguage concomitants of the affect being measured. These aspects of speech also provide signals by means of which an affect can be detected and measured. We are assuming that the increments in affect experienced and communicated by these particular paralanguage variables are roughly proportional to the affect experienced and communicated via verbal content variables alone. We have some evidence to support this assumption. In one study (Gottschalk *et al.*, 1966), we found our anxiety scores to be similar on an ordinal scale when the scorer used only a typescript of speech as compared to when both the typescript was read and a tape-recorded transcription was played. In another study (Gottschalk and Frank, 1967), we found that only negligible information was lost with respect to assessing magnitude of anxiety if typescripts of speech alone were used without listening to sound recordings of the speaker's voice while reading the typescripts (see Chap. IX, pp. 250 ff.). Paralanguage variables probably serve to clarify and emphasize quantitative differences in the emotional feelings occurring, rather than to differentiate them. One of the most important reasons that paralanguage variables are not useful in systematically assaying the magnitude of affective reactions in spoken language is that no one has yet been able to devise a reliable method to measure paralanguage variables (see, e.g., the investigations of Dittmann and Wynne, 1961).

(*b*) On the basis of verbal content alone, the magnitude of any one affect at any one period of time is directly proportional to three primary factors: (1) The frequency of occurrence of categories of thematic statements. (2) The degree to which the verbal expression directly represents or is pertinent to the psychological activation of the specific affect (e.g., to say that one is killing or injuring another person or wants to do so is regarded as a more direct representation of hostile aggression than to say that one simply disapproves of another person). (3) The degree of personal involvement attributed by the speaker to the emotionally relevant idea, feeling, action, or event.[2]

(c) The degree of direct representation (also called *centrality* by H. Sargent, 1961) of the specific affect in the verbal expression (b2 above) and the degree of personal involvement attributed by the speaker (b3 above) can be represented mathematically by a weighting factor. Higher weights have tended to be assigned to scorable verbal statements which communicate affect that, by inference, is more likely to be strongly experienced by the speaker. Completely unconscious or repressed affect of any kind is considered, by our method of weighting, not to signify affect of high magnitude, but rather to amount to zero or no affect. This numerical weight, which is assigned to each thematic category, designates roughly the relative probability that the thematic category is associated with our construct of the affect. Initially, weights have been assigned deductively on the basis of common sense (as in the example b2 above) or from clinical psychoanalytic judgment (as in d below). Subsequently, the weights have been modified and revised whenever further empirical evidence has been sufficient to warrant such a change (Gottschalk et al., 1961a, 1963, 1964a).

(d) The occurrence of suppressed and repressed affects may be inferred from the content of verbal behavior by noting the appearance of a variety of defensive and adaptive mechanisms. We assume that the verbal content of spontaneous speech, like dream content, contains the workings of primary and secondary process thinking, though speech employs presumably different proportions of these kinds of thinking than the dream. Thus, the immediate magnitude of an affect is considered to be approximately the same, whether the affectively toned verbal thematic reference is expressed in the past tense, present tense, or future tense, as an intention, as a conditional probability, or as a wish. Some of the defensive and adaptive mechanisms signaling the presence of suppressed and repressed affect in language are: (1)

---

[2] By inspection, one can see that the affect scales we are using (see Schedules 2.1, 2.2, 2.3, and 2.4, pp. 23 ff.) have used principles (b2) and (b3) in somewhat varying proportions. For example, the hostility scales do not employ principle (b3) to the extent that the anxiety scale does.

affect or its associated ideation or behavior attributed to other human beings; (2) affect or its associated ideation or behavior occurring in subhuman animals or in inanimate objects; (3) affect and its equivalents repudiated or denied; and (4) affect and its equivalents acknowledged but reported to be present in attenuated form.

(e) The product of the frequency of use of relevant categories of verbal statements and the numerical weights assigned to each thematic category provides an ordinal measure of the magnitude of the affect.

In other words, the greater the specific kind of affect of a speaker over a given unit of time, the more verbal references will be made, as compared to thematic statements of all types, to experiences or events of the types that we have classified in relevant categories with varying weights. Thus, multiplying the weight for the category by the number of references in the verbal sample classified in that category, and then summing up all the content categories pertinent to the specified affect, provides an ordinal index of the intensity of the feeling state. (See Schedules 2.1, 2.2, 2.3, and 2.4, pp. 23–24, 33–35, for examples of thematic categories and weights.)

(f) Individuals differ considerably in rate of speech, and the same individual may vary in rate of speech from one unit of time to another. Since our numerical indices of magnitude of emotion can vary with the number of words spoken per unit time, the numerical score derived from one verbal sample may be compared to the score derived from another verbal sample composed of a different number of words by using a correction factor which expresses the affect scores of speakers in terms of a common denominator, namely, the score per 100 words. We have learned that affect scores are essentially the same proportionately, whether we express the scores per number of clauses (thematic references of all types) or per number of words.

In previous studies, we have made this correction by dividing the total raw score by the number of words spoken and multiplying by 100. Recently we have investigated correcting all raw scores for correlation with number of words spoken by using as the corrected score the difference between the observed score and the score linearly predictable from the number of words. Such differences, suitably scaled, give a more continuous distribution than does a simple ratio score, when the raw scores include many zeros (signifying no relevant content items were spoken). But unless the correlation is determined separately for each sample studied, correlations still persist between the corrected affect score and number of words in some samples. We have finally decided that the most satisfactory and simplest way to take into consideration rate of speech is by adding 0.5 to the raw score, multiplying by 100, and dividing by the number of words spoken. This method avoids the discontinuity occurring whenever no scorable items have occurred in some verbal samples. It also provides a uniform transformation over all samples and, with rare exceptions, reduces the correlation between the affect score and number of words essentially to zero.

A further transformation, using the square root of the corrected score, is made to obtain the final score. This transformation is intended to reduce the skewness of the score distributions, thus making the measure more amenable to parametric statistical treatment. The square-root transformation tends to make the ordinal scale approximate the characteristics of an interval scale.

The mathematical formula we are using to derive the magnitude of an emotion is: Magnitude of an emotion per 100 words =

$$\left[\frac{100 \ (f_1 w_1 + f_2 w_2 + f_3 w_3 \ \ldots \ f_n w_n + 0.5)}{N} \right]^{1/2}$$

where f_n is the frequency per unit of time of any relevant type of thematic verbal reference, w_n is the weight applied to such verbal statements, and N is the number of words per unit time. The weights are based on the degree of direct representativeness or centrality to the specific affect indicated in the verbal content and/or on the degree of personal involvement implied.

The Measurement of Anxiety from Verbal Samples [3]

OTHER MEASURES AND CONCEPTS OF ANXIETY

There are relatively few objective measures of immediate, labile emotional states, such as anxiety. Most psychological tests

---

[3] Excerpted, with some alterations and additions, from G. C. Gleser, L. A. Gottschalk, and K. J. Springer, "An anxiety scale applicable to verbal samples," A.M.A. Arch. Gen. Psychiat., 5: 593–605, 1961—with permission of the publisher.

have been designed to measure general traits or typical behavior and thus are fairly insensitive to small changes in labile emotional response. Moreover, such tests can seldom be used in longitudinal studies because of a tendency for the responses evoked in the testing situation to become learned or stereotyped.

The fact that there is a paucity of objective indices of immediate psychological states makes difficult the development of a method of measuring such variables, since no direct criteria are available. Thus, it is necessary to proceed by slow and tedious steps, using various indirect methods of assessing validity. In this and subsequent sections, we shall attempt to present the steps we have taken in developing a measure for assessing in small speech samples the potentially labile psychological state known as anxiety.

Despite the centrality of the concept of anxiety in psychological theory, it is only within the last decade that attempts have been made to measure anxiety objectively. One of the earliest objective measures, the Taylor Manifest Anxiety Scale (MAS) (Taylor, 1953), developed within the context of learning theory, has been a great spur to clinical research. After its appearance, attempts were made to relate the MAS to previously known or assumed indices of anxiety. Thus a vast literature has arisen on the relation of the MAS to task performance, to clinical ratings of anxiety, and to physiological measurements. A comprehensive review of this literature can be found in articles by Sarason (1960) and Krause (1961). We will summarize briefly here some of the points of interest relevant to our own efforts.

The MAS, because it requires a recognition by the subject of his feelings and behaviors, has been considered subject to bias in both a positive and negative direction. Further, it evaluates the typical reaction of an individual rather than his specific reaction under different conditions. This lack of specificity of the anxiety measured by the MAS may account for the variability in results when the MAS is related to task performance. In order to measure the anxiety pertinent to specific situations, a number of scales have been developed, such as the Test Anxiety Questionnaire of Mandler and Sarason (1952).

Variations in the correlation of the MAS with clinical ratings of anxiety have brought about further refinements in thinking about the nature of anxiety and its measurement. In particular it became evident that differences among clinical ratings may arise from variations in the theoretical construct of anxiety (see, e.g., Lauterbach, 1958).

Partly because of the inherent difficulties in the psychological measurement of anxiety, assessment by means of assumed physiological concomitants has become increasingly prevalent. Physiological signs, such as the galvanic skin response (GSR), heart rate, respiration, blood chemistry, and so forth, have the advantage of being easy to quantify and being sensitive to small and rapid changes in intensity. Since, however, individuals vary in their pattern of autonomic response to stress, no single index has been found sufficient as a general indicator of emotional arousal (Lacey, 1959). Further, while some promising work has been done toward this end (Ax, 1953; Schachter, 1957; Gottschalk et al., 1965b), the problem of identifying distinctive patterns which will discriminate specific emotions, such as anxiety from anger, has not been resolved.

Verbal report has been widely used as a source of information regarding an individual's emotional state. Despite this fact, it has been only quite recently that the analysis of speech structure and content has been approached objectively. Two rather different uses of structural characteristics have been provided by the Type-Token Ratio (TTR) and the Speech Disturbance Ratio. The TTR measures the ratio of different words (types) to total words (tokens). Recently, the TTR, in small segments of speech, has been related to variations in emotional states (Jaffe, 1958). Like physiological signs, however, the TTR provides only minimal discrimination of specific emotions. The Speech Disturbance Ratio makes use of a disturbance in such structural properties of speech as stuttering, repetitions, etc., to provide an index of transient anxiety (Mahl, 1956). One advantage of using such structural characteristics is that categories can be defined with reasonable clarity and objectivity, thus reducing scoring unreliability. The question may be raised, however, whether disturbances in the structural properties of speech relate more to physiological tension than to anxiety. Independent studies by Boomer and Goodrich (1961) have raised a serious question whether Mahl's Speech Disturbance Ratio is a valid measure of anxiety. In the investigations of Boomer and Goodrich, changes in the Speech Disturbance Ratio during psychotherapeutic interviews were not correlated significantly with clinical ratings of anxiety.

The application of objective scoring systems to the content of speech has focused primarily on small-group interactions (Bales, 1950) and psychotherapy (Murray, 1956; Leary, 1957; Leary and Gill, 1959; Dollard and Auld, 1959; Pool, 1959; Lorr *et al.*, 1961; Marsden, 1965; Lorr and McNair, 1966; Chance, 1966; Auld and Dollard, 1966). Very little attention has been given to developing scoring systems for specific emotional states such as anxiety. The systems have varied as to the definition of content units and as to the amount of inference which must be made in categorizing the data. The Discomfort Relief Quotient (Dollard and Mowrer, 1947), for example, is based on small units and confined to manifest content, and thus decisions in assigning statements to categories is fairly objective. Other approaches involve analyses of large portions of interview material by means of interpretive judgments of trained clinicians. One recent attempt to combine these approaches, that of Dollard and Auld (1959) and Auld and Dollard (1966), is of particular pertinence here. Directed toward the analysis of psychotherapy interviews, it deals specifically with anxiety as one of the major variables. The approach in general is an attempt to apply systematic scoring to latent as well as manifest content. In formal structure (division of material into small units, quantification on the basis of frequency, and categorization of anxiety into types), it has some similarity to the approach to be described here. In contradistinction, however, it requires scorers trained in the theory on which the system is based, that is, in psychoanalytic theory, for it is the scorer who makes the interpretive decision as to the applicability of the score.

THEORETICAL AND DESCRIPTIVE FEATURES OF THIS ANXIETY SCALE

The type of anxiety that we are attempting to measure is what might be termed "free" anxiety in contrast to "bound" anxiety, which manifests itself in conversion and hypochondriacal symptoms, in compulsions, in doing and undoing, in withdrawal from human relationships, and so forth. It is likely that some aspects of bound anxiety are registered by our scale, particularly by means of those content items in the scale which involve the psychological mechanisms of displacement and denial. So far as we know at this time, such bound anxiety is preconscious, is relatively readily accessible to consciousness, and is capable—along with grossly conscious anxiety feelings—of activating autonomic nervous system and central nervous system signs of arousal. There is evidence, in fact, which will be given in detail later (see Chapter V), that our anxiety scores reflect not only the subjective awareness of anxiety from the conscious and the preconscious level, but also the level of relevant autonomic arousal and postural and kinesic activity.

We have classified anxiety, on the basis of clinical experience, into six subtypes: death, mutilation, separation, guilt, shame, and diffuse or nonspecific anxiety (see Schedule 2.1). We recognize, of course, that the nature and sources of anxiety may be classified in other ways. Furthermore, we know that the categories we are using are not always discrete and unique, but this circumstance is consistent with the impression that people may be experiencing different kinds of anxiety simultaneously. We should also note that we have not attempted to differentiate between fear and anxiety in any of our categories, since we believe it is impossible to make this distinction on the basis of verbal content alone.

Fear of death has been singled out by existentialists as the origin of all human anxiety (Horney, 1945; Kierkegaard, 1944; Tillich, 1944), but in our classification we have included only those items dealing directly with death and destruction. Mutilation fear and anxiety, as we have conceptualized the term, is synonymous with castration anxiety, and the descriptive items on our scale pertaining to this type of anxiety are derived from psychoanalytic psychology (Freud, 1936; May, 1950). The concept of separation anxiety and the descriptive items designating what references in speech are to be counted under this heading have also been derived from psychoanalytic psychology, and specifically from Bowlby (1960) and others. In our descriptive items differentiating between shame and guilt anxiety, we have leaned on the work of Piers and Singer (1953).

Actually, the categories for our anxiety scale were selected by one of us (L. A. G.) by listening to many people who were considered to be anxious and not anxious and noting that these were categories of anxiety that were both relatively frequently present and readily identifiable. Further crystallization of the ideas for the descriptive features of the content items under each category heading came from listening to tape recordings of hypnotically induced anxiety states.[4] In the tape recordings, student nurses told stories in reaction to the same TAT cards while in a hypnotic trance and before and after it was suggested that each hypnotized subject was very anxious. The categories and descriptive details in Schedule 2.1 give the content items eventually selected.

SCHEDULE 2.1

Anxiety Scale*

1. Death anxiety—references to death, dying, threat of death, or anxiety about death experienced by or occurring to:

   a. self (3).
   b. animate others (2).
   c. inanimate objects (1).
   d. denial of death anxiety (1).

2. Mutilation (castration) anxiety—references to injury, tissue or physical damage, or anxiety about injury or threat of such experienced by or occurring to:

   a. self (3).
   b. animate others (2).
   c. inanimate objects destroyed (1).
   d. denial (1).

3. Separation anxiety—references to desertion, abandonment, ostracism, loss of support, falling, loss of love or love object, or threat of such experienced by or occurring to:

   a. self (3).
   b. animate others (2).
   c. inanimate objects (1).
   d. denial (1).

4. Guilt anxiety—references to adverse criticism, abuse, condemnation, moral disapproval, guilt, or threat of such experienced by:

   a. self (3).
   b. animate others (2).
   d. denial (1).

5. Shame anxiety—references to ridicule, inadequacy, shame, embarrassment, humiliation, overexposure of deficiencies or private details, or threat of such experienced by:

   a. self (3).
   b. animate others (2).
   d. denial (1).

---

[4] The tape recordings were lent to L. A. Gottschalk by Levitt, Persky, and Brady, who made them in connection with an investigation of anxiety (1964).
* Numbers in parentheses are the weights.

SCHEDULE 2.1 (contd.)

6. Diffuse or nonspecific anxiety—references by word or phrase to anxiety and/or fear without distinguishing type or source of anxiety:

    a. self (3).
    b. animate others (2).
    d. denial (1).

NOTES:

1. In the above scale, the reference is not scored if the speaker is the agent and the injury, criticism, etc. is directed to another.

2. When "we" is used, score as "I."

3. Death, injury, abandonment, etc. may come from an external source or situation.

4. In any of above, the weight should be increased by 1 if the statement of anxiety or fear is modified to indicate that the condition is extreme or marked.

5. The following is a list of words of the kind that may be scored in Category 6 if the type of anxiety is not explicitly stated and in any one of the other categories if the stimulus source of the reaction is denoted. Any grammatical form of the word may be scored, whether it is an adjective, noun, adverb, or verb, and so forth. The list is not intended to be complete but merely to provide examples of scorable word concepts.

ADJECTIVES	NOUNS	ADVERBS	VERBS
fearful	fear	fearfully	to fear
frustrated	frustration	frustratedly	to frustrate
tense	tension	tensely	to tense
worried	worry	worriedly	to worry
shaky	....	shakily	to shake
desperate	desperation	desperately	to despair
agitated	agitation	agitatedly	to agitate
irritable	irritation	irritably	to irritate
trembling	tremble	tremblly	to tremble
scared	....	scarily	to scare
dangerous	danger	dangerously	to endanger
troubled	trouble	....	to trouble
jittery	jitters	....	....
panicky	panic	....	to panic
upset	upset	....	to upset
terrified	terror	....	to terrorize
frightened	fright	frightfully	to frighten
overwhelmed	....	overwhelmingly	to overwhelm
threatened	threat	threateningly	to threaten
eerie	eeriness	eerily	....
weird	weirdness	weirdly	....
rattled	....	....	to rattle
anxious	anxiety	anxiously	....
timid	timidity	timidly	....
nervous	nerves	nervously	....

The weights for each subcategory were assigned on the basis of the principles discussed previously in the section of this chapter entitled *The Quantification of Affects* (pp. 12 ff.), namely, on the basis of the degree of personal involvement and the degree of direct representation. The reader should refer to that section also for specific information regarding all the assumptions we have made in order to convert verbal statements uttered by an individual into an anxiety score. These weights are, of course, approximations, and they are on an ordinal, rank-order scale. Various construct validation studies (to be described in Chapter V) have provided some evidence that the weights are justifiable approximations. The square-root transformation of the anxiety scores in our various validation studies appears to provide a scaling of anxiety by this verbal behavior approach which has some earmarks of an interval scale. For example, when parametric statistics are used as well as nonparametric statistics in evaluating the relationship of our anxiety measures to other psychological, physiological, biochemical, and pharmacological variables, a comparison of the statistical indices usually shows negligible differences.

An example follows of a fragment from each of two verbal samples. The examples illustrate our system of scoring those clauses that have scorable anxiety items, with appropriate symbols designating each category in the anxiety scale (Schedule 2.1). The numbers in parentheses indicate the weights assigned to each scorable content item. The diagonal marks indicate grammatical clauses. A detailed description and discussion of scoring procedures, with many examples, is provided in a *Manual of Instructions for Using the Gottschalk-Gleser Content Analysis Scales* (Gottschalk, Winget, and Gleser, 1969).

FEMALE PATIENT

The most interestin' part of my life is / what's happening to me / and
$$3a(3)$$
why my sister and them so interested in my life. / Why did they want
$$3a(3)$$
to put me away / and why they want my kids away from me? / And
$$1b(2)$$
it all started / back when my mother died / and up until now it's getting worser and worser. / And at times when I get in these raves like this / I just want to go off / and I wants to start drinking / and at times I don't pay the kids any attention. / I don't leave them in the
$$3a(3)$$
house or nothing. / But it just seem that they far off from me / and
$$3a(3)$$
I can't reach them. / And I do / all I can for my sisters and them /

5a(3)   5a(3)

and they just say / I'm crazy / and they makes fun of me / and they

3a(3)   3a(3)

don't want me around them. / And so that's why / I guess / I started

6a(4)

this / and it's beginning to bother me worser and worser and worser
and worser.

MEDICAL STUDENT

Well, the uh experience (I'd like to tell you about today) is a dramatic one. / It happened to me this summer / when I was in charge of the waterfront at a uh athletic camp. / And uh it was a fairly rough day / but it was warm / and we had a lot of kids down. / We had, / I think / there was about 120 or so in. / Uh and uh the guy screwed up the count, the the counselor. / It wasn't a waterfront counselor / and uh he wasn't too methodical about it. / And it wasn't so much / that he screwed it up / as that he just kind of forgot / whether he was dealing with odd or even numbers. / And uh so he he uh I I told him, / I says, / make sure / that you get this count

1b(2)

right / because some kid's life may depend on it. / And just think /

1b(2)   1b(2)

if if it's your kid / or it's a kid in your cabin. / What are you going

4b(2)   4b(2)

to say to the parents / when uh you're the one / that's responsible /

1b(2)

for that kid uh losing his life or something like that? / I think /

4b(2)   4b(2)

that scared him pretty much and uh, / maybe that scared him too much, / I don't know and uh. /

The Measurement of Hostility from Verbal Samples[5]

OTHER MEASURES AND CONCEPTS OF HOSTILITY

In reviewing the literature on the measurement of hostility, it becomes apparent that a conceptual and semantic problem exists which makes comparison and evaluation of various measures difficult. The construct of hostility, as used by many investigators, is a global one embracing many conceptually different factors. Even the concept of hostility directed outward includes at least

[5] Excerpted, with minor alterations and additions, from L. A. Gottschalk, G. C. Gleser, and K. J. Springer, "Three hostility scales applicable to verbal samples," *A.M.A. Arch. Gen. Psychiat.*, 9: 254–279, September, 1963—with permission of the publisher.

four interrelated factors, any one of which may be equated by one investigator or another with the total construct: (a) a behavioral act, either physical or verbal, called "aggression" [6] and interpreted as having a destructive function by an outside observer; (b) a self-reported attitude of dislike, resentment, or suspicion toward the world or objects in it, sometimes called "hostility"; (c) a subjective experience of an affect called "anger," with physiological concomitants; (d) a dispositional or potential state (rather than an ongoing phenomenon) earmarked by graded tendencies to be aroused to "hostility" or "aggression." Any particular measure may focus on one or more aspects of this aggression-hostility-anger complex, often without explicit indication by the investigator of the meaning intended. Furthermore, the level of awareness of the hostility, ranging from conscious to unconscious, is another dimension which may be involved in the construct of hostility without being made explicit.

The concept of hostility directed toward the self, also called "hostility inward," is likewise frequently undefined or confused. Sometimes it is not differentiated from hostility directed away from the self. Sometimes it is regarded as a dispositional state rather than an ongoing experience. On other occasions, it is equated with the syndrome of depression or considered to be the psychodynamic precursor of depression. And quite commonly it is used synonymously with the term "masochism."

Which aspect of hostility is emphasized depends partly on the theoretical position, partly on the goals of the investigator, partly on the kinds of subjects being observed (e.g., human beings or subhuman animals), and partly on the kind of technique from which the assessment of hostility has been made (e.g., projective tests, inventories, or observer rating scales). This ambiguity in definition or emphasis has resulted in puzzling findings of low positive or even negative relationships between observations obtained from different techniques all aiming to measure "aggression" or "hostility."

Not only has the nature of the construct called "hostility" varied, but also different extraneous factors have entered into its

---

[6] To complicate matters further, "aggression" is used by some writers to include both constructive and destructive polarities on the plausible grounds that active, vigorous movements and ideation can be expressive of an organizing, nurturing, socializing, and creative process as well as of a disorganizing and disruptive process.

measurement depending on the technique used to obtain "hostility" scores. Projective methods, for example, have been plagued with the problem that different results are obtained depending on the stimuli used and scores are often not predictive of behavior or responses in contexts other than the test situation. Self-report or inventory techniques have had to cope with the question of varying levels of awareness of hostile attitudes, as well as the subject's unwillingness to admit, during such self-reporting, to what are culturally considered to be unacceptable characteristics. When physiological measures have been used, there still has remained the unsolved problem of deriving and differentiating affects (e.g., anger, sadness, and fear) on the basis of such measures. Still another difficulty has been that of arousing a single specific affect (such as hostility outward) rather than a different one (say, anxiety) or a conglomeration of affects, when a presumptively hostility-arousing situation has been used in an experimental situation.

It is not feasible in this chapter to present a comprehensive review of all the approaches to the measurement of the aggression-hostility-anger complex or the depression-hostility-in-masochism complex. Extensive discussions and evaluations can be found in *The Psychology of Aggression* by Buss (1961), *The Phenomena of Depressions* by Grinker *et al.* (1961), and *Affective Disorders*, edited by Greenacre (1953). A detailed review of Rorschach and Thematic Apperception Test (TAT) hostility scales has been made by Hafner and Kaplan (1960). Perhaps it will suffice to mention here some of the techniques used in the context of the problems mentioned above.

Inventory measures of hostility-aggression have been constructed with items derived both from the MMPI (Cook and Medley, 1954; Schultz, 1954; Fischer, 1956; Siegel, 1956; Lorr *et al.*, 1961) and from independent sources (Bass, 1956; Buss *et al.*, 1956; Guilford, 1959; Lorr *et al.*, 1961). Some of these measures consist of items chosen on the basis of face validity (Moldawski, 1953; Cook and Medley, 1954; Siegel, 1956), and others have been selected by virtue of their empirical relationship to clinical ratings of aggressiveness (Schultz, 1954; Fischer, 1956). The inventories have been compared with projective techniques, learning tasks, and clinical and self-ratings, with varying degrees of success (Dinwiddie, 1954; Smith, 1954; Buss *et al.*, 1956; Buss,

1961). In general, it has been found that the more similar the criterion measure was to self-report, the better was the correlation between criterion and inventory. Factor analysis of some of these inventories (Bass, 1956; Guilford, 1959) has indicated two sub-classes of items, labeled "aggression" and "hostility," but the distinction in items usually has not been maintained in the final scores derived from these inventories. In the most recent and most carefully worked out of the MMPI derived inventories, that of Buss (1961), these subclasses have been considered meaning-fully distinct and thus have been maintained in the final score.

All inventories, including the various adjective checklists (Nowlis and Nowlis, 1956; Gleser, 1960; Oken, 1960; Zuckerman, 1960; Clyde, 1961) commonly used to assess affect level or pre-vailing mood, since based on self-report, primarily tap conscious attitudes acceptable enough to the subject to be acknowledged. They would seem to be of limited usefulness, therefore, in studying relationships in which suppressed or repressed anger may play a major part.

Projective tests, such as the Rorschach and TAT, have tradi-tionally provided evaluations of deeper, more enduring personality traits, but in this role the tests have been somewhat unwieldy to manipulate and difficulty to quantify. Thus, in the last decade, quite a bit of effort has been directed toward developing hostility content scales to overcome these difficulties (Elizur, 1949; Walker, 1951; DeVos, 1952; Finney, 1955; Gluck, 1955a, 1955b; Mur-stein, 1956; Stone, 1956; Wirt, 1956). Some of the scales are divided into an overt and a covert portion and include weights reflecting the intensity of the hostility expressed. Hafner and Kap-lan (1960) found a differing relationship between the overt and covert portions of their hostility scales, depending on whether applied to the Rorschach or the TAT. The overt and covert por-tions showed a high positive correlation on the Rorschach but a significant negative one on the TAT. Further, there was no cor-relation between the hostility scores on the Rorschach and TAT. A difference in the meaning of hostility scores on the Rorschach and TAT was also noted by Buss when comparing his inventory with the two projectives. Inventory scores correlated with a modi-fied, multiple-choice form of the TAT (Hurley, 1955) but not with Rorschach scores.

Out of the vast array of conflicting results obtained from

studies relating hostility scales derived from projective tests to overt behavioral aggression, Buss found certain general trends appearing. He noted that (a) hostile content scales yield a direct relationship to overt behavior; (b) gross weights are as successful as more highly differentiated weights in this regard; and (c) correlations are higher when less ambiguous stimuli are used and when subjects are more aware of their hostile feelings. These findings have led Buss to suggest that inventories provide as good a measure of aggressive behavior as projectives.

In none of the measures mentioned so far has a distinction been made as to the direction of hostility, toward or away from the subject. Both kinds of hostility have been included often in the final scores. In our hostility scales, we have seriously attempted to separate these different factors, for we believe they represent qualitatively different psychological variables. The Rosenzweig Picture-Frustration Test (Rosenzweig et al., 1947; Rosenzweig, 1950) is the one projective technique which includes an explicit division of direction of hostility, specifically into extrapunitive, intrapunitive, and impunitive categories. Some difficulty has occurred with this test in obtaining responses representative of the subject's actual rather than his ideal self (Bjerstedt, 1965; Rosenzweig, 1963).

The measurement of transient affect, such as that created in the laboratory, is not satisfactorily handled by either projectives or inventories. The AC Personal Audit Inventory of Lorr et al. (1963) does include a section reflecting the subject's level of hostility on the particular day, but most measures of transient affect have been created for a specific experimental situation. For example, the Oken Scale (1960) was developed within the context of a psychophysiological study of hypertensives. This scale consists of clinical ratings of the affect level of subjects in whom anger has been aroused by experimental procedure. Since Oken and his collaborators were interested in a measure of suppressed anger, they rated both verbally and physically expressed aggression and consciously experienced hostility, an estimate of the amount of suppression being derived from the difference between the aggression observed and the hostility reported. It is interesting to note that the investigators had difficulty in eliciting pure affects such as fear, depression, and anger. When an affective response occurred, it was rarely without traces of other affects as well.

One final mention will be made of other kinds of material to which a hostility scale has been applied. Saul *et al.* (1954) developed a six-point scale of hostility for quantitative analysis of the dreams of hypertensive patients and found a significant relationship between such dream content and hypertension. This scale provided a background for some of the early approaches to the construction of our hostility scales.

THEORETICAL AND DESCRIPTIVE FEATURES
OF OUR HOSTILITY SCALES

We have not thought of our approach as a direct measure of aggressive behavior. Since we have been primarily interested in assessing immediate and changing levels of affect, it is the anger portion of the hostility concept which has invited our attention. In particular, we have focused our interest on the direction of hostility, distinguishing between hostility directed away from the self, hostility directed toward the self, and ambivalently directed hostility.[7] The last of our three hostility scales appears to include a peculiar combination of inwardly and outwardly directed hostility, measuring a phenomenon comparable to the sadomasochistic as well as the paranoid syndrome described in clinical psychiatry. A means of making quantitative inferences of the level of hostile affect from the content of language has been built into our three scales, which are based upon psychoanalytic theory and clinical experience. The scales are applied to language elicited in a relatively unstructured and permissive situation that provides minimal cues to the subject as to what spontaneous verbal responses are considered of evaluative significance. We believe that our method of assessing affects does not tend to give the subject much opportunity to present himself in a distortedly favorable light; our method of assessment is more similar to a projective test than to a self-rating test.

Most comparable to our work is the recent attempt by Dollard and Auld (1959) (see also Auld and Dollard, 1966) to apply an objective scoring system to the content of psychotherapy

---

[7] Originally, we labeled this type of hostility "covert hostility" inward because the kinds of verbal statements scored on this scale are all themes about destructive, injurious, critical thoughts and actions of others to the self. Later, we changed the name of the type of hostility measured by this scale when we learned in our validation studies that the scores derived from such themes were correlated with measures of either hostility outward, hostility inward, or both.

interviews. Their approach also includes hostility as one of the major variables. It is similar to ours in its attempt to score systematically latent as well as manifest content. One major difference, however, lies in the level of training required of the scorer. In their system, the interpretive decision as to the applicability of the score is made by the scorer, whereas in ours, that decision is built into the specific items of the scale.

In order to convert our categorical information about verbal statements into a scale presumed to measure the amount of hostility experienced by the individual in a given interval of time, we have made a series of assumptions. These have been enumerated in detail in the previous section entitled *The Quantification of Affects* (pp. 12 ff.).

In reviewing various concepts of hostility, we have indicated that some of the problems in measuring hostility or comparing scores obtained by different assessment procedures have evolved from inadequate definition of the construct being evaluated. Let us, therefore, give our working definition of hostility and indicate in more detail how it is measured.

We have developed a set of three hostility scales derived from spoken or written verbal samples. The scales have been designed to assess the relative magnitude of transient, rather than sustained, affect. The three types of hostility scales that have been developed are based on the direction of the impulse. Our hostility directed outward scale (see Schedule 2.2) measures the intensity of adversely critical, angry, assaultive, asocial impulses and drives toward objects outside oneself. The hostility directed inward scale (see Schedule 2.3) measures degrees of self-hate and self-criticism and, to some extent, feelings of anxious depression and masochism. The ambivalent hostility scale (see Schedule 2.4), though derived from verbal communications suggesting destructive and critical thoughts or actions of others to the self, measures not only some aspects of hostility directed inward but at the same time some features of hostility directed outward. For several reasons, discussed in the chapter on hostility scales, validation studies (Chapter VI), it appears to deserve separate classification from the other two scales. All three hostility scales assign higher weights to scorable verbal statements communicating hostility that, by inference, is more likely to be strongly experienced by the speaker; whereas, completely repressed hostility is not scored.

SCHEDULE 2.2

Hostility Directed Outward Scale: Destructive, Injurious, Critical Thoughts and
Actions Directed to Others

(I) Hostility Outward—Overt

Thematic Categories

a 3* Self killing, fighting, injuring other individuals or threatening to do so.

b 3 Self robbing or abandoning other individuals, causing suffering or anguish to others, or threatening to do so.

c 3 Self adversely criticizing, depreciating, blaming, expressing anger, dislike of other human beings.

a 2 Self killing, injuring or destroying domestic animals, pets, or threatening to do so.

b 2 Self abandoning, robbing, domestic animals, pets, or threatening to do so.

c 2 Self criticizing or depreciating others in a vague or mild manner.

d 2 Self depriving or disappointing other human beings.

a 1 Self killing, injuring, destroying, robbing wildlife, flora, inanimate objects or threatening to do so.

b 1 Self adversely criticizing, depreciating, blaming, expressing anger or dislike of subhuman, inanimate objects, places, situations.

(II) Hostility Outward—Covert

Thematic Categories

a 3* Others (human) killing, fighting, injuring other individuals or threatening to do so.

b 3 Others (human) robbing, abandoning, causing suffering or anguish to other individuals, or threatening to do so.

c 3 Others adversely criticizing, depreciating, blaming, expressing anger, dislike of other human beings.

a 2 Others (human) killing, injuring, or destroying domestic animals, pets, or threatening to do so.

b 2 Others (human) abandoning, robbing, domestic animals, pets, or threatening to do so.

c 2 Others (human) criticizing or depreciating other individuals in a vague or mild manner.

d 2 Others (human) depriving or disappointing other human beings.

e 2 Others (human or domestic animals) dying or killed violently in death-dealing situation or threatened with such.

f 2 Bodies (human or domestic animals) mutilated, depreciated, defiled.

a 1 Wildlife, flora, inanimate objects, injured, broken, robbed, destroyed or threatened with such (with or without mention of agent).

b 1 Others (human) adversely criticizing, depreciating, expressing anger or dislike of subhuman, inanimate objects, places, situations.

* The number serves to give the weight as well as to identify the category. The letter also helps identify the category.

SCHEDULE 2.2 (contd.)

(I) Hostility Outward—Overt

Thematic Categories

c 1 Self using hostile words, cursing, mention of anger or rage without referent.

(II) Hostility Outward—Covert

Thematic Categories

c 1 Others angry, cursing without reference to cause or direction of anger; also instruments of destruction not used threateningly.

d 1 Others (human, domestic animals) injured, robbed, dead, abandoned or threatened with such from any source including subhuman and inanimate objects, situations (storms, floods, etc.).

e 1 Subhumans killing, fighting, injuring, robbing, destroying each other or threatening to do so.

f 1 Denial of anger, dislike, hatred, cruelty, and intent to harm.

SCHEDULE 2.3

Hostility Directed Inward Scale: Self-Destructive, Self-Critical Thoughts and Actions

I. Hostility Inward

Thematic Categories

a 4* References to self (speaker) attempting or threatening to kill self, with or without conscious intent.

b 4 References to self wanting to die, needing or deserving to die.

a 3 References to self injuring, mutilating, disfiguring self or threats to do so, with or without conscious intent.

b 3 Self blaming, expressing anger or hatred to self, considering self worthless or of no value, causing oneself grief or trouble, or threatening to do so.

c 3 References to feelings of discouragement, giving up hope, despairing, feeling grieved or depressed, having no purpose in life.

a 2 References to self needing or deserving punishment, paying for one's sins, needing to atone or do penance.

b 2 Self adversely criticizing, depreciating self; references to regretting, being sorry or ashamed for what one says or does; references to self mistaken or in error.

c 2 References to feelings of deprivation, disappointment, lonesomeness.

a 1 References to feeling disappointed in self; unable to meet expectations of self or others.

---

* The number serves to give the weight as well as to identify the category. The letter also helps identify the category.

SCHEDULE 2.3 (contd.)

I. Hostility Inward   Thematic Categories

b 1   Denial of anger, dislike, hatred, blame, destructive impulses from self to self.

c 1   References to feeling painfully driven or obliged to meet one's own expectations and standards.

SCHEDULE 2.4

Ambivalent Hostility Scale: Destructive, Injurious Critical Thoughts
and Actions of Others to Self

II. Ambivalent Hostility

Thematic Categories

a 3*   Others (human) killing or threatening to kill self.

b 3   Others (human) physically injuring, mutilating, disfiguring self or threatening to do so.

c 3   Others (human) adversely criticizing, blaming, expressing anger or dislike toward self or threatening to do so.

d 3   Others (human) abandoning, robbing self, causing suffering, anguish, or threatening to do so.

a 2   Others (human) depriving, disappointing, misunderstanding self or threatening to do so.

b 2   Self threatened with death from subhuman or inanimate object, or death-dealing situation.

a 1   Others (subhuman, inanimate, or situation), injuring, abandoning, robbing self, causing suffering, anguish.

b 1   Denial of blame.

The following examples illustrate our systems of scoring on the three hostility scales. These fragments of verbal samples have been broken down into their component grammatical clauses (complete or elliptical), and those clauses which are scorable on one or more of the scales are marked with the appropriate symbols. The first symbol, a Roman numeral, indicates the type of hostility; the second symbol, a single small letter, indicates a subcategory of verbal items; the third symbol identifies the weight assigned to the thematic category scored. In the following examples, hostility inward scoring is designated with a I, ambivalent hostility is designated with a II, and all scoring on the hostility directed outward scale is enclosed in parentheses, the (I) denoting overt hostility outward and the (II) denoting the covert portion of the scale.

A detailed description of our scoring procedures for these three hostility scales, with many examples, is provided in our *Manual*.

---

* The number serves to give the weight as well as to identify the category. The letter also helps identify the category.

Example 1. Army veteran: Note especially the ambivalent hostility.

$\qquad\qquad\qquad\qquad\qquad\qquad$ IId3 $\qquad$ (Ic3)

". . . And this one man that caused me nothing but hell through the rest of my army career / was made a captain. / He was so efficient /
$\qquad\qquad\qquad\qquad\qquad\qquad\qquad\qquad\qquad$ IId3
that I was the first man / that was busted from the rank of a sergeant to a private / since that outfit was activated for not coming to
$\qquad\qquad\qquad\qquad\qquad\qquad\qquad\qquad\qquad\qquad$ Ib1
attention while working on Saturday morning / when we were off duty. / And all through my army career I was transferred from company to company / and invariably he was always transferred to be the commanding officer. / And I could be / maybe I'd last a month
$\qquad\qquad\qquad\qquad\qquad\qquad\qquad\qquad\qquad$ IId3
or two. / I'd be broken to a private and transferred again. / So finally, I transferred to the paratroopers. / And I had the misfortune
$\qquad\qquad\qquad\qquad\qquad\qquad$ (Ib1)
of running into him again in Africa. / I was selected as a scout to
$\qquad\qquad\qquad\qquad\qquad\qquad$ (IIa3)
take his troops forward into combat on Hill 609. / And in the mean-
$\qquad\qquad$ IIc3
time I had been courtmartialed / for leaving the base on a class B
$\qquad\qquad$ IIc3
pass / and was sentenced to / I think / it was / the best I remember /
$\qquad\qquad\qquad\qquad$ IId3 $\qquad\qquad\qquad\qquad\qquad$ IId3
it was sixty days in the guardhouse. / I'd been kicked out of the
$\qquad\qquad\qquad\qquad\qquad\qquad\qquad\qquad\qquad$ IIc3
aviation cadets. / And he told me, / well, first he called me a sonofa-
$\qquad\qquad\qquad\qquad$ IIc3 $\qquad\qquad\qquad\qquad\qquad\qquad$ (IIc1)
bitch / which I could do nothing about. / And he beat his fist on
$\qquad\qquad\qquad\qquad\qquad\qquad$ (IId1)
the desk / till blood bounced on my uniform. / And he said: / 'If
$\qquad$ (IIa3) $\qquad\qquad\qquad\qquad\qquad$ IIa3
we were on the battlefield, / I'd shoot you.' / And I reminded him of
$\qquad$ IIa3 $\qquad\qquad\qquad\qquad\qquad\qquad\qquad\qquad\qquad$ (Ia3)
that, of *that* statement / when we were going to the front that night. / I asked him, / I said: / 'When we start out tonight, Captain, / you
$\qquad$ (Ic3) $\qquad\qquad\qquad\qquad\qquad\qquad\qquad\qquad\qquad$ IIa3
be damn sure / that you're in front of me / because I don't want to be shot in the back.' " /

Example 2. Woman psychiatric inpatient: Note especially hostility inward.

"The most interesting part of my life is / why my sister and them
$\qquad$ IId3 $\qquad\qquad\qquad\qquad\qquad\qquad$ IId3
want to put me away / and why they want to take my kids away

(II*d*1)

from me. / It all started back / when my mother died / and it's get-

(I*b*1)

ting worser and worser. / When I want to start drinking / I don't

(I*d*2)   (II*f*1)

pay the kids any attention. / I don't leave them alone in the house

II*c*3

or nothing. / My sisters and them, they just say / I'm crazy / and

II*c*3   II*d*3

make fun of me. / And they don't want me around them. / I want

II*d*3

them to let my life alone / and let me be happy / and don't make

I*b*2

me miserable / I want to get all this drinking and stuff out of me. /

II*d*3   (I*c*2)   I*b*2

They keep bothering me. / I got away from them once / and stopped

I*b*2

drinking / and I was doing real good / and then I started drinking

again / and that just kept getting worser. / And sometimes I get to

I*c*3   I*a*4

the place / I just don't care. / Sometimes it seems / like I want to

I*a*4   I*b*1

take my life / and I done tried that three times / and I don't want that

to happen anymore / because I got my kids to raise up. / And I'm

I*c*3

just in misery / and there's something / that I just want to get away

II*a*1

from all the time. /

Example 3. Male high school student: Note especially hostility out.

(I*b*1)

"This pledging period you go through / is kind of stupid. / Take for

II*b*3   (II*a*3)

instance last Sunday / when they beat us up. / I can't see / what they

(I*c*2)   (II*a*3)

accomplish / when they take someone / and give him five or ten

(I*b*1)

swats. / And some of the stupid things they make you do / like run-

ning around a car / when you're at a red light / is very dangerous. /

(II*e*2)

Somebody can get killed / when they pull some of these stunts off. /

(I*b*1)

So I didn't feel in too pleasant a mood / when I answered that ques-

(I*b*1)

tionnaire; / and I put down every way / I felt sore / that I could. /

(I*b*1)

That's the way / I felt. / And coming down here to take this test is an example. / I wanted to come. / But before I came in this room /
(II*a*3)   II*b*3   (II*f*1)
the guys take us / and we get punched again and all. / I didn't
(I*b*1)   (I*c*3)
mind / but what the heck's the sense of it. / It's not their right / to
(II*a*3) II*b*3
kick you through the floor, every time they feel like it. / Because you
I*b*1 (I*c*3)
have as much right on this earth / as they do." /

The Measurement of Relative Degree of Social Alienation and Personal Disorganization (the Schizophrenic Scale) from Verbal Samples [8]

The speech of man is one aspect of his behavior which distinguishes him from other mammals, including primates. It communicates his moods, his emotions, his sensory experiences, his memories, his plans, and his assessments of objects around him. It exemplifies man's sustained dependence on and involvement with other human beings throughout his life, for it is a behavioral function that is learned and ordinarily carried on between two or more people instead of alone.

That the verbal behavior of an individual suffering from a mental disorder is relatively distinctive—both in form and in content—has been obvious to those who listen to the conversations of people with personality disorders. The depressed person is laconic and talks about self-depreciatory and morose topics. The manic person is verbose and tends to talk extravagantly about achievements and frequent, superficial contacts with people. The hysteric and schizophrenic are quite variable in the duration of their remarks, and they, too, have characteristic thematic and structural features in their speech.

We have attempted to go beyond the clinical observation that there are certain qualitative peculiarities in the verbal behavior of people who have severe personality disorders. We have entertained the hypothesis that, perhaps, the degree of personal and social disorganization of an individual can be quantitatively

[8] Excerpted, with considerable alterations and additions, from L. A. Gottschalk, G. C. Gleser, R. Daniels, and S. Block, *J. Nerv. Ment. Dis.*, 127: 153–166, 1958, and from L. A. Gottschalk, G. C. Gleser, E. B. Magliocco, and T. D'Zmura, *J. Nerv. Ment. Dis.*, 132: 101–113, 1961—with permission of the publishers.

assessed, at any one time, from the frequency of occurrence of a cluster of speech habits and themata which have pertinence to the individual's subjective experience.

GENERAL INFORMATION ABOUT THE PECULIARITIES OF LANGUAGE IN SCHIZOPHRENIA

The verbal behavior of the schizophrenic patient has been an area of special interest and attention to other investigators as a source of information about the phenomenology and psychopathology of schizophrenia. Some writers have described ways in which the form and structure of language behavior are diagnostic of the schizophrenic syndrome (Bleuler, 1911; Mittenecker, 1951; Lorenz, 1953, 1955; Lorenz and Cobb, 1954; Mirin, 1955). For example, the content of the patient's communications has been found difficult to understand or quite unintelligible. The language has been seen as ambiguous, with a tendency to diffusion or generalization. The words, themselves, have been noted to be used inexactly, and frequently there is frank incoherence or disjunction. Elliptical statements may occur. The sentences may have frequent self-contradictions and euphemisms, and they may contain many self-references and impersonal constructions (Mittenecker, 1951; Rosen, 1955; Gottschalk et al., 1957, 1958a, 1961a).

From the psychopathologic point of view, schizophrenic language has been noted to be concretistic and "paleologic" (White, 1949; Arieti, 1950, 1954), and the initial distortion in language has been ascribed to a confusion of the word symbol with the symbolized object (Arieti, 1948) in which the usual meaning becomes ignored and the language becomes private (Arieti, 1950; Jenkins, 1952; Klages, 1954; Cameron et al., 1956).

Goodstein (1951) has summarized, interpreted, and attempted to integrate the various theoretical positions regarding schizophrenic language. Kasanin (1946) has edited a book in which eight leading investigators of schizophrenic behavior have provided theoretical considerations on the language and thinking processes in schizophrenia, and Bellak and Benedict (1958) have provided an up-to-date review and discussion of the subject in their recent volume.

Our attention is centered on the speech of schizophrenic patients, not to try to amplify further the already substantial knowledge and theoretical considerations regarding the thinking and communication disturbances in schizophrenia. Rather, we are trying to exploit what is empirically known about the peculiarities of the schizophrenic mode of verbal communication for the purpose of developing a means of quantifying the relative severity of social alienation and personal disorganization among people in general and among schizophrenic individuals in particular. The values of such an aim are, broadly speaking, twofold: (1) to gain knowledge applicable to a general method of quantifying psychological and behavioral patterns; and (2) to take another step toward developing useful tools in clinical psychiatric research—a means, for example, of assessing the effects of various hopefully therapeutic activities or medications on the ebb and flow of schizophrenic manifestations occurring in the language behavior of patients.

THEORETICAL AND DESCRIPTIVE FEATURES OF OUR (SCHIZOPHRENIC) SCALE OF SOCIAL ALIENATION AND PERSONAL DISORGANIZATION

The initial approach of our investigations of schizophrenic speech was to analyze verbal productions of schizophrenics over a period of time according to certain structural, emotive, and informative categories believed to have high relevance to the schizophrenic pattern of relating to the environment. Furthermore, it was planned to test whether the frequency of occurrence of themata in these categories was quantitatively related to the degree of personal disorganization, social alienation, and isolation of the schizophrenic patients.

Our concept of the schizophrenic syndrome has been that it is composed of different subgroups featuring somewhat different types of thinking disorders, such as described by Wynne and Singer (1963a, 1963b, 1965) and by different phenomenological subgroups, as exemplified by those of Kraeplin (1904), Bleuler (1911), and the current nosological classification of the American Psychiatric Association. The common denominators of the schizophrenic syndrome have been considered to be disturbances in the coherence and logicality of thinking processes and disturbance in human relationships especially in the form of withdrawal, avoidance, and antagonism. Another principal characteristic of our working concept of the schizophrenic syndrome has been that it is a phenomenon quantitatively describable, that is, that there are relative degrees of severity of schizophrenia and that, in some schizophrenic individuals, the severity can fluctuate considerably from day to day. This concept of the schizophrenic syndrome is, of course, in opposition to the viewpoint expressed in such statements as "once a schizophrenic always a schizophrenic."

Our working concept of the schizophrenic syndrome, in fact, holds that the principal and characteristic features of schizophrenia—social alienation and personal disorganization—are present to varying extents in nonschizophrenic individuals but not in such a continuous and/or extreme fashion. Some supportive empirical evidence for this concept has been previously reported (Gottschalk et al., 1964a) and will be reviewed later in this book (Chapter VII, pp. 186 ff.).

The assumptions and principles upon which we have based our verbal behavior method of measuring the severity of the schizophrenic syndrome are:

1. The severity of the schizophrenic syndrome can be validly estimated from the typescript of the speech of an individual without recourse to other channels of communication, such as linguistic, paralinguistic, kinesic, and postural. The major part of the variance in the degree of social alienation and personal disorganization can be accounted for by variations in certain lexical and structural features in the content of verbal communications. (Some evidence to support this position is available in Gottschalk et al., [1966a] and Gottschalk and Frank [1967].)

2. The smallest communication unit conveying information in our language about process, agent, and object is the grammatical clause, a combination of subject and predicate. In some utterances, as with interjections, either one or both of these elements are omitted but understood through conventional usage by speaker and audience. Lexical and structural content per clause, with only a few exceptions, will suffice to provide a satisfactory quantitative estimate of the schizophrenic syndrome.

3. The magnitude of the schizophrenic syndrome is directly proportional to:

    a. The frequency of occurrence in a language sample of verbal themata listed in our schizophrenic scale.

    b. The degree to which the verbal expression—lexical or structural content—indicates alienation from the self or others and/or impairment of cognitive function.

This degree, for different subcategories of content, has been first roughly estimated from clinical experience and has then been checked with further empirical studies. It has been represented as a weighting factor, and each weight designates roughly the relative probability that the thematic or structural speech category is associated with our conception of the schizophrenic syndrome.

4. The weights applied to the categories of our schizophrenic scale are considered to be the same whether the thematic (lexical content) references are expressed in the past, present, or future tense, as a conditional probability, as a wish, or as a report of a dream. This is similar to the procedure used with our affect scales. It is based on the idea that primary process thinking is an indicator of the intensity of a current psychological state.

5. The frequency of use of relevant verbal categories (from the schizophrenic scale) multiplied by the numerical weight assigned to the category and, finally, the summation of these products, provides an ordinal index of the intensity of the schizophrenic syndrome.

In Schedule 2.5, there are listed the form and content categories of speech that constitute the scale of social alienation and personal disorganization. In developing this method, one of the investigators (L. A. G.) set down all the thematic and formal characteristics of the verbal activities of schizophrenic patients which he believed might vary in frequency of occurrence with the

SCHEDULE 2.5

Content Analysis Scale of (Schizophrenic) Social Alienation and
Personal Disorganization

Scores (Weights)		Categories and Scoring Symbols ‡
Modified*	Original†	
		I. Interpersonal references (including fauna and flora).
		A. To thoughts, feelings or reported actions of avoidance, leaving, deserting, spurning, not understanding of others.
0	+1	1. Self avoiding others.
+1	+1	2. Others avoiding self.
		B. To unfriendly, hostile, destructive thoughts, feelings, or actions.
+1	+1	1. Self unfriendly to others.
+⅓	+1	2. Others unfriendly to self.
		C. To congenial and constructive thoughts, feelings, or actions.
−2	−1	1. Others helping, being friendly towards others.

SCHEDULE 2.5 (contd.)

Scores (Weights)		Categories and Scoring Symbols ‡
Modified*	Original†	
−2	−1	2. Self helping, being friendly towards others.
−2	−1	3. Others helping, being friendly towards self.
		D. To others (including fauna, flora, things and places).
0	+1	1. Bad, dangerous, low value or worth, strange, ill, malfunctioning.
−1	−½	2. Intact, satisfied, healthy, well.
		II. Intrapersonal references.
		A. To disorientation-orientation, past, present, or future. (Do not include all references to time, place, or person, but only those in which it is reasonably clear the subject is trying to orient himself or is expressing disorientation with respect to these. Also, do not score more than one item per clause under this category.)
+2	+1	1. Indicating disorientation for time, place, or person or other distortion of reality.
0	−½	2. Indicating orientation in time, place, person.
0	+½	3. Indicating attempts to identify time, place, or person without clearly revealing orientation or distorientation.
		B. To self.
0	+1	1a. Physical illness, malfunctioning (references to illness or symptoms due primarily to cellular or tissue damage).
+1	+1	1b. Psychological malfunctioning (references to illness or symptoms due primarily to emotions or psychological reactions *not secondary* to cellular or tissue damage).
0	+1	1c. Malfunctioning of indeterminate origin (references to illness or symptoms not definitely attributable either to emotions or cellular damage).
−2	−½	2. Getting better.
−1	−1	3a. Intact, satisfied, healthy, well; definite positive affect or valence indicated.
−1	−1	3b. Intact, satisfied, healthy, well; flat, factual, or neutral attitudes expressed.
+½	+½	4. Not being prepared or able to produce, perform, act, not knowing, not sure.
+½	+1	5. To being controlled, feeling controlled, wanting control, asking for control or permission, being obliged or having to do, think, or experience something.
+3	+½	C. Denial of feelings, attitudes, or mental state of the self.
		D. To food.
0	+1	1. Bad, dangerous, unpleasant or otherwise negative; interferences or delays in eating; too

SCHEDULE 2.5 (contd.)

| Scores (Weighs) | | Categories and Scoring Symbols‡ |
Modified*	Original†	
		much and wish to have less; too little and wish to have more.
0	−½	2. Good or neutral.
		E. To weather.
−1	−½ §	1. Bad, dangerous, unpleasant or otherwise negative (not sunny, not clear, uncomfortable, etc.).
−1	−1	2. Good, pleasant or neutral.
		F. To sleep.
0	+1	1. Bad, dangerous, unpleasant or otherwise negative; too much, too little.
0	−½	2. Good, pleasant or neutral.
		III. Miscellaneous.
		A. Signs of disorganization.
+1	+1	1. Remarks or words that are not understandable or inaudible.
0	+1	2. Incomplete sentences, clauses, phrases; blocking.
+2	+1	3. Obviously erroneous or fallacious remarks or conclusions; illogical or bizarre statements.
		B. Repetition of ideas in sequence.
0	+½	1. Words separated only by a word (excluding instances due to grammatical and syntactical convention, where words are repeated, e.g., "as far as," "by and by," and so forth. Also, excluding instances where such words as "I" and "the" are separated by a word).
+1	+1	2. Phrases, clauses (separated only by a phrase or clause).

New Items

+1	0	IV. A. Questions directed to the interviewer.
+½	0	B. Other references to the interviewer.
+1	0	V. Religious and biblical references.

* These weights are a revision of the weights described in our 1961 publication so as to indicate the findings obtained in the study herein reported. These weights are more sensitive and discriminatory in cross-sectional studies and studies involving the task of differentiating schizophrenics from nonschizophrenics. They can be used satisfactorily in longitudinal investigations. Note that categories signifying evidence of the schizophrenic syndrome are given positive weights and vice versa.

† Described in our 1958 publication. These weights may be more sensitive in longitudinal studies. Note that the direction of scoring is reversed as compared to the weights given in our 1958 publication to conform with the modified weights.

‡ For the rules for scoring the categories, see our manual (Gottschalk *et al.*, 1969).

§ Scored +½ for the first two in a verbal sample and thereafter this item is scored −1.

relative levels of integration and operational perspective of a schizophrenic person. One group of categories chosen covered statements about how the patient perceived the relationships between other people or between others and himself. The categories included avoidance propensities, hostile or adversely critical propensities, and friendly approaching tendencies. One group of categories covered information about the speaker's subjective experiences, such as orientation or disorientation, disturbances of emotion or functioning within the self, and feelings of improvement or well-being. One category covered references—whether good, bad, or neutral,—to various common conversational topics, such as the weather, food, or sleep. Another group of categories covered certain structural aspects: the form, clarity, and accuracy of the verbal activity, such as repetitions of words or phrases, bizarre or unintelligible remarks, and obviously fallacious remarks. In a series of validation studies over a period of ten years (Chap. VII, pp. 186 ff.), some of these content categories have been discarded, modified, or added to as empirical evidence pertaining to reliability and validity has warranted this. The "original" weights refer to those arrived at after our initial validation study (Gottschalk *et al.*, 1958a); the "modified" weights are based on subsequent validation studies (Gottschalk *et al.*, 1961a, 1964a). The verbal categories in the schedule are by no means considered an exhaustive collection of the content and structural speech characteristics of schizophrenic patients. There are undoubtedly many other classifications of the speech of schizophrenics which might be of pertinence and usefulness in such an endeavor. Hopefully, further research by others and ourselves may serve as a guide to what other categories might be added and how some of our subcategory weights might be advantageously altered. Furthermore, there are a number of categories, especially those not pertaining to thought disorder, which are not specific for schizophrenia but relate more generally to psychopathological and physical maladaptation. The frequency of these categories contributes to the capacity of this scale to measure severity of illness and malfunctioning in general. The inclusion of these categories, as a matter of fact, makes the scale not only a measure of the severity of the schizophrenic syndrome but also a measure of psychiatric morbidity (for further details, see Chap. IV, pp. 84–93). In this respect, the scale has usefulness as a general measure of transient changes in the psychiatric health-sickness dimension. Furthermore, it can be expected to give unusually high scores with people acutely ill from physical or mental disturbances that in no respect can be considered congruent with schizophrenia (e.g., Gottschalk *et al.*, 1967). In such instances, the scores are obviously false positives for schizophrenia, but they do correctly reflect the degree of general morbidity. However, the nosological classification we call "schizophrenia" is a heterogeneous collection of attitudes, traits, and behaviors central to which are certain peculiarities of thought. There is no evidence that the nonschizophrenic population is devoid of at least transient deficiencies in thinking processes of the kind typifying schizophrenics and, furthermore, it is apparent that the nonschizophrenic population of individuals does have the capacity to behave, if only briefly, like the schizophrenic. Indeed, the evidence suggests that schizophrenic disorders involve a set of behaviors distributed on a continuum in the general population and that the people we label schizophrenics are simply manifesting the characteristic features of the syndrome more continuously and at a more prominent level than the nonschizophrenics (see also Wynne and Singer, 1963*a*, 1963*b*, 1965) and the "borderline" or "schizoid" groups. In this sense, one would expect that everyone could obtain some score on a schizophrenic scale, but that only those consistently receiving higher scores would be diagnosed as having schizophrenia.

An example follows of a fragment of a five-minute verbal sample actually produced by a schizophrenic patient: the example illustrates our system of scoring those clauses that have scorable items, with appropriate symbols designating each category. Italicized words indicate repetitions; unintelligible or inaudible words are indicated in parentheses. No assignment of weights is implied by the numbers in the code symbols; the numbers help designate subcategories (see Schedule 2.5 for key to scoring symbols and weights).

Example

IIIB2

In the morning I *clean my* teeth / *clean my* gums and all that / *clean*
IIIB2   IIIA1
my teeth and tongue and all that / (2 words) said that. / Spoke about
IID2   ID1
it upstairs. / And after I eat breakfast / all that white scum comes

         IIB4   IIB4   IIIB2

on 'em again. / *I don't know* what from. / *I don't know* whether /
       IIIA1   IIB1c

it's from fermenting from my ear, / but I got a stone in it out
       IIB1c   IIB1c

here. / Never was removed, / whether it's from that or what. / Looks
IIB1*b*   IIB1*b*   IIIA1

awful bad. / I'm ashamed to show it to anybody. / The funniest rays
IIIA1   IA2   IIIA1

(3 words) / but I been losing friends by it. / These rays (3 words) /
       IB2   IIB4

incriminating against them / and they innocent people. / I don't
                 IIB4   IIIB2

know / *why that is.* / I can't understand / *why that is* either, at
       IIIA1   IIIA3

all. / Don't (2 words) / it breaks right through my body or my sys-
             IA2   IIB4

tem like. / Been losing friends by it. / Don't know why it is. / My
IIB1*a*   IIIB2

lips are always *real dry* like, *real dry.* / Months now. / My folks are
ID2   IIB4   IIIA1   ID2

all good people too. / I can't understand / (3 words) / They good. /
       IIB1c   IC3

When my health failed, / why then my folks asked for me not to do
any work. . . .

The Measurement of Other Psychological States from Verbal Samples—Theoretical Assumptions and Hypotheses

The approaches for quantifying such psychological states as affects and the schizophrenic syndrome from speech can be generalized and applied to any psychological state. The recommended steps are as follows:

1. An operational definition of the psychological state is decided upon. This definition, to be useful to others, must describe the psychological state in terms of its broadest current accepted usage.

2. All of the lexical cues are enumerated that enable the listener to infer, with some modest level of probability, that a speaker is experiencing the psychological state in question. These cues must, then, be classified into categories that are minimally overlapping.

3. An estimate is made as to how directly and specifically each content category signifies the psychological state being measured. This estimate should take the form of a comparison, on an

approximate basis, of the relative potency of any one content category as an indicator of this psychological state as compared to all other content categories. Our experience indicates that it is better not to make too many fine distinctions at this point. Possibly only two or three levels suffice. These estimates are, then, transformed into tentative weights, and the weights may be used in the calculation of scores employed in initial validation studies (as described under the measurement of affects and the measurement of social alienation and personal disorganization).

4. The frequency of occurrence of the specific lexical content categories multiplied by the weights assigned to each content category is summated. Mathematical transformation of the raw scores may be found advantageous to obtain indices in terms of a score per 100 words and to make the distributions of scores more amenable to parametric statistical evaluation.

5. Preliminary testing of reliability of scoring such a content scale by someone other than the originator of the scale will clarify those categories that are ambiguous or in some other respect difficult to score. Modification of the content categories at this point in their evolution in the direction of more reliably scored categories is an advisable practice. Subsequent interscorer reliability studies should be carried out using the new scale and a reliability coefficient of .80 to .85 should be sought. If such a level of reliability is not obtained, either further training of scorers is necessary or content categories on which scorers have poor consensus should be eliminated or further revised.

6. Construct validation studies should be carried out and criterion measures—clinical rating scales, psychological tests, and any other relevant procedures that provide even an approximate measure of the psychological construct—should be used. After doing such validation studies, an item analysis should be carried out to determine what content categories are contributing to the concordance of verbal behavior scores with the criterion measures. The possibility should be kept in mind that the a priori weights assigned to the categories may need modification to obtain better concordance with appropriate criterion measures. Whenever weights are changed on the basis of such empirical studies, further empirical studies should, ideally, be undertaken to check whether the modified weights provide scores that correlate better with the criterion scores.

CHAPTER III
Reliability and Generalizability Studies

SOURCES OF ERROR VARIANCE IN PROCESSING AND SCORING SPEECH SAMPLES

There are many points in the processing of the raw data of speech samples and converting them into scales measuring a psychological construct at which distortion and random error may occur. Errors arise as a result of fluctuations in the fidelity of recording of speech samples, distortions or misinterpretations in processing the typescript, variations in interpreting coding categories and applying them to the verbal content, and slips in the tabulation and computation of final scores. Such processing errors limit the interpretability of scores, regardless of the decision purposes for which measures are obtained, and hence should be reduced to a minimum by introducing various controls and checks.

Poor recordings can be minimized by keeping recorders in good condition, using sensitive microphones that can record voices at varying distances, obtaining speech samples in relatively quiet surroundings, and making certain that the interviewer knows how to use the recording instrument properly. The skill of the interviewer in this respect is of utmost importance, since the exigencies of a particular research study may necessitate taking recordings under less than optimal environmental conditions. We have obtained successful recordings from bedridden patients and from patients in large wards by careful placement of the microphone and volume controls. On the other hand, little can be done to salvage an inaudible recording.

It may seem surprising to some readers that distortions and misinterpretations of the verbal record can occur during transcription. People have a propensity to react to external signs and symbols in terms of the private meanings they are reminded of, and these meanings may bias the perceptive process so that false perceptions occur. Thus the typist in preparing a typescript often

49

distorts what was said in the record, particularly when the recording is poor or the speaker is difficult to understand. To minimize these kinds of errors in our laboratory, one typist routinely transcribes the tape-recorded verbal samples we obtain and another typist or research technician "proof-listens" to the transcript to catch errors.

Scoring errors, that is, the discrepancies that occur when technicians code the content of a clause in one scoring category of a scale rather than another or fail to code a clause that others code, are somewhat different than the processing errors previously mentioned. Variations in coding can occur because of ambiguities in the formulation and delineation of the content categories, idiosyncratic expressions used by the speaker, variations among technicians in their understanding of the content categories, and fluctuations in the mental state of the technician. Thus, coding errors can only be minimized, not eliminated, by the developer of content scales. The user must introduce his own controls in terms of training and the design of scoring procedures (including multiple scoring) that can reduce error variance arising from this source to a size suitable for his purposes.

In the development of the content scales presented in this book, we have expended considerable effort in clarifying the definition of each category to reduce ambiguity. Content categories of a new scale are given preliminary trials to determine whether the description and definition of each category is readily understandable and capable of differentiation from other categories in the scale. In the preliminary trials, interscorer consensus is examined at the level of the clause and for each code separately. Content categories that contain ambiguities resulting in poor consensus are reworded or eliminated. If difficulties encountered with certain types of content can be resolved by examples and guidelines, these have been recorded for future use.

After the initial trials, interscorer reliability studies are carried out using the final transformed score, and a reliability coefficient of .85 or above is sought. This requires, of course, not only reasonably clear and scorable content categories, but also technicians who are well trained in the scoring procedures. As has been previously indicated, the method does not require any psychoanalytic or psychodynamic expertise on the part of the scorer. The theoretical inference has already been built into the scales.

The principal requirement of the scorer is to be able to classify and place the content of what is being scored literally, rather than figuratively, into the content categories of the scale.

The scales that have been used over the longest period of time, namely, the anxiety and hostility scales and the scale of social alienation–personal disorganization, have revealed by this time where difficulties and disagreements are likely to appear during the coding process. Guidelines with examples have been collected and are available in the form of a scoring manual (Gottschalk *et al.*, 1969).

From time to time, we have obtained estimates of the error variance attributable to coders and to occasion of scoring for each of our scales in order to determine whether any shift has occurred with the passage of time in the way categories are interpreted. In this way, we have attempted to maintain a "quality control" of the final scores used in our substantive research. We have further reduced error variance due to scoring in most such studies by using the average of two independent scorings of each verbal sample.

ESTIMATES OF ERROR VARIANCE IN SCORING SPEECH SAMPLES

Anxiety Scale—Reliability Studies

Studies have been undertaken to determine the variance in anxiety scores attributable to differences among scorers in samples of verbal material obtained from several populations of subjects. In the eight years or more that this scale has been in use, six different coding technicians have been employed in our laboratory to score the anxiety scale, and several persons in laboratories other than our own have also been trained in its use. Extent of scoring agreement has been determined using different combinations of scorers and, in general, has yielded consistent estimates of the scoring reliability of the total anxiety scale using trained personnel.

We have chosen three recent studies for which estimates of scoring variance on the subscales are available to indicate the range and extent of agreement obtained on different samples. Results are presented in Table 3.1. The first column under each sample heading indicates the estimated variance of subjects'

TABLE 3.1

Estimates of Scoring Reliability for Anxiety Subscales and Total Anxiety Scale

Subscales	Psychiatric outpatients N = 50				Mixed psychiatric inpatients N = 65				Medical patients N = 82			
	V_{M_p}*	V_e†	ρ^2_{XM}‡	$\rho^2_{\bar{X}M}$§	V_{M_p}	V_e	ρ^2_{XM}	$\rho^2_{\bar{X}M}$	V_{M_p}	V_e	ρ^2_{XM}	$\rho^2_{\bar{X}M}$
Death	.167	.027	.86	.93	.148	.048	.75	.86	.205	.044	.82	.90
Mutilation	.115	.017	.87	.93	.224	.045	.83	.91	.104	.027	.79	.88
Separation	.247	.117	.68	.81	.205	.144	.59	.74	.177	.101	.64	.78
Guilt	.308	.081	.79	.88	.341	.094	.78	.88	.071	.047	.60	.75
Shame	.236	.236	.50	.67	.431	.265	.62	.77	.367	.085	.81	.90
Diffuse	.342	.101	.77	.87	.283	.040	.88	.94	.258	.092	.74	.85
Total scale	.480	.122	.80	.89	.537	.200	.73	.84	.417	.067	.86	.93

* Estimated population variance of person's universe score.
† Estimated error variance.
‡ Estimated reliability of scores using any one scorer.
§ Estimated reliability of average scores of any two independent scorers.

scores if averaged over a universe of scorers (V_{Mp}). The second column (V_e) is the estimated variance of scores obtainable on any one subject's verbal sample using different scoring technicians. The latter variance, which includes differences among technicians in their average level of scoring for the entire sample, is also error variance under the assumption that scores provided by any technician will be used interchangeably with those provided by any other technician. The third column (ρ^2_{xM}) is the estimated reliability of scores using any one coder for any verbal sample, and $\rho^2_{\bar{x}M}$ is the estimated reliability of the average of two such codings (Cronbach et al., 1963). It is this latter estimate that applies to our validity studies reported below, since we routinely average the scores obtained from two independent codings.

It is evident from the table that for most subscales, somewhat less error variance occurs in coding the medical patients' and psychiatric outpatients' verbal samples than in coding psychiatric inpatients. Many of the latter samples were short, a circumstance which contributes to unreliability. Considering all three groups of records, the least reliable subscales are those for separation and shame anxiety. The reliability of the total scale ranges from .84 to .93 for the average of two codings. The error variance of such averages ranges from .03 to .10.

A more complete study of the variance attributable to coders was performed on a sample of 30 verbal records obtained from chronic schizophrenics. These were each coded twice by two technicians, the interval between codings being approximately two years. Our purpose in making this study was to determine to what extent coders change their concept of the scales from time to time and hence contribute error to the interpretation of scores obtained in studies done at different periods of time (Gleser et al., 1965b). The analysis of variance for the total anxiety score is shown in Table 3.2. Coders differ very little in their average level of scoring from time to time ($V_{C \times O}$) or in their overall average (V_C). Coders differ from each other consistently to some extent in their coding of specific verbal samples ($V_{P \times C}$), and there is some consistent change in their scoring of particular verbal samples from one period of time to another ($V_{P \times O}$), possibly attributable to further learning. There is also a difference over and above these two-way interactions in the coding of any specific sample from time to time by any one technician. These sources of variance all

TABLE 3.2

Analysis of Variance of Anxiety Scores Each Coded Twice by Two Technicians*

Source	df	MS	Variance estimates
Protocols (P)	29	1.046	.234
Occasion of scoring (O)	1	.005	.000
Coder (C)	1	.006	.000
P × O	29	.063	.021
P × C	29	.070	.024
O × C	1	.002	.000
P × O × C	29	.022	.022

* Reliability of single scoring $= \dfrac{.234}{.301} = .78$.

* Reliability of average of two independent scorings $= .84$.

contribute to error in the interpretation of the anxiety scores obtained on a verbal sample by any one coder at any particular time. Thus, the total estimated error variance is .066. This yields an estimate of .78 for the reliability of a single coding on any one scoring occasion and a reliability of .84 for the average of two independent scorings whether obtained by two different technicians or by one technician on two widely separated occasions. These results are very similar to those obtained in a study reported previously (Gleser et al., 1961) using 20 protocols from a nonpatient sample. In the latter study, the estimated reliability of a single coding on any occasion was .76 and that for the average of two scores using different technicians was .86.

Another study of scoring reliability involved a comparison of the scores of four different technicians, each coding verbal samples obtained on 19 male and female students each tested on two occasions. In this study, the reliability of a single scoring was estimated to be .84 and that for the average of any two scorings was .91. As might be expected, there was no interaction between occasions of testing and coders, indicating that these two sources of error can be treated independently. In general, then, the generalizability of scores on the total anxiety scale as coded by a single technician is about .80, and that for the average of two independent scorings is about .90.

Hostility Scales—Reliability Studies

In Table 3.3, we have indicated the between-person variance (V_{M_p}), the error variance (V_e), the reliability of a single score

TABLE 3.3

Estimates of Scoring Reliability of Hostility Scales

Groups	No.	Hostility Outward												Ambivalent hostility				Hostility inward			
		Overt				Covert				Total											
		V_{M_p}*	V_e†	ρ^2_{XM}‡	$\rho^2_{\bar{X}M}$§	V_{M_p}	V_e	ρ^2_{XM}	$\rho^2_{\bar{X}M}$	V_{M_p}	V_e	ρ^2_{XM}	$\rho^2_{\bar{X}M}$	V_{M_p}	V_e	ρ^2_{XM}	$\rho^2_{\bar{X}M}$	V_{M_p}	V_e	ρ^2_{XM}	$\rho^2_{\bar{X}M}$
Psychiatric outpatients	50	.142	.073	.66	.80	.226	.037	.86	.92	.246	.068	.78	.88	.172	.053	.76	.87	.262	.032	.89	.94
Mixed psychiatric inpatients	65	.107	.056	.66	.79	.279	.011	.96	.98	.306	.047	.87	.93	.250	.020	.92	.96	.312	.062	.83	.91
Nonpsychiatric V.A. inpatients	43	.110	.058	.65	.79	.161	.035	.82	.90	.237	.061	.80	.89	.228	.022	.91	.95	.151	.042	.78	.88

* Estimated population variance of person's universe score.
† Estimated error variance.
‡ Estimated reliability of scores using any one scorer.
§ Estimated reliability of average scores of any two independent scorers.

(ρ^2xm), and that of the average of two scores (ρ^2x̄m) for each of our hostility scales as found in three separate samples of individuals. The reliability estimates are based on the supposition that scores obtained by different technicians will be used interchangeably, that is, the difference in mean scoring level from one scorer to another is included in the error variance.

The scoring reliability of the hostility scales is generally satisfactory. The scoring reliability of the overt hostility outward subscale is, however, sometimes a little low. This appears primarily due to the relatively small "true score" variance for the subscale, although the error variance estimates are also somewhat larger than those obtained for the covert subscale.

From these data, we can estimate the standard error of an obtained score based on the average of two scorings. The values are approximately .17 for the total hostility outward scale, .13 for the ambivalent hostility scale, and .15 for the inward hostility scale. These standard errors, although apparently small, indicate that differences in individual hostility scores of less than about .40 (twice the standard error of the difference) should be interpreted only with extreme caution.

The correspondence of hostility scores obtained by different technicians at different times was examined for a sample of 30 male and 30 female chronic schizophrenic patients. Two technicians scored the samples during the time that a research project was underway with these subjects and again about two years later. The results of the study are shown in Table 3.4.

TABLE 3.4

Estimates of Variance of Hostility Scales Attributable to Protocols, Coders, and Occasions of Scoring

| | Hostility outward | | | Hostility inward | Ambivalent hostility |
Estimate	Overt	Covert	Total		
$V_{\text{Protocols (P)}}$	.154	.098	.234	.176	.255
$V_{\text{Occasion of scoring (O)}}$ ..	.001	.000	.000	.000	.004
$V_{\text{Coders (C)}}$	.000	.000	.000	.001	.001
$V_{\text{P} \times \text{O}}$	.020	.016	.009	.010	.001
$V_{\text{P} \times \text{C}}$	.056	.015	.041	.005	.009
$V_{\text{O} \times \text{C}}$	.000	.001	.002	.000	.000
$V_{\text{P} \times \text{O} \times \text{C}}$	.023	.024	.034	.020	.014
ρ^2 *	.606	.636	.731	.830	.898

* Estimate of generalizability of scoring to a universe of coders and occasions of coding for data scored by any qualified coder.

The data indicate that there has been practically no variation in the general level of scores over the past two years in the laboratory as a whole (V_{Occasion}) or per any individual coder ($V_{o\times c}$). Technicians vary somewhat in their coding of a specific protocol from time to time ($V_{P\times o}$) but the largest variance arises from differences in their perception of the scoring categories as applied to a particular protocol ($V_{P\times c}$) and in their specific set at any one time in coding a specific protocol ($V_{P\times c\times o}$). Thus the use of the average scoring by two coders reduces the largest sources of error and efficiently increases generalizability. For example, the estimated generalizability of the average score for total hostility outward becomes .833. The overt and covert subscales are still somewhat less reliable than we should like them to be.

Social Alienation–Personal Disorganization (Schizophrenic) Scale—Reliability Studies

For most of the studies we have undertaken with the schizophrenic scale, only one coder has been used. The relationships we obtained between our scores and an outside criterion for samples of schizophrenic patients (see Chapter VII) were high enough to indicate that scoring reliability was adequate, at least when the scale was applied to verbal samples obtained on a schizophrenic population.

In a more recent study, in which longitudinal data were obtained over a nine-week period on 35 male and 39 female chronic hospitalized schizophrenics, two coders were employed. For the preliminary (baseline data), the two sets of scores were compared, and correlations of about .90 were found between coders. The larger discrepancies, however, were examined to determine sources of unreliability in the category definitions.

As a final check on scoring reliability, the two sets of verbal samples obtained from each patient in the fourth week of the study were analyzed. At this time, all the patients were on placebo. Several of the more disturbed patients were mute on one or both occasions, so that two verbal samples were available for only 27 males and 36 females. The sexes were treated separately, using analysis of variance. The variance estimates are shown in Table 3.5. It may be noted that the variance estimates for subjects and for subjects $\times$ occasions are much larger for the males than for the females. This corresponds to other data, indicating that the extent and range of severity of symptomatology was greater for the males than for the females. It was for this reason that the data for the two sexes were analyzed separately.

TABLE 3.5

Estimates of Variance Attributable to Subjects, Occasions, and Coders on the Social Alienation–Personal Disorganization Scale for a Male and a Female Sample of Chronic Hospitalized Schizophrenics

Source	Variance estimates	
	Males (N = 27)	Females (N = 36)
Subjects (S)	56.53	22.73
Occasions (two samples within a week) (O) ..	.00	.34
Coders (C)	.10	.00
S × O	16.31	7.80
S × C	.00	.00
O × C	.00	.00
S × O × C	.70	1.48

It is evident from Table 3.5 that there was very little, if any, systematic difference in coding between the two technicians; the estimated variance for coders is .10 and .00 respectively in the two samples. Furthermore, there was no tendency for coders to differ in their overall evaluation of the verbal samples for any particular patient ($V_{S \times C}$) or in their coding of samples obtained early in the week as compared to those taken later. The primary source of error in scoring stems from differences in the interpretation of coding as applied to a specific verbal sample ($V_{S \times C \times O}$). This variance estimate is considerably larger for the female than for the male sample, probably because many of these samples entailed more subtle evidences of bizarre thinking and contained more interpersonal references, whereas many of the male samples were obviously bizarre and repetitious.

Assuming that decisions will be made on the absolute score value, our data yield estimates for the standard error of measurement of 0.9 and 1.2 scale units for males and females respectively. The error variance of coding is small relative to the variance of scores on any one occasion for these samples (observed score variance), so that the coefficient of generalizability is .95 for the females and .99 for the males. If this scale is used on other than a schizophrenic population, however, it is likely that the ratio of error variance to total variance would range considerably higher and that the scoring reliability would be correspondingly lower. Thus, for the nonschizophrenic psychiatric patients reported in Chapter IV, if we assume the same error variance for coding as indicated for the female sample in Table 3.5, the reliability of a single scoring is estimated as approximately .84. Even this estimate is of the order of reliability that we obtain using the average of two scorings with our affect scales.

GENERALIZABILITY OF SCORES FOR INDIVIDUALS OVER INTERVALS OF TIME AND IN RESPONSE TO DIFFERENT STIMULI

In order for a measurement to be useful in scientific research or clinical practice, it must be representative of some larger class of observations that might have been made on the subject. Since our scales are intended to be measures of immediate affect, the span of time to which they might be expected to generalize is rather narrow. We should not expect a single five-minute score to yield an estimate of the individual's typical scores over a period of days. We should, however, expect that under usual circumstances (lack of traumatic interactions or experimental intervention), such a sample would be representative of a time period somewhat longer than five minutes and that the scores would be generalizable over different interviewers and for somewhat different stimuli or instructions than we generally use.

The assessment of generalizability is essentially that of determining the relative stability of a measure over those types of situations and periods of time for which a general interpretation is intended. A single answer to such questions is unlikely, however, where measurement of affect is concerned, since different individuals may be expected to differ considerably in the variability of their affect. Some people are characterized by lability of affect from one time and situation to another, whereas others are not. Moreover, persons may be more labile affectively when they are ill than when they are functioning normally. Thus, the extent to which it is possible to generalize the level of an individual's affective state from a single score is likely to depend on both the person and his total situation as well as on such matters as the amount of time which has elapsed, the difference between interviewers, and the nature of the stimulus eliciting the speech.

It is extremely difficult to obtain an estimate of the generalizability of verbal scales over short intervals of time without introducing considerable artificiality into the situation. There are no units such as items or other discrete stimuli that might be used to obtain an estimate of internal consistency within the "test" itself. On first thought, one might consider the response categories or subscales as units for this purpose. However, they function quite differently from test items in that they are not independent units of behavior but rather mutually exclusive response alternatives that are assumed to be manifestations of the same affect or state. The continuity of speech is such that only relatively few response categories are likely to characterize any one protocol. Thus, a person who has a high score on death or mutilation anxiety may have no score on shame or guilt anxiety. Correlations among categories, therefore, are likely to be zero or negative. Whatever such correlations would be, they give no information on the appropriateness of our assumptions or the generalizability of the resulting score.

The only unit that might be correlated meaningfully in a verbal sample would be randomly sampled clauses or short intervals of speech from the total five-minute sequence. To split the sample into two or more contiguous parts would not be an adequate solution, since the parts would then be mutually dependent. While a random sampling method could have been devised, we have usually obtained estimates of generalizability by determining the consistency of two or more five-minute verbal samples taken at intervals of from one-half hour (during a single experimental session) to two or three weeks.

We have obtained considerable information on the generalizability of our measures, although it is certainly not as complete as we should like. We have usually controlled the effect of the interviewer by using the same interviewer for all subjects in a single study and for all samples in a longitudinal study. We have also used standardized instructions in most cases. Our findings vary considerably from sample to sample, depending on the type of subject, the setting, the subject's perception of any change in the situation, and the time elapsed. Variance estimates are often more inconsistent from study to study than are generalizability coefficients. For most subjects, however, it is evident that our method of affect measurement is generalizable over different stimuli and over a short range of time.

Anxiety Scale—Generalizability

The anxiety scores we have derived from the coding of verbal productions are primarily conceived of as indicating the psychological state of the individual on a particular occasion, that is, for only a short interval of time. Variance in anxiety from time to time under these circumstances is, therefore, considered to be true variance. Anxiety, however, is often considered to be a trait variable. To the extent that a general level of anxiety contributes to the affect measured by a verbal sample, it may be expected that the amount of anxiety displayed by a person on one occasion should be somewhat related to the amount displayed on other occasions. Thus, some generalization to the typical anxiety level of the individual should be possible. When scores are intended for this purpose, variations in a person's score from occasion to occasion contributes to error variance and reduces generalizability (Cronbach et al., 1963; Gleser et al., 1965b).

In order to investigate the extent to which one can generalize from the score on a single verbal sample, designed to provide a measure of immediate anxiety, to the typical anxiety level of an individual over different intervals of time, we have analyzed several small samples from different populations for which more than one verbal sample had been obtained. In all cases, the same investigator obtained all samples on any one individual. These studies are summarized in Table 3.6. It is evident from the table that the estimates of variance among individuals (V_{M_p}) differ considerably from one sample to another, the highest value occurring for delinquent boys. These boys were taking part in an experimental procedure in which their galvanic skin response was obtained under various conditions of rest and stimulation (Fox et al., 1965). The two verbal samples were taken during an adaptation and testing period prior to attaching GSR equipment. Thus, the variance among persons probably represents individual differences in anticipatory anxiety. The resulting generalizability coefficient of .43 indicates that 43 percent of the variance of observed scores may be attributed to individual differences in reaction to the situation. Thus, interpretation of a single score as representing the individual's anxiety in a specific type of situation can be made only with considerable caution. On the other hand, this study most nearly represents multiple sampling of a sustained

TABLE 3.6

Estimates of Variance and Generalizability of Anxiety Scores over Various Intervals of Time

Time interval	Type of subject	Number of subjects	Observations per subject	Variance estimates		Generalizability of single score
				V_{Mp}*	V_e†	
30 min.	Male students and V.A. patients in an experimental procedure	20	2	.095	.200	.32
45 min.	Delinquent boys 15 to 16 years of age in experimental situation	43	2	.350	.468	.43
1 day	7 male and 9 female dermatological patients on placebo	16	5	.180	.510	.26
1 week	10 male and 9 female students	19	2	.059	.246	.19
2–3 weeks	Medically ill male V.A. patients in testing situation	16	2	.149	.242	.38
2–3 weeks	Hypertensive women on placebo	9	3	.251	.520	.33

* Variance of person's universe scores.
† Error variance.

immediate affect. Thus, the coefficient of .43 is probably a lower bound estimate of the generalizability of verbal scores as a measure of immediate affect.

The value of .32 obtained in the first study listed in Table 3.6 is not as suitable an estimate for this purpose, since the first verbal sample was obtained during a period when the subject had a catheter in the vein of his arm from which blood was drawn at intervals, whereas the second sample was obtained at the end of the study after the catheter was removed. Thus, the situation was somewhat different for the two occasions of sampling. The other studies all involved testing on discrete days in a situation more nearly approximating an interview.

In a somewhat different type of study, we applied the anxiety scale to verbatim stories obtained on nine TAT cards. The subjects were 24 men, women, and their adolescent offspring who were members of five families. The resulting scores were analyzed using a two-way variance analysis. The average intraclass correlation between scores on any two cards was .25. The response to any card, however, was considerably shorter than our usual verbal sample. The average anxiety score for all nine cards had an estimated generalizability of .79 to a universe consisting of any randomly sampled nine-card set, provided the same cards were used for all subjects. The mean anxiety score for subjects differed very significantly from one card to another, indicating that the nature of the stimulus was a factor in overall score level.

From our data, it is evident that no simple statement can be made regarding the extent to which scores on a single occasion can be interpreted as representing a trait measure of anxiety. The estimate depends on the type of population being tested, the interval involved, and the type of situation under which the individual is tested or the stimulus used to elicit verbalization. Some generalizability is indicated in every sample, but the situation of testing is fairly uniform over the occasions sampled in any one study, so that one cannot estimate how well the scores for any individual might represent his anxiety level in other situations. For this purpose, most of the coefficients we have obtained are overestimates. It might be expected that verbal anxiety scores obtained on any one occasion would correlate rather poorly with paper-and-pencil tests of trait anxiety, such as the Cattell anxiety scale (1961) or the Taylor Scale of Manifest Anxiety (1953). At least five to ten verbal samples taken under somewhat varied circumstances would be needed for this purpose.

Hostility Scales—Generalizability

A study that gave some evidence of the generalizability of our hostility outward measure over short intervals of time was obtained by allowing one male subject to tape-record his free associations for a period of 15 to 30 minutes with no one else present in the room. We obtained a total of 39 such recordings. Two hundred word segments were scored for hostility outward. Scores for the first 600 words of each protocol (roughly equivalent to a five-minute sample) were correlated with the score on the remainder of the protocol. The correlation was .68, indicating that the affect score for the early portion was fairly representative of the general level of affect over the total period.

Several other small samples of data have given us some idea of the generalizability of scores over various periods of time. These results are tabulated in Table 3.7, which indicates the estimated within-person variance (V_{WP}), the estimated between-persons variance (V_{MP}), and the coefficient of generalizability for each scale as obtained in several samples.

In one study, 28 dermatological patients were tested daily for three to eight days while they were on placebo in connection with some drug studies. The hostility scores for the first three of these daily samples were analyzed separately for males and females to determine the average variance over a three-day period for an individual. In both outward and ambivalent hostility, the males were significantly more variable from day to day than the females, whereas their average level varied somewhat less from patient to patient V_{MP} so that the coefficient of generalizability of scores on one occasion for both these scales are smaller for males than for females. On the inward hostility scale, the males were more variable than the females over both occasions and persons, so that the resulting coefficients of generalizability are about comparable.

Two other small samples, one of men and one of women, give some indication of the generalizability of hostility scores over a somewhat longer period of time. The samples are drawn from different populations and hence cannot be directly compared. The first consisted of 16 males, ranging in age from 30 to 72 years,

TABLE 3.7

Generalizability of Hostility Scores for Groups of Subjects over Intervals of Time

Time interval	Type of subjects	Sex	Number of subjects	Observations per subject	Total hostility outward			Ambivalent hostility			Inward hostility		
					V_{wp}	V_{Mp}	ρ^2_{XM}	V_{wp}	V_{Mr}	ρ^2_{XM}	V_{wp}	V_{Mp}	ρ^2_{XM}
½ hour	Students in experimental procedure	M	20	2	.11	.07	.39	.11	.04	.27	.06	.00	.00
¾ hour	Delinquent boys	M	43	2	.45	.18	.28	.56	.33	.37	.17	.00	.00
3 days	Dermatological patients	M	15	3	.15	.07	.30	.19	.07	.27	.13	.16	.55
3 days	Dermatological patients	F	13	3	.07	.10	.59	.09	.14	.61	.09	.06	.40
2–3 weeks	Medically ill V.A. patients	M	16	2	.17	.03	.15	.10	.07	.40	.10	.11	.52
2–3 weeks	Hypertensive women	F	9	3	.12	.08	.38	.14	.12	.46	.15	.16	.51

who were hospitalized for various medical illnesses. Each gave two verbal samples spaced from two to three weeks apart. The scores for inward and for ambivalent hostility on one occasion showed a moderate degree of generalizability, but scores for hostility outward were extremely variable over occasions relative to the variability over persons. The second sample consisted of eight hypertensive women and one nonhypertensive control, who were tested once a week for three weeks during their scheduled visit to a clinic and while on a placebo. For these women, the scores on all three scales were fairly consistent over occasions relative to the variability between persons, although the generalizability of the outward hostility scale was somewhat less than that for the other two scales. These data suggest that the average of from three to five verbal samples suitably spaced over a limited interval of time should give a fairly dependable indication of the typical level of inward or ambivalent hostility for most subjects. A somewhat larger number of verbal samples would be needed to obtain the typical level of hostility outward, particularly for males.

In interpreting these results, it should be noted that while the tests covered a particular interval of time, they were not random occasions, since in each case the persons were interviewed under similar circumstances and in the same locale. It is conceivable that hostility scores would vary considerably more if they were taken under different circumstances and at different times of the day. Another factor that should be noted is that all verbal samples in these generalizability studies were obtained by male interviewers. Possibly the results would be different if female interviewers had been used.

In the study mentioned previously (pp. 63 f.), our outward hostility scale was applied to stories obtained from TAT cards. The average hostility outward score on nine TAT cards (for which responses were available for all subjects) significantly differentiated the subjects (p < .001) and had an estimated coefficient of generalizability of .74 to a universe of such stimuli. The mean scores on the TAT cards also differed significantly from each other, indicating that the nature of the stimuli is a factor in overall score level. Hostility inward and ambivalent hostility cannot be scored on the TAT by our method, unless one is willing to assume that the subject is identifying himself with a specific character in his story.

Social Alienation–Personal Disorganization (Schizophrenic) Scale—Generalizability

The scale of social alienation–personal disorganization, unlike our affect scales, is intended to measure a relatively enduring psychological state; hence a single measure might be expected to represent potential scores over some interval of time. That this is actually the case, at least for a population of chronic schizophrenics, is evidenced by the fact that a correlation of .63 was obtained in one study between scores on a five-minute verbal sample and clinical ratings of the patient's behavior during the previous three-day period.

More direct evidence of the generalizability of these scores for a chronic schizophrenic population is presented in Table 3.5. For these data, two verbal samples were obtained from each subject approximately three days apart during the fourth week of a study, involving 35 male and 39 female schizophrenics, all of whom had been placed on placebo for the interim. Two verbal samples were available for only 27 males and 36 females, since some of the patients were mute on one or both occasions. Whereas the variance in scores over subjects was much greater for the males than the females in this study, their variance from one occasion to the other was also greater ($Vs \times o$). These variance estimates are fairly large, indicating considerable fluctuation in scores from one occasion to another. The estimates, however, account for only 23 to 29 percent of the total observed variance. Thus, considerable stability is indicated for the scores on social alienation–personal disorganization as a measure of the relative standing of an individual in the group. The coefficient of generalizability of a set of scores on one occasion to a universe of possible scores during the week as scored by a single coder is estimated to be .77 for the males and .71 for the females.

Reliability and Number of Words per Verbal Sample

We recommend using only verbal samples of at least 70 or more words because the smaller the number of words in the verbal sample, the less the adequacy or reliability of the sample as a true measure of any psychological variable. A choice of a minimum of 70 words has been arrived at as a rough compromise between reliability of sampling and loss of research data.

CHAPTER IV
Normative Studies and
Intercorrelations of Scores

By providing normative or standardization data for non-psychiatric and psychiatric subjects, we are not implying that ideal standards for emotions or other psychological states can be established on a statistical basis. We are not using the term normal or normative in the sense of ideal or preferred, but rather in the sense of the typical or average for a group of people in some situation. Percentile scores are provided for our scales in order to answer the question frequently asked us: What is a high or low score for this or that modality using these content analysis scales?

When one is dealing with any measuring instrument, it is necessary to have some basis for interpreting the scale values obtained. Such meaning is acquired through knowledge of the range of possible values of the measure and the probability of a value occurring in any particular range for some class of objects under known conditions of measurement. Thus, to many persons the quantity 175 centimeters conveys little meaning. Telling them that the average American male is 175 centimeters tall and that most men are between 150 and 195 centimeters in height would give them some basis for interpreting lengths within this range.

Measurements are usually interpreted in a relative rather than absolute manner. Thus, 200 centimeters is small for the height of a room and large for that of a man. Similarly, psychological measures obtained by a particular procedure must be interpreted with respect to some population of persons or events or both. The choice of populations for which separate standardization data is needed is by no means a simple or obvious one. Any factor that can affect the central tendency or range of values can provide a basis for classification and differential interpretation for some purposes of testing. Thus, the distribution of scores might vary as a function of the subject's age, sex, race, socioeconomic class, medical condition, and relationship to examiner or as a function of any combination of these factors. In the following section, we examine the effect of some of these factors on the central tendency of scores we obtain by means of the content analysis scales. Minor differences are ignored in the interest of stability and for the purpose of giving more information on the total distribution of scores. For most scales, we have presented separate standardization data for three classifications only: nonpsychiatric subjects, psychiatric outpatients, and psychiatric inpatients. For the affect scales, data on medically ill patients have been combined with those for students and employed personnel, since these groups were found to differ only slightly in their overall distribution. On the other hand, medical patients are tabulated separately for the scale of schizophrenic alienation and personal disorganization, as are also the scores for acute and chronic schizophrenics, since notable differences in distribution were evidenced among all these groups for this scale.

We suspect that the range and distribution of scores on our affect scales are much more a function of the situation under which the verbal sample is obtained than of demographic variables per se. Material in subsequent sections tends to corroborate this statement. The score distributions presented in this section were all obtained under interview conditions and all were the first verbal sample provided by that individual.

ANXIETY SCALE—NORMATIVE STUDIES AND INTERCORRELATIONS OF SCORES

In an early normative study, anxiety scores were derived from verbal productions of 94 gainfully employed white males and females between the ages of 20 and 50. The characteristics of this sample of individuals, most of whom were employed by the Kroger Company, has been described elsewhere (Gleser et al., 1959). The distribution of their total anxiety scores was highly skewed, with 14 percent zeros and raw scores ranging up to 12.80. Because a distribution of scores with somewhat less skewness is better from the standpoint of statistical manipulation, a mathematical tranformation was made to the square root of the obtained anxiety scores. The distributions of scores using this transformation were presented in 1961 (Gleser *et al.*). Subsequently, 0.5 was added to raw frequency scores before dividing by the number of words and taking the square root. This was done to allow for the fact that persons obtaining zero scores with long verbal samples have a greater probability of actually being very low in anxiety than those having short verbal samples. The zero values are thus spread out over a range that has the added advantage of avoiding a buildup of zero scores.

The square-root score corrected for discontinuity at zero, then, is the score used herein for norms and for all statistical comparisons. The overall percentile scores for several nonpsychiatric patient samples combined (N = 282)[1] and also for 107 psychiatric outpatients and 107 psychiatric inpatients are shown in Table 4.1. From these distributions and from a validity study (see Chapter V), it was decided that a score of 2.2 indicates moderate anxiety, and a score of 3.0 or more is indicative of the presence of pathological anxiety.

TABLE 4.1

Percentile Scores for the Total Anxiety Scale in Three Groups

	Nonpsychiatric employees, students, medical inpatients (N = 282)[1]	Psychiatric outpatients (N = 107)	Psychiatric inpatients (N = 107)
95	2.65	3.40	3.25
90	2.40	3.20	2.77
85	2.20	3.02	2.52
80	2.05	2.83	2.35
75	1.90	2.50	2.20
70	1.78	2.27	2.07
60	1.58	1.97	1.80
50	1.45	1.78	1.60
40	1.28	1.59	1.41
30	1.10	1.40	1.22
25	.98	1.31	1.10
20	.85	1.22	.98
15	.68	1.13	.83
10	.53	1.02	.70
5	.35	.82	.50
Mean	1.46	1.92	1.68
s.d.	.71	.82	.81

[1] The samples used were the Kroger sample (N = 94), undergraduate college students (N = 87), psychiatric residency applicants (N = 22), Veterans Administration hospital medical inpatients (N = 29), and Jewish Hospital medical inpatients (N = 50).

In comparing these distributions, one needs to keep in mind that they represent scores of unscreened individuals. Thus the nonpsychiatric group includes many persons who might have needed psychiatric help and who certainly may have been quite anxious at the time the verbal samples were taken. Similarly, the psychiatric outpatients include persons with diagnoses of psychological and sociological trait disturbances as well as neuroses. Thus, whereas the two distributions differ significantly, they are not as distinctly different as would be obtained if the samples were drawn from screened normal and neurotic subjects.

Anxiety and Intelligence

Ninety members of the Kroger sample could be fit into a two-way classification on the basis of sex and intelligence with 15 subjects per cell. Intelligence (I.Q.) was stratified on the basis of the Wonderlic Test (1945)—dull normal, bright normal, and superior. An analysis of variance of the verbal anxiety scores for the 90 individuals revealed no difference between males and females in average anxiety, but a significant negative trend in anxiety with I.Q. level (p < .05), the lowest I.Q. group having the highest anxiety score (r = −.28). The cell averages are shown in Table 4.2. This difference is probably not due to I.Q. itself or

TABLE 4.2

Analysis of Variance of Total Anxiety Scores for Employed Personnel
(Kroger Sample) Stratified as to Sex and I.Q.

		Average verbal anxiety scores			
Sex	N	Low I.Q. 80–100	Medium I.Q. 101–115	High I.Q. 116 and up	Combined
Males	45	1.72	1.28	.99	1.33
Females	45	1.54	1.48	1.24	1.42
Combined	90	1.63	1.38	1.12	1.38

Variance analysis

Source	DF	Sum of squares	Mean square	F
Sex	1	.185	.185	....
I.Q.	2	4.001	2.000	3.85*
Sex × I.Q.	2	.838	.419	....
Residual	84	43.601	.519	....

* p ≤ .05.

to educational level, which also correlated —.27 with anxiety, but rather to the likelihood that individuals of lower I.Q. and/or education felt more stress in the test situation because they sometimes felt inadequate giving a five-minute monologue in the presence of another person. This is suggested by the fact that when the scores in different categories of anxiety were analyzed separately, those for shame anxiety were found to be contributing most to this trend, the mean shame anxiety scores correlating significantly with I.Q. level (r = —.28). On the other hand, while guilt anxiety was only infrequently scored, the high I.Q. group was found to be significantly higher on this category (r = .22, p = .05).

A follow-up study was obtained on the Kroger sample three years later, at which time subjects still available (42) gave a second five-minute verbal sample. For the repeat sample, there was no evidence of a correlation between I.Q. and total anxiety. This finding supports the belief that intelligence is not intrinsically related to anxiety as scored from verbal samples. It is likely, however, that subjects of lesser intelligence or education may become somewhat more anxious when faced for the first time with a request to speak for five minutes. Apparently, such "first-time" anxiety tends to be allayed somewhat with practice or experience.

The only other study we have undertaken in which a measure of I.Q. was available was that of 43 delinquent adolescents of ages 14 to 16 who were being detained at the Hamilton County (Ohio) Juvenile Detention Center. Their I.Q. scores—obtained by a Wechsler Adult Intelligence Scale, a Wechsler Intelligence Scale for Children, or a Stanford-Binet—averaged 95.65 ± 10.70. In this group of subjects, there were no significant correlations between I.Q. and total anxiety (r = .02) or any of the anxiety subscores. However, guilt anxiety (averaged over three five-minute verbal samples) correlated .17 with I.Q., and shame anxiety correlated —.13, thus corroborating to some extent the trends in the Kroger sample.

Anxiety and Sex Differences

While there was no significant sex difference for overall anxiety in the Kroger sample, some interesting differences did occur in the type of anxiety expressed as indicated by the separate category scores for anxiety. When these were analyzed separately, again using the square-root transformation, it was found that females had significantly lower average scores than males in the categories for "death" and "mutilation" anxiety and significantly higher average scores on "shame" anxiety. For females, in fact, shame anxiety was by far the most important category scored; whereas for the males, death, mutilation, and shame were scored with about equal average frequency.

Sex differences in subscale scores were reexamined using the total normative sample of 173 males and 109 females. For the larger sample, the females had significantly higher mean scores on separation and shame anxiety and significantly lower scores on death anxiety. Since subscale scores are highly skewed, despite the square-root transformation, the distribution of scores for each subscale was obtained separately for males and females. Selected percentile scores are shown in Table 4.3. Using the median test, the difference in medians for shame and separation anxiety are significant, the median for females being higher. Males, however, have considerably more high scores in death anxiety, so that the difference is significant (p < .05) at the 75th percentile. There is also a tendency for males to have higher mutilation anxiety.

Sex differences in the subscales were also examined in samples of 107 psychiatric outpatients and 107 psychiatric inpatients. For outpatients, the females again had significantly higher mean scores on separation and shame anxiety. The females were also significantly higher on diffuse anxiety. In the median test, the sexes differed significantly only on shame and diffuse anxiety. There were no significant differences between the sexes in the inpatient sample.

Anxiety and Age

We have examined the relationship between age and anxiety in several samples of adults. There is no evidence of a linear relationship, product-moment correlations in all samples yielding nonsignificant coefficients. If there is a trend in anxiety with age, it is probably of a curvilinear form, increasing up to some age and then decreasing. However, the variance in anxiety scores accounted for by the age of the subject would be quite small at most.

One subscale of anxiety, however, evidently increases consistently with age. In three separate samples we have found cor-

TABLE 4.3

Percentile Score for Anxiety Subscales by Sex

Nonpsychiatric subjects (males 173, females 109)

Percentile	Death		Mutilation		Separation		Guilt		Shame		Diffuse	
	M	F	M	F	M	F	M	F	M	F	M	F
90	1.09	.70	1.09	.92	.98	1.20	1.16	1.04	1.33	1.90	1.08	1.20
75	.61	.09	.65	.41	.63	.75	.65	.71	.74	1.15	.62	.81
50	.07	.06	.08	.07	.08	.21*	.07	.08	.08	.61*	.08	.09
25	.04	.03	.04	.04	.04	.05	.04	.04	.04	.08	.04	.05
Mean	.29	.17†	.35	.27	.29	.41*	.30	.30	.41	.69*	.34	.44
s.d.	.51	.34	.55	.51	.46	.52	.49	.47	.57	.70	.46	.63

Psychiatric outpatients (males 44, females 63)

Percentile	Death		Mutilation		Separation		Guilt		Shame		Diffuse	
	M	F	M	F	M	F	M	F	M	F	M	F
90	.88	1.06	.72	1.07	1.12	2.05	1.76	1.89	1.26	1.57	1.26	2.04
75	.40	.52	.40	.35	.93	1.08	1.30	1.31	.90	1.16	.77	1.36
50	.08	.08	.08	.07	.30	.45	.30	.69	.45	.81*	.20	.73*
25	.04	.04	.04	.04	.05	.07	.05	.08	.07	.42	.05	.37
Mean	.22	.29	.20	.27	.41	.66*	.66	.78	.49	.78*	.42	.87*
s.d.	.36	.47	.30	.51	.49	.75	.80	.74	.48	.58	.56	.75

TABLE 4.3 (contd.)

Psychiatric inpatients (males 41, females 66)

Percentile	Death		Mutilation		Separation		Guilt		Shame		Diffuse	
	M	F	M	F	M	F	M	F	M	F	M	F
90	.67	.92	1.24	1.02	.89	1.47	1.14	1.25	1.40	1.58	1.29	1.35
75	.42	.51	.72	.37	.55	.77	.65	.65	1.05	.91	.73	.82
50	.08	.07	.09	.07	.08	.09	.08	.09	.32	.38	.25	.10
25	.04	.03	.04	.03	.04	.04	.04	.04	.06	.09	.05	.05
Mean	.22	.25	.40	.26	.34	.45	.44	.37	.58	.69	.43	.51
s.d.	.32	.43	.53	.58	.48	.60	.63	.53	.67	.74	.53	.68

* Females significantly higher.
† Males significantly higher.

relations of .25, .24, and .28 between age and death anxiety (see Table 4.4). Such a relationship makes considerable sense, since death appears increasingly important and threatening as one grows older. It is interesting that such a trend can be found in our data, inasmuch as death anxiety is one of the more infrequently scored subcategories of the total anxiety scale. Some additional evidence that the death anxiety score relates to the increased risk of dying is provided by the study of Miller (1965), who found significantly higher scores on death, separation, shame, and diffuse anxiety scores in a group of medical outpatients who had suffered a myocardial infarction as compared to such scores from a group of outpatients with other medical diseases.

TABLE 4.4

Correlations between Anxiety Subscale Scores Derived from Verbal Samples and Age of Subject

Subscale	Employed personnel (Kroger sample) (N = 94)	Psychiatric outpatients (N = 50)	Psychiatric inpatients (N = 43)
Death	.25	.24	.28
Mutilation	—.07	—.05	.09
Separation	.11	—.03	—.03
Guilt	—.09	.09	—.23
Shame	.10	.09	—.21
Diffuse	.04	.07	—.05
Total scale	.19	.13	—.17
Age			
Mean	30.7	30.7	37.7
s.d.	8.9	11.5	13.3

Anxiety and Race

There is no evidence in our data of any difference between Negro and white subjects in total anxiety score. The average anxiety score for 43 female white psychiatric inpatients was 1.71, and that for 23 female Negro patients was 1.75. For 21 female white outpatients, the mean was 1.95, as compared to 1.75 for Negro patients. The male samples contained too few Negroes for adequate comparison, but no systematic trend was evident.

With regard to the subscales, there was some consistent indication in our patient samples that the Negroes were more concerned with separation anxiety and less with death anxiety than were the white patients. However, more carefully controlled studies would be needed to determine the meaning and significance of these trends.

Intercorrelations among the Anxiety Subscales

Table 4.5 presents the intercorrelations among the anxiety subscales in three separate samples. For the most part, these subscales tend to be uncorrelated and hence may be assumed to measure independent psychological components of anxiety.

In the light of classical psychometric theory, one might question whether it is meaningful to combine such noncorrelated scores into a single score, let alone to speak of the resulting scale as measuring a single construct, anxiety. We have not assumed, however, that scores on the separate subscales represent the same dimension or kind of anxiety, but rather that they are interchangeable with regard to the intensity of anxiety. Thus, it might be noted that our total anxiety score can be conceptualized as the resultant magnitude of anxiety, that is, the square root of the sum of squares of the intensities on the separate subscales. We have so far ignored the direction of this resultant, which would depend on the relative magnitude of the separate subscores. Our choice makes it evident that we believe that the physiological and biochemical concomitants of immediate anxiety relate to the overall intensity, rather than to the kind of anxiety, that a person is experiencing.

HOSTILITY SCALES—NORMATIVE STUDIES AND INTERCORRELATIONS OF SCORES

Preliminary normative data for the hostility scales was derived from five-minute verbal productions of 94 gainfully employed white males and females between the ages of 20 and 50, most of whom worked for the Kroger Company. A more complete description of this sample has been published elsewhere (Gleser et al., 1959). These data were supplemented, approximately three years after the first study, by additional recordings of speech obtained on 29 of the male and 15 of the female subjects of the sample. Additional normative data were obtained on 40 male and 47 female white college students, 21 male psychiatric residents, 28 male medical inpatients from a Veterans Administration hospital, and 34 male and 15 female private hospital medical inpatients.

Percentile scores for each of the three hostility scales and for

TABLE 4.5

Intercorrelations among Scores from Anxiety Subscales in Several Samples of Subjects

Subscale	Mean	s.d.	Mutilation	Separation	Guilt	Shame	Diffuse	Total Scale
Employed personnel (Kroger sample), males and females (N = 94)								
Death	.23	.51	.04	.10	.00	−.16	.02	.34
Mutilation	.27	.56		.11	.06	.03	.06	.52
Separation	.27	.44			−.05	.04	.00	.33
Guilt	.15	.36				−.07	.08	.14
Shame	.66	.73					.00	.58
Diffuse	.19	.38						.21
Total scale	1.35	.73						
Psychiatric outpatients, males and females (N = 50)								
Death	.26	.42	.26	.13	.10	−.16	.04	.26
Mutilation	.20	.35		.18	.09	−.44	.04	.10
Separation	.38	.56			.11	.01	.32	.48
Guilt	.42	.60				−.03	.51	.62
Shame	.65	.59					.20	.47
Diffuse	.57	.63						.74
Total scale	1.64	.73						
Medical inpatients (Veterans Administration hospital), males only (N = 39)								
Death	.29	.49	.38	.08	−.20	−.18	.11	.42
Mutilation	.50	.63		.02	.02	−.18	.05	.61
Separation	.38	.50			.17	−.07	−.04	.31
Guilt	.29	.45				−.02	.18	.19
Shame	.32	.52					.46	.40
Diffuse	.42	.54						.53
Total scale	1.53	.69						

the overt and covert subscales of hostility outward were obtained from the above-mentioned samples. These are shown in Table 4.6. It may be noted that all of the distributions are somewhat skewed despite the square-root transformation and correction for continuity. This indicates that comparisons between small groups might better be based on medians than on means. Scores above 1.00 for hostility inward, 1.20 for ambivalent hostility, and 1.70 for hostility outward are rare ($<$ 10%) in this normative sample.

TABLE 4.6

Percentile Scores for Verbal Hostility Scores in Nonpsychiatric Subjects (N = 322)

Percentile score	Hostility outward			Hostility inward	Ambivalent hostility
	Overt	Covert	Total		
95	1.45	1.52	1.95	1.26	1.45
90	1.21	1.30	1.67	1.00	1.20
80	.96	.97	1.35	.83	.86
70	.83	.83	1.17	.69	.67
60	.70	.68	1.04	.59	.58
50	.62	.58	.91	.52	.49
40	.54	.49	.78	.44	.40
30	.46	.42	.63	.36	.35
20	.38	.35	.51	.30	.30
10	.30	.28	.40	.25	.25
5	.25	.24	.30	.22	.22
Mean	.69	.70	.96	.59	.61
s.d.	.36	.42	.50	.35	.39

Hostility and Sex Differences

A further breakdown was made of the score distributions to determine whether men and women differed on these scales. The medians, means, and standard deviations of these distributions are shown in Table 4.7 for the combined samples of employed personnel, students, and medical patients separately and for the total male and female samples. There is no significant difference between the sexes in the mean or medians for hostility inward or ambivalent hostility scores in any of these samples. However, the mean score on hostility outward for the sample of employed men (.90) is higher than that for the women (.67) at the .03 level of significance. The medians are also significantly different by a χ^2 test. The mean hostility outward score for the male students is slightly higher than that for female students and likewise for patients, although these differences are not significant. The median

TABLE 4.7

Male and Female Scores on Hostility Outward in Normative Samples

Hostility outward subscale	Employed personnel (Kroger) original and repeat sample		College students (including psychiatric resident applicants)		Medical inpatients		Total group	
	Male (N = 76)	Female (N = 62)	Male (N = 61)	Female (N = 47)	Male (N = 61)	Female (N = 15)	Male (198)	Female (124)
Overt								
Median	.53	.54	.75	.73	.63	.57	.63	.61
Mean	.60	.60	.80	.82	.72	.65	.70	.69
s.d.	.33	.31	.39	.41	.33	.29	.36	.36
Covert								
Median	.62	.50	.64	.59	.61	.48	.62*	.52
Mean	.73	.60	.76	.71	.71	.59	.73†	.64
s.d.	.44	.38	.44	.44	.41	.28	.43	.40
Total								
Median	.90	.67	1.10	1.04	.92	.82	.98*	.82
Mean	.92	.79	1.11	1.09	.97	.83	1.00	.91
s.d.	.48	.46	.49	.55	.49	.35	.49	.50

* $\chi^2 = 3.79$, p = .06.
† p = .05.

hostility outward score for men is higher than that for women at the .06 level of probability; the means differ at the .05 level. This difference, though small, suggests that sex should be treated as a factor in studies involving the outward hostility scale.

Hostility and Age, Education, and Intelligence

No definite relationships have been found between our three hostility scales and such variables as age, educational level, and intelligence (Table 4.8). The one exception to this generalization has occurred with our hostility inward scores. These appear to increase slightly with age and principally in females rather than males, judging from analyses we have made with several samples of subjects studied, such as the normative sample ($N = 94$), psychiatric outpatient sample ($N = 50$), and a sample of V.A. medical inpatients ($N = 30$). This trend was not confirmed, however, in two small samples of psychiatric inpatients ($N = 24$ and 19).

Hostility and Race

The subjects in our normative samples were all white. It occurred to us that one might obtain a somewhat different distribution of hostility scores from Negro subjects, because Negroes as a minority group may have had to learn early to inhibit the expression of hostile aggression or because they might be more inhibited in their verbal responses when interviewed by white personnel (the only racial group we have thus far used to collect verbal samples). To check this possibility, we examined the scores obtained in a mixed sample of psychiatric patients obtained through various studies. The group consisted of 50 psychiatric clinic outpatients (including 21 white females, 9 Negro females, 18 white males, and 2 Negro males) and 107 hospitalized psychiatric patients (including 42 white females, 23 Negro females, 34 white males, and 8 Negro males). Ages ranged from 14 to 69, and diagnoses included psychoses, neuroses, and character disorders.

The median scores for Negro patients and white patients were .76 and .62 on inward hostility and .63 and .56 on ambivalent hostility. In neither case were the differences significant.

The median scores on total hostility outward were .87 for the white males and .94 for the white females as compared to

TABLE 4.8

Correlations* among Verbal Hostility Measures and Demographic Variables

Employed personnel (N = 94)

Variable	Mean	s.d.	Hostility inward	Ambivalent hostility	Hostility outward			Age	Education	I.Q.
					Total	Overt	Covert			
Number of words	543.4	217.8	-.34	-.11	.07	-.08	.03	-.12	.29	.20
Hostility inward	.47	.20		.09	.08	.23	.00	.20	-.14	-.07
Ambivalent hostility	.55	.34			.41	.34	.32	.13	-.06	.09
Total hostility outward	.89	.40				.61	.85	.13	.13	.09
Overt	.61	.32					.15	.02	.13	.12
Covert	.69	.45						.13	.06	.00
Age	30.7	8.9							-.21	-.06
Education	12.0	3.5								.74
I.Q.	108.0	12.3								

Psychiatric outpatients (N = 50)

Variable	Mean	s.d.	Hostility inward	Ambivalent hostility	Hostility outward			Age		
					Total	Overt	Covert			
Number of words	531.1	226.6	-.19	-.09	-.05	-.19	-.06	.13		
Hostility inward	.76	.53		.48	.13	.50	-.26	.18		
Ambivalent hostility	.68	.44			.31	.41	.06	.09		
Total hostility outward	1.06	.53				.68	.79	-.04		
Overt	.80	.42					.14	-.10		
Covert	.72	.46						.00		
Age	30.7	11.5								

* Certain correlations are underlined for emphasis.

.60 and .71 for the Negro males and females respectively. The median score for combined white patients was .90 and for combined Negro patients was .69. The difference in medians was not significant for the males but was significant at less than the .01 level for the females and at the .001 level for the males and females combined. Therefore, it would appear that, at least for patients, there is a definite racial difference in scores on the hostility outward scale, the white patients obtaining higher scores.[2] One might have expected that this difference would have arisen primarily from differences in the overt hostility subscale, but an examination of the data did not reveal a significant difference for either subscale taken separately.

A confirmatory trend with regard to race difference in hostility outward scores was noted in another sample, consisting of 7 Negro and 8 white male and 8 Negro and 5 white female inpatients on the Dermatologic Service of the Cincinnati General Hospital, for each of whom three verbal samples on successive days had been obtained. These patients were on placebo in connection with a psychoactive drug study (Gottschalk *et al.*, 1960*b*). The median score for the white patients was 1.05 and for the Negro patients .83.

Intercorrelations among Hostility Measures

From Table 4.8, it may be noted that only the ambivalent hostility scale and the outward hostility scale are substantially correlated in a normative sample of individuals (.41). There is, however, a small positive correlation (.23) between scores on hostility inward and scores on overt hostility outward. In the sample of psychiatric outpatients (Table 4.8) outward hostility and ambivalent hostility are again correlated, and the overt hostility outward subscale is substantially correlated with hostility inward. Hostility inward and ambivalent hostility scores are also highly correlated in this sample. Also, in a sample of 74 chronic schizophrenic patients (see Table 4.13), intercorrelations among hostility scores were even higher than they were among the psychiatric outpatients. These findings do bear out, as suggested by the name, that ambivalent hostility may be associated with either outward

---

[2] All of our studies have been carried out using Caucasian interviewers, which may be a factor contributing to these racial differences.

or inward hostility, or both, particularly where some psycho-pathological process is present.

SOCIAL ALIENATION AND PERSONAL DISORGANIZATION (SCHIZOPHRENIC) SCALE—NORMATIVE AND COMPARATIVE STUDIES

The scale of social alienation and personal disorganization was designed to measure a somewhat more enduring psychological state than those measured by our affect scales, a state particularly characteristic of the schizophrenic patient. While other types of psychiatric patients, general medical patients, and even nonpatients may at times exhibit some degree of social alienation and personal disorganization, particularly under stressful conditions such as medical illness, their score distributions would be expected to vary considerably from those obtained on a schizophrenic sample. Furthermore, it would be hoped that such a scale would differentiate psychiatric patients who do not exhibit schizophrenic symptoms from those patients diagnosed as schizophrenics.

In a study (Gottschalk and Gleser, 1964a) excerpted in part in this section,[3] we determined in what respects and to what extent the verbal behavior items categorized in our schizophrenic scale can differentiate groups of known schizophrenic individuals from the patient groups mentioned above and also from a group of non-patients. This study was primarily directed toward validation and refinement of our scale and resulted in a few minor changes in the weights given to certain subclasses of references to produce the scale that is presently in use. In general, the findings indicated that our scale of social alienation and personal disorganization is capable of discriminating verbal samples of schizophrenic patients from those patients with other psychiatric illnesses but not from those of brain-damaged patients.

Method

The subjects were groups of schizophrenic and nonschizophrenic individuals who spoke 45 words or more under the cir-

---

[3] Excerpted in part from L. A. Gottschalk and G. C. Gleser, "Distinguishing characteristics of the verbal communications of schizophrenic patients," in *Disorders of Communication A.R.N.M.D.* (Baltimore: William and Wilkins, 1964), 42: 400–413—with permission of the publishers.

cumstances of our procedure for eliciting speech. All of the groups except one, the brain-syndrome group, were composed of subjects from whom verbal samples had been previously obtained in connection with other studies.

Table 4.9 gives a summary description of each sample of subjects. The Longview State Hospital schizophrenic sample was composed of 113 schizophrenic patients—most of whom were chronic rather than acute. The General Hospital schizophrenic sample of 29 patients was composed largely of acute cases. The sample of other mixed psychiatric patients consisted of patients from the psychiatric wards of the Cincinnati General Hospital whose psychiatric diagnosis did not include schizophrenia or a brain syndrome. The brain syndrome sample of patients was obtained from different wards—psychiatric, medical, surgical— of the Cincinnati General Hospital and the Cincinnati Veterans Administration Hospital.

The psychiatric diagnoses of the above groups of patients had been arrived at by psychiatric teams, albeit different teams, including psychiatrists and psychologists at the different hospitals. The other groups of subjects had not been routinely examined psychiatrically, but they were included as either contrasts or complements to the known schizophrenic samples. The general medical sample, for example, was composed of patients of similar socioeconomic background to the General Hospital and Longview schizophrenic samples, but these patients were seen as inpatients or outpatients at the Cincinnati General Hospital for general medical rather than psychiatric reasons. The "normal" employed sample was composed of 60 subjects, 30 men and 30 women, having intelligence quotients ranging from low to high average (85 to 115), who were in good medical health and who had been gainfully employed in various capacities at the Kroger Company for at least a year.

Although verbal samples were elicited from the different groups by different "interviewers," our previous studies indicate that the verbal variables we are assessing here are not appreciably modified by this factor, because the standardized instructions and procedures for eliciting speech samples minimize the personality of the "interviewer" as a stimulus in the situation and maximize the subject's personal contribution to the content and structure of his verbal output (however, see pp. 259 f.).

TABLE 4.9

Groups Used in the Study of the Social Alienation–Personal Disorganization Scale

Group	Source	Medical or psychiatric status	Race and Sex				Age	
			Men		Women			
			Negro	White	Negro	White	Mean	Standard deviation
Chronic schizophrenic ...	Longview State Hospital	Subacute and chronic schizophrenic reactions	4	17	18	74	44.4	13.8
Acute schizophrenic	Cincinnati General Hospital psychiatric wards	Acute schizophrenic reactions	2	11	7	9	35.9	11.9
Brain syndrome*	V.A. and Cincinnati General Hospital inpatient services	Acute and chronic brain syndromes	6	11	0	1	55.1	13.7
Psychiatric nonschizophrenic	Cincinnati General Hospital psychiatric wards	Neurotic reactions, character disorders, and psychotic depressions	2	8	5	11	36.9	12.2
General medical	Cincinnati General Hospital nonpsychiatric inpatient and outpatient services	Chronic medical conditions including cardiovascular, genito-urinary, respiratory and endocrine disorders	10	8	20	10	48.9	16.1
"Normal" employed	Industrial firm	Employed personnel I.Q. range 85 to 115	0	30	0	30	32.0	10.6

* This group included the following diagnoses: generalized cerebral arteriosclerosis (3 cases), cerebral artery thrombosis (4 cases), head injury with subarachnoid hemorrhage (2 cases), basilar artery insufficiency (1 case), bilateral carotid artery obstruction (1 case), brain abscess (1 case), brain tumor (1 case), senile brain syndrome (1 case), brain damage due to paraldehyde intoxication (1 case), brain damage due to chronic alcoholism (3 cases).

Procedure

The typescripts of the tape-recorded, five-minute, free-associative monologues of the subjects were scored by technicians who coded each clause pertinent to any of the categories used in the schizophrenic scale previously published (1961a). One refinement, however, was made in this scale to make it more specific and discriminatory in the assessment and scoring of verbal statements about one's own illness or general dysfunction. This modification involved category IIB1—references to self, injured, ailing, deprived, malfunctioning, getting worse, bad, dangerous, low value or worth, and strange. An additional breakdown was made subclassifying whether such verbal statements indicated the malfunctioning involved: references to illness or symptoms due primarily to cellular or tissue damage (IIB1a), references to illness or symptoms due primarily to emotions or psychological reactions not secondary to cellular or tissue damage (IIB1b), and references to illness or symptoms not definitely attributable to either emotions or cellular damage (IIB1c). This refinement of categorization was made in order to see whether, from such brief verbal samples, a breakdown of this kind might not facilitate discrimination of the primary diagnostic classification of the patient; for example, the distinguishing of psychiatric illness from general surgical or medical illness.

The frequency of usage for each category on the scale was calculated for each subject relative to the total number of words in each verbal sample.

Results

In the previous study (1961a), we assigned a set of "modified" weights to each category of verbal items on our schizophrenic scale on the basis of several item analyses. Verbal items found to signify evidence of the schizophrenic syndrome were given positive weights, and items associated with more healthy, nonschizophrenic behavior were given negative weights. Items that made no consistent contribution to prediction of criterion scores were given zero weights. The total weighted frequency score was corrected for number of words spoken but not otherwise transformed.

In Table 4.10 we have listed, according to the different kinds

TABLE 4.10

Comparison of Diagnostic Groups on Categories of Verbal Expression Used in the Social Alienation–Personal Disorganization Scale

Verbal expression categories	Chronic schizophrenic (113)		Acute schizophrenic (29)		Brain syndrome (18)		Psychiatric nonschizophrenic (26)		General medical (48)		"Normal" employed (60)	
	% giving response	Sample average*	% giving response	Sample average*	% giving response	Sample average*	% giving response	Sample average*	% giving response	Sample average*	% giving response	Sample average*
Categories scored with positive weights (schizophrenic responses)												
IA2, others avoiding self	22.1	.15	27.6	.11	22.2	.10	23.1	.08	12.5	.06	10.0	.02
IB1, self unfriendly to others	21.3	.16	20.7	.07	11.1	.02	15.4	.08	4.2	.02	13.3	.03
IB2, others unfriendly to self	37.2	.27	34.5	.18	22.2	.10	30.8	.18	6.2	.03	8.3	.02
IIA1, disorientation	8.0	.07	0.0	.00	22.2	.07	7.7	.04	0.0	.00	0.0	.00
IIIB1a, physical illness, malfunctioning	15.3	.17	24.2	.10	22.2	.20	15.4	.07	50.0	.57	13.3	.04
IIIB1b, psychological malfunctioning	76.6	1.03	75.9	.78	72.2	1.11	92.3	1.01	56.2	.59	58.3	.29
IIIB1c, malfunctioning of indeterminate origin	28.8	.26	51.8	.40	44.4	.26	50.0	.30	64.6	1.31	13.3	.03
IIB4, unsure, unable to perform	85.0	1.53	75.9	.73	72.2	.74	61.5	.60	62.5	.96	71.7	.40
IIB5, needing or wanting control	54.0	.44	51.8	.23	33.3	.19	57.7	.21	39.6	.27	36.7	.11
IIC, denial of feelings, affect	30.1	.10	24.2	.05	22.2	.17	19.2	.04	14.6	.05	10.0	.02
IIIA1, words inaudible	51.3	1.08	6.9	.06	44.4	.84	23.1	.16	22.9	.15	8.3	.05
IIIA2, erroneous or bizarre statements	54.9	.56	55.2	.37	44.4	.34	26.9	.12	16.7	.08	11.7	.02
IIIA3, repetition of phrases, clauses	85.8	1.74	86.2	1.19	88.9	1.85	96.2	.93	87.5	1.06	88.3	.66
IVA, questions to interviewer	45.1	.64	51.8	.47	44.4	.76	46.2	.27	35.4	.21	31.7	.16
V, religious and biblical references	15.9	.24	34.5	.55	11.1	.18	23.1	.13	27.1	.20	5.0	.01

TABLE 4.10 (contd.)

Verbal expression categories	Chronic schizophrenic (113)		Acute schizophrenic (29)		Brain syndrome (18)		Psychiatric nonschizophrenic (26)		General medical (48)		"Normal" employed (60)	
	% giving response	Sample average*	% giving response	Sample average*	% giving response	Sample average*	% giving response	Sample average*	% giving response	Sample average*	% giving response	Sample average*
Categories scored with *negative* weights (nonschizophrenic responses)												
IC, self, others, friendly, helpful, loving	81.4	1.14	75.9	1.32	72.2	1.05	96.2	1.47	79.2	1.28	90.0	1.22
IIB2, self improving, better	27.4	.12	20.7	.04	5.6	.06	26.9	.14	39.6	.31	6.7	.01
IIB3, self well, adequate	62.8	.78	75.9	.85	66.7	1.14	84.6	.86	70.8	.95	91.7	1.36
Categories weighted zero												
IA1, self avoiding others	25.7	.14	20.7	.11	16.7	.10	30.8	.11	8.3	.03	10.0	.02
ID1, others bad, ill, strange	61.1	.75	58.6	.40	66.7	.52	84.6	.75	54.2	.38	75.0	.60
ID2, others well, achieving adequate	45.1	.34	58.6	.41	55.6	.51	80.8	.80	54.2	.48	85.0	.88
IID1, food bad, interference with eating	8.8	.05	3.4	.01	5.6	.03	11.5	.04	18.8	.08	10.0	.02
IID2, food good, adequate	16.8	.13	17.2	.08	11.1	.02	23.1	.15	27.1	.18	33.3	.14
IIE1, weather bad	5.3	.02	3.4	.01	5.6	.02	3.8	.05	8.3	.08	21.7	.07
IIE2, weather good	2.7	.01	0.0	.00	5.6	.02	7.7	.03	8.3	.06	10.0	.03
IIF1, sleep bad, dangerous	2.7	.01	10.3	.02	5.6	.01	11.5	.04	10.4	.04	3.3	.01
IIF2, sleep good, sufficient	8.0	.04	6.9	.02	5.6	.01	11.5	.04	10.4	.04	3.3	.01
IIIA2, blocking	61.1	.40	75.9	.49	77.8	.74	76.9	.43	33.3	.19	53.3	.17
IIIB1, repetition of words	69.0	1.04	93.2	1.11	83.3	.65	73.1	.57	64.6	.59	78.3	.49
IVB, references to interviewer	52.2	.60	44.8	.21	27.7	.07	11.5	.17	10.4	.04	13.3	.06

* Average frequency (per 100 words) of verbal references scored in each category.

of weights (positive, negative, zero) assigned to the verbal categories, the percentage of subjects in each group making verbal references codeable in the separate categories of our scale of social alienation and personal disorganization, together with the average score for each group. This latter score indicates the average frequency (per 100 words) of verbal references scored in the designated category and hence represents the unweighted contribution that the category would make to each group's average score on the schizophrenic scale.

Of the 15 types of statements given a positive weight on our schizophrenic scale, five occurred more frequently in both the acute and chronic schizophrenic groups than in any of the other groups. These are self unfriendly to others (IB1), others unfriendly to self (IB2), unsure and unable to perform (IIB4), denial of feelings or affect (IIC), and erroneous or bizarre statements (IIIA3). Four additional categories occurring most frequently in either the acute or the chronic schizophrenic group were others avoiding self (IA2), words inaudible (IIIA1), questions to interviewer (IVA), and religious and biblical references (V). Of the six remaining categories, verbal remarks manifesting disorientation (IIA1) occurred most frequently among the brain-damaged subjects. References to needing or wanting control (IIB5) occurred typically with schizophrenic patients and miscellaneous nonschizophrenic psychiatric patients and less frequently in the groups of patients with brain syndromes, other medical conditions and "normal" controls. Repetition of phrases or clauses (IIIB2) was about equally common in the verbal samples from all the different groups; both the chronic schizophrenics and the brain-damaged patients, however, tended to have more such repetitions in their verbal records as evidenced by their higher average scores. References to physical ailments (IIB1a) and malfunctioning of indeterminate origin (IIB1c) occurred considerably more frequently in the verbal samples of the general medical patients than in any other samples; whereas, references to psychological malfunctioning (IIB1b) were most prevalent in the group of psychiatric nonschizophrenic patients, although they were also high for the schizophrenic and brain-damaged patients.

Of the three scores given a negative weight (as indicating the relative absence of the schizophrenic syndrome), only references to the self as well or adequate (IIIB3) were least prevalent in the chronic schizophrenics, and these kinds of statements were most prevalent in the "normal" employed group. The latter subjects seldom spoke of themselves as improving or better (IIB2), a verbal content category frequently used by the medically ill patients. It was typical of all groups to speak of self and others being friendly or helpful (IC), but this category was used least frequently by the brain-damaged patients.

Of the verbal categories weighted zero, as a result of previous item analyses for capacity to predict differences in degree of illness among schizophrenic patients, some interesting findings occurred indicating that several of these categories are of value in discriminating schizophrenics from nonschizophrenic groups. The category of others well, achieving, adequate (ID2) occurred least frequently among chronic schizophrenic patients. References to the weather, bad (IIE1) and good (IIE2), although they occurred infrequently in general, appeared rarely in acute schizophrenics and with greatest frequency in the speech samples of the medical patients and the "normal" controls. Repetition of words (IIIB1) occurred most frequently in the acute schizophrenic records but was also quite prevalent in many other groups. References to the interviewer (IVB), however, were considerably more prevalent in both the chronic and acute schizophrenic speech samples than in the speech of any of the other groups.

On the basis of the above findings, modifications were made in the weights of verbal categories in the schizophrenic scale to increase the discriminative power of the scale with respect to the schizophrenic-nonschizophrenic dimension. The categories and the weight changes are as follows: (1) References to illness or malfunctioning of definitely physical origin (IIB1a) or of indeterminate origin (IIB1c) have now a weight of zero. Thus, only references to psychological symptoms, feelings of strangeness, inadequacy, deprivation, rejection or worthlessness (IIB1b) have a weight of +1. (2) References to the investigator (IVB) have a weight of +½. (3) References to the weather as being bad (IIE1) and as good or neutral (IIE2) have a weight of —1. (4) References to others as well, achieving, adequate (ID2) have a weight of —1 (see Schedule 2.5).

The distribution of total scores on the scale of social alienation–personal disorganization and the cumulative percentages for each of the six groups of subjects are shown in Table 4.11. Using

TABLE 4.11

Distribution of Scores on the Social Alienation–Personal Disorganization Scale by Groups

Score interval	Chronic schizophrenic		Acute schizophrenic		Brain syndrome		Psychiatric nonschizophrenic		General medical		"Normal" employed	
	Frequency	Cumulative %	Frequency	Cumulative %	Frequency	Cumulative %	Frequency	Cumulative %	Frequency	Cumulative %	Frequency	Cumulative %
18.0 or greater	4	100.0			1	100.0						
16.0 to 18.0	7	96.5			0	94.5						
14.0 to 16.0	1	90.3			0	94.5						
12.0 to 14.0	1	89.4			1	94.5						
10.0 to 12.0	4	88.5			1	88.9			1	100.0		
8.0 to 10.0	11	85.0	4	100.0	0	83.3			0	97.9		
6.0 to 8.0	9	75.2	2	86.2	1	83.3	1	100.0	1	97.9		
4.0 to 6.0	14	67.3	7	79.3	2	77.8	2	96.2	2	95.8		
2.0 to 4.0	16	54.9	6	55.2	6	66.7	3	88.5	7	91.7	1	100.0
0.0 to 2.0	14	40.7	3	34.5	1	33.3	4	76.9	6	77.1	4	98.3
−0.1 to −2.0	15	28.3	4	24.1	3	27.8	5	61.5	11	64.6	16	91.7
−2.0 to −4.0	11	15.0	0	10.3	0	11.1	6	42.3	9	41.7	19	65.0
−4.0 to −6.0	3	5.3	1	10.3	0	11.1	2	19.2	7	22.9	11	33.4
−6.0 to −8.0	1	2.7	1	6.9	1	11.1	2	11.5	0	8.3	8	15.0
−8.0 to −10.0	1	1.8	1	3.4	0	5.6	1	3.8	2	8.3	0	1.7
−10.0 to −12.0	1	0.9	1	0.0	0	5.6	0	0.0	1	4.2	0	1.7
−12.0 to −14.0	0	0.0	0	0.0	1	5.6	0	0.0	1	2.1	0	1.7
−14.0 to −16.0	0	0.0	0	0.0	0	0.0	0	0.0	0	0.0	1	1.7
Total	113		29		18		26		48		60	
Median	3.3		1.5		3.0		−1.2		−1.3		−2.9	

a cutting score of zero, the chronic schizophrenics have a significantly greater proportion of scores above this value than do the normal subjects, the medical patients, or the miscellaneous psychiatric patients (P < .01), but they do not differ from the acute schizophrenics or the brain-damaged patients. Both the acute schizophrenics and the brain-damaged patients have a significantly greater proportion of scores above this value (P < .05) than do the medical patients or the normal subjects.

We have developed a scale from the content categories of the social alienation–personal disorganization scale which gives maximal weights to those verbal characteristics distinguishing brain damage or functional impairment from schizoid or schizophrenic malfunction. This scale, the cognitive and intellectual impairment scale, is described and discussed in detail in Chapter VIII.

OTHER RELATIONSHIPS AMONG VERBAL THEMATIC CONTENT SCORES

Relationships between Measures of Anxiety and Hostility

Product-moment correlations of the total anxiety scores and the anxiety subscale scores with the several hostility measures for two samples are presented in Table 4.12. It may be noted that total anxiety is only moderately correlated with total hostility outward, hostility inward, and ambivalent hostility in the sample of employed personnel. The total anxiety score is somewhat more highly correlated with hostility inward and with ambivalent hostility in the sample of psychiatric outpatients. Whereas the correlation between anxiety and total hostility outward is about the same in the two samples, it stems from a correlation between anxiety and covert hostility in the sample of employed personnel— the higher correlation is between anxiety and overt hostility in the patient group.

Looking at the subscales, it appears that at least part of this shift may be due to the fact that guilt is positively correlated with overt hostility in the patient group but not in the group of employed personnel. Furthermore, shame anxiety is significantly negatively correlated with covert hostility in the patient sample. In this regard it is interesting to note that shame is significantly correlated with hostility inward in both samples, whereas guilt is highly correlated with hostility outward (see pp. 164 f. for a further discussion of these latter relations).

(see pp. 164 f. for a further discussion of these latter relations).

TABLE 4.12

Correlations* between Anxiety Subscales and Hostility Scales Derived from Verbal Samples

				Hostility outward		
Anxiety subscales	Number of words	Hostility inward	Ambivalent hostility	Total	Overt	Covert
Employed personnel (N = 94)						
Death	.06	−.01	.28	.23	−.10	.35
Mutilation	−.01	.08	.18	.46	.04	.55
Separation	.12	.16	.18	.15	.16	.06
Guilt	.22	−.09	.05	.26	−.15	.38
Shame	−.31	.43	.02	−.09	.15	−.13
Diffuse	.16	−.03	.07	.18	.16	.11
Total anxiety scale	−.18	.35	.34	.39	.10	.46
Psychiatric outpatients (N = 50)						
Death	.28	−.10	.16	.36	.08	.38
Mutilation	.19	−.28	−.02	.11	−.24	.32
Separation	.29	.36	.41	.06	.07	−.04
Guilt	.05	.37	.46	.56	.30	.43
Shame	−.23	.43	.02	−.10	.21	−.32
Diffuse	.06	.54	.38	.07	.16	−.13
Total anxiety scale	−.06	.64	.55	.35	.32	.13

* Higher correlations are underlined for emphasis.

Relationships among Affect and Social Alienation—Personal Disorganization Scores in a Schizophrenic Sample

Two or three verbal samples were obtained within a week's time on a sample of 74 chronic schizophrenic subjects in connection with a study of phenothiazine withdrawal (see pp. 215 f. for additional details of study). These were scored on the affect scales and also for social alienation and personal disorganization. The scores on each scale were averaged for the verbal samples obtained from each patient and correlations were obtained among these average scores. These are shown in Table 4.13. The main affect scores are even more highly intercorrelated than were those for the psychiatric outpatients. Furthermore, all types of hostility except covert hostility outward and hostility inward are significantly correlated with the scores for social alienation–personal disorganization (Gottschalk *et al.*, 1968).

TABLE 4.13

Correlations among Verbal Behavior Measures* for a
Sample of Chronic Schizophrenics (N = 69)

Verbal measure	2	3	4	5	6	7	8
1. Number of words	−.12	.15	.18	.32	−.06	.22	.01
2. Anxiety	....	.44	.36	.51	.51	.62	.35
Hostility outward
3. Overt	....	....	.23	.84	.48	.69	.52
4. Covert	....	....	....	.67	.10	.25	.06
5. Total	....	....	....	....	.37	.64	.40
6. Hostility inward	....	....	....	....	....	.42	.10
7. Ambivalent hostility	....	....	....	....	....	....	.32
8. Social alienation–personal
disorganization	....	....	....	....	....	....	....

* The average of scores on two or three verbal samples taken within an interval of a week while patients were on one of the phenothiazine pharmacologic agents.

CHAPTER V
Anxiety Scale—Validation Studies

Construct validation is a step-by-step process that requires repeated reexamination and retesting, in new situations, of the constructs being evaluated. After initial validation studies were completed for our measures of the constructs of anxiety, hostility outward, hostility inward, ambivalent hostility, and social alienation–personal disorganization (the "schizophrenic syndrome"), a large variety of additional investigations were carried out using these verbal behavior measures. These have provided considerable data on the ways in which such verbal behavior scores relate to other relevant measurable phenomena. The data afford growing evidence as to how the constructs measured by these verbal behavior measures "fit" with other empirical data.

Our formulation of these psychological constructs has been deeply influenced by the position that psychological states have biological roots. Both the definition of each separate construct and the selection of the specific verbal content items used as cues for inferring each construct were influenced by the decision that whatever psychological state was measured by this content analysis approach should—whenever possible—be associated with some biological characteristic of the individual in addition to some psychological manifestation or to some social situation. Hence, not only psychological but also physiological, biochemical, and pharmacological studies could all provide further construct validation. Let us, then, describe validation studies, our own and those of others, which round out the understanding of what is measured by our content analysis procedure.

PSYCHOLOGICAL STUDIES

Correlations between Clinical Ratings of Verbal Samples Using the Overall-Gorham Anxiety Scale and Anxiety Scores from the Gottschalk-Gleser Scale

For a verbal content scale to be used as a measure of an emotional construct, such as anxiety, it is important to demonstrate that the scale relates to what is commonly accepted professionally as designated by the construct. Thus, a minimal requirement of an anxiety scale based on a verbal sample is that it yield values consistent with professional judgment as to the extent of anxiety the individual is evidencing in the sample. To determine this, we selected from our files a set of 12 five-minute tape recordings of speech scored previously on anxiety by our method of verbal content analysis. Samples were chosen to represent a fairly wide range of scores. Sixteen judges (11 psychiatric residents in training and 5 graduate psychologists) were asked to rate the magnitude of anxiety in these five-minute speech samples using the Brief Psychiatric Rating Scale of Overall and Gorham (1962). The raters first read the typescripts of the verbal samples and rated the intensity of anxiety; then, at least a month later, the raters listened to the tape recordings of the speech samples while reading the typescripts and again rated the magnitude of anxiety. The product-moment correlations between anxiety scores derived from typescripts by the verbal content analysis method and the average Overall-Gorham anxiety scale ratings of 16 judges was .74 (p $\leq$ .01) when typescripts alone were used and .84 (p $\leq$ .001) when typescripts and sound recordings were used in obtaining the Overall-Gorham ratings (Gottschalk and Frank, 1967). When these anxiety scores were corrected for attenuation (Gulliksen, 1950) in order to obtain an estimate of the correlations of the Gottschalk-Gleser scoring method with perfectly reliable ratings, the correlations became respectively .78 and .86. The latter correlation is not much greater than the square root of the scoring reliability of our content analysis scales; thus correcting for attenuation due to unreliability of scoring verbal anxiety would produce a correlation approaching 1.00. This fact indicates that our content analysis method of assessing anxiety is yielding scores which (except for scaling) coincide with a consensus of psychiatric judgment. These findings also tend to indicate that negligible information is lost in assessing the magnitude of anxiety from content analysis of speech and by using typescripts alone, without listening to the accompanying vocal variables (see pp. 250 f. for a fuller discussion of this aspect of the study).

Group Comparisons of the Magnitude of Anxiety

One evidence of validity is the ability of a measure to differentiate among samples known to come from different populations with regard to the attribute being measured. In an early study we compared the distribution of anxiety scores for 24 psychiatric patients (a mixed group of schizophrenic and neurotic patients all seen shortly after hospitalization) to that of a medically and psychiatrically healthy sample of people. The difference in means (.98) was significant beyond the .001 level. Only 20 percent of the normals had a score of 2.0 and above as compared to 50 percent of the patients.

Furthermore, the mean anxiety of 1.92 for a sample of 107 psychiatric outpatients (see Table 4.1) was very significantly higher than that of the normative sample of 94 people for which the mean anxiety was 1.46 ($t = 5.17$, $p < .001$). A group of 107 psychiatric inpatients, most of whom were on tranquilizers, had a mean anxiety of 1.68, which was between that of the normals and psychiatric outpatients and significantly different ($p < .05$) from both.

In another study, ten patients with essential hypertension who were being treated at the Cincinnati General Hospital outpatient medical clinic were compared to a group of ten nonhypertensive patients attending the clinic for other ailments. Each group consisted of five men and five women, ranging in age from 25 to 74. Seventeen of the 20 patients were Negro. The primary purpose of the study was to examine the relationship between hostility and hypertension (Kaplan et al., 1961), but we also compared the groups with respect to their anxiety scores. Using a two-tailed t-test, it was found that the average anxiety score for the hypertensive group was significantly higher than that of the non-hypertensive group ($p = .02$). The average score for the non-hypertensives was slightly lower than for our normative group, and that of the hypertensives was somewhat higher, but neither of these differences was significant. Separation anxiety was notably high for the hypertensive females, whereas death and mutilation anxiety were high for the hypertensive males.

Correlations of Verbal Content Analysis Scores with Ratings of Anxiety Obtained from Clinical Psychiatric Interviews

Each of the 24 acute schizophrenic and neurotic psychiatric inpatients mentioned above was independently rated on a clinical scale of anxiety by two resident psychiatrists just prior to the time the patient gave a five-minute verbal sample. This clinical scale (see Table 5.1), which was devised by one of us (L. A. G.), was designed to provide a rating of the magnitude of immediate anxiety evidenced in current motor and autonomic activity as well as by the patient's verbalization of symptoms of anxiety (Maas *et al.*, 1961). The scale yields an overall rating of anxiety ranging from 0 to 6.

TABLE 5.1

Clinical Rating Scale of Anxiety

FREE ANXIETY SCALE   Score _____

I. Motor and sensory signs (voluntary nervous system)

  6   viz., extreme hyperactivity, pacing or marked restlessness, rapidly shifting glances, startle reactions, tremors, great pressure of speech, or tense muscular rigidity as if defending against imminent attack; marked paresthesias
  5
  4
  3   moderate—viz., "fidgety" in chair, transient tremors, mild motor defensive posturing, or mild pressure of speech
  2
  1
  0   viz., usual motor and sensory activity

II. Autonomic signs (involuntary nervous system)

 A. Skin signs
  6   viz., marked sweating, paleness, redness, blotchy discoloration: *acute* epidermal changes such as edema (other than with obvious organic disease), urticaria, or piloerection
  5
  4
  3   viz., moderate palmar perspiration, or cold and clammy hands and feet; epidermal changes such as active acne vulgaris, acute contact dermatitis, recently *weeping* atopic eczema, evanescent flushing, etc.
  2
  1
  0   normal skin

 B. Eye signs
  6   marked mydriasis or miosis
  5
  4
  3   moderate
  2
  1
  0   normal

TABLE 5.1 (contd.)

C. Cardiovascular signs

6   marked tachycardia, arrhythmias, extra-systoles, weak or bounding pulse, systolic blood pressure elevated with lesser diastolic elevation and widened pulse pressure; vertigo, syncope

5

4

3   moderate

2

1

0   cardiovascular actions within normal limits

D. Respiratory signs

6   marked hyperventilation or dyspnea

5

4

3   moderate

2

1

0   normal respiration

E. Genitourinary and gastrointestinal signs

6   viz., loss of bladder or anal sphincter control; vomiting or abdominal cramping

5

4

3   moderate—viz., hyperperistalsis, or frequent flatus, or polyuria, or diarrhea

2

1

0   normal

III. Mental signs

A. Subjective signs (in patient)

6   marked feelings of apprehension, impending doom; marked feelings of fear related to environment and/or to externalized threats as perceived in hallucinations, or illusions, or delusions; fear related to internal perception of impending loss of contact with reality

5

4

3   moderate

2

1

0   none

B. Signs in content of verbalizations

6   marked apprehension about estrangement and/or alienation from others, things or places; marked fear related to confusion about identity (personal, sexual, etc.) of self, of others, or changes in body image; marked sleep disturbances, particularly difficulty falling asleep

5

4

3   moderate

2

1

0   none

TABLE 5.1 (contd.)

C. Interpersonal signs

6   marked fluctuations in patient's ability to maintain intellectual (cognitive) and emotional contact with observer; marked anxiety provoked in observer by patient

5

4

3   moderate

2

1

0   none

Summary of ratings

I. Motor and sensory signs ...._____

II. Autonomic signs

   A. Skin signs_____

   B. Eye signs_____

   C. Cardiovascular signs_____

   D. Respiratory signs_____

   E. Genitourinary and gastrointestinal signs_____
$$A + B + C + D + E \text{ (average)}_____$$

III. Mental signs

   A. Subjective signs_____

   B. Verbal content signs_____

   C. Interpersonal signs_____.......................$A + B + C$_____

Total anxiety score_____

Using a Pearson product-moment correlation, the verbal behavior anxiety score was correlated with the average clinical rating of the two psychiatrists. The resulting value, .66, was significant beyond the .001 level. Correlations of the verbal behavior scores with the clinical anxiety ratings were equally high in the motor, autonomic, and psychologic subscales of the clinical rating scale of anxiety. For the separate categories of anxiety compared to the clinical rating, the highest correlation was obtained with diffuse (nonspecific) anxiety ($r = .63$). The only other category which correlated significantly with the ratings for this sample was that of "separation" anxiety ($r = .47$) (see Table 5.2).

TABLE 5.2

Correlations of Anxiety Scores with Clinical Ratings of Psychiatric Patients

Anxiety category	Correlations with clinical rating (N = 24)
Death	.16
Mutilation	.03
Separation	.47
Guilt	.20
Shame	.20
Diffuse	.63
Total anxiety scale	.66

Two other types of psychiatric ratings have been employed in validating the anxiety scale—namely, the Wittenborn Psychiatric Rating Scale (1955) and the Mental Status Schedule (Spitzer, 1965; Spitzer *et al.*, 1964, 1965, 1967). Both of these instruments are multidimensional in nature and have been developed using factor-analytic and other psychometric techniques.

For a sample of 19 psychiatric inpatients, a correlation of .65 was found between acute anxiety as defined by the Wittenborn Scale (and rated by the psychiatric resident in charge of the patients) and anxiety as determined from a five-minute verbal sample. Death, separation, guilt, and shame anxiety all contributed to the correlation. Verbal anxiety scores also correlated .55 with scores from Wittenborn's phobic-compulsive scale, which in turn was highly correlated (r = .76) with Wittenborn's Scale of acute anxiety in this sample. Hostility in, as measured by the verbal samples, correlated .74 and .45 with the Wittenborn acute anxiety and phobic-compulsive scales, respectively, and .70 with anxiety scores derived from speech.

As part of a longitudinal study of 74 chronic schizophrenic hospitalized patients, each patient was interviewed by a psychiatrist using the standardized interview and Mental Status Schedule (Spitzer, 1965; Spitzer *et al.*, 1964, 1965, 1967). In addition, each patient was seen on two or three occasions over an interval of a week by a nonprofessional assistant who obtained standard five-minute verbal samples. The average scores on anxiety from these verbal samples were correlated with scores obtained from the Mental Status Schedule. A significant correlation of .24 was obtained between the average anxiety scores from the verbal samples and the anxiety-depression subscale of the Mental Status

Schedule. There was also a correlation ($r = .23$) between average anxiety and the somatic preoccupation subscale of the Mental Status Schedule.

Correlations with Anxiety Scores Derived from Self-Report Procedures

INVENTORIES

Most self-report inventories of anxiety are designed to measure anxiety considered as a trait variable. As such, they attempt to tap the typical reaction of the individual in a wide variety of situations. The verbal behavior measure of anxiety, on the other hand, is intended to measure the intensity of the momentary anxiety in a specific situation, that is, the immediate affect being experienced at the time of reporting. If it is presumed that more stable individual differences in anxiety also exist among persons, so that some persons react with more anxiety than others under a great variety of circumstances, then the scores on immediate anxiety would contain some variance attributable to this general trait in addition to the variance attributable to the specific response in the particular situation. Only by combining scores from speech samples obtained under different conditions over a period of time could one expect to obtain an average score having considerable congruence with trait measures. Even then, the amount of overlap would depend on the similarity of the situations sampled by the items of the self-report inventory to those in which verbal productions are obtained, that is, ordinary interpersonal situations, stress situations, and so forth (Endler et al., 1962). That there tends to be a typical verbal anxiety level for an individual is evidenced by our generalizability studies. As we have noted previously (p. 62), however, the typical anxiety component accounts for only 19 to 43 percent of the observed variance in a single situation. Hence, correlations of verbal anxiety with trait measures of anxiety can be expected to be positive but small, except when several independently sampled verbal measures are averaged.

Minnesota Multiphasic Personality Inventory (MMPI)

MMPI scores were available for two small groups of subjects on whom verbal samples were obtained. One group consisted of

14 patients hospitalized primarily for some type of dermatological disease. These patients had produced three to eight (usually five) five-minute verbal samples each over a period of from one to two weeks while they were on a placebo in connection with a study of the effects of perphenazine (a major tranquilizer) and/or prednisone (a glucocorticosteroid hormone) on emotions. The average anxiety score on the verbal samples obtained while the patient was taking a placebo was used as the verbal measure of anxiety. This score was correlated with the standardized psychasthenia scale (Pt) of the MMPI corrected for K. This scale was chosen as the best measure of manifest anxiety among the primary MMPI scores, since it has been found to correlate .93 with the Taylor anxiety scale (Welsh and Dahlstrom, 1956) and to have a factor loading of .85 on the anxiety dimension (A) proposed by Welsh (1956). The Pt scores for this group ranged from 46 to 78, with a mean of 60.9 and a standard deviation of 10.4. The product-moment correlation between our verbal anxiety scores and the MMPI psychasthenia (Pt) scores was .51, which is significant at the .03 level by a one-tailed "Student's" t-test. The correlations for the separate anxiety categories were: death, .11; mutilation, .17; separation, .08; guilt, .11; shame, .20; and diffuse, .37.

The Welsh A factor anxiety scores derived from the MMPI on the group of 14 dermatological patients correlated .68 with the average verbal anxiety score (p < .01). Mutilation, shame, and diffuse anxiety again yielded the highest correlations for the separate categories (Table 5.3).

The second group for which MMPI scores were available consisted of 20 residency applicants in psychiatry. For this group,

TABLE 5.3

Correlation of Anxiety Scores with MMPI Scales

Anxiety category	Pt scale MMPI dermatological pts* (N = 14)	Welsh A-scale MMPI dermatological pts* (N = 14)
Death	.11	—.07
Mutilation	.17	.56
Separation	—.08	—.11
Guilt	.11	.13
Shame	.20	.26
Diffuse	.37	.33
Total anxiety scale	.51	.68

* Verbal scores based on the average of 3 to 8 verbal samples per subject.

the average Pt scores was 54.3, with a standard deviation of 5.99. The product-moment correlation between these scores and the single verbal anxiety score available was .18. The much smaller correlation obtained for this group as compared to that of the dermatitis patients was not surprising, for two reasons. First, the range of Pt scores for the latter group was extremely restricted, being only about 60 percent of that for the dermatitis group and of the *population in general*. Such restriction of range has the effect of attenuating correlations. Second, only one verbal sample was available for the resident sample, and, as mentioned above, the score obtained on one occasion is not very representative of the averages of several measures and hence of the general anxiety level of the individual over time.

IPAT (Cattell and Scheier)

Sholiton *et al.* (1963) obtained five-minute verbal samples, according to our standardized procedure, on 28 male medical patients with various lung or heart diseases in a Veterans Administration hospital. The correlation between the anxiety scores derived from the verbal samples and the total IPAT anxiety scale (Cattell and Scheier, 1961) was 0.41 (p $\leq$ .05). The correlation was .47 with overt anxiety and .32 with covert anxiety as measured by the IPAT.

Three five-minute verbal samples were obtained from 43 juvenile delinquent boys (14 to 16 years old) over a two-hour period as part of a psychophysiological study of the galvanic skin response. The boys had notably high anxiety scores (mean = 1.99, s.d. = .63), primarily attributable to high scores on guilt anxiety (mean = 1.20). The IPAT was administered approximately 30 minutes after the first verbal sample and just prior to the second verbal sample. During the intervening 30 minutes, the subject was allowed to rest. Polygraph recordings were made during the period between the second and third verbal sample. In this study, the correlation between the IPAT and the average total anxiety score was only .08. The correlation was .28 between verbal anxiety and the covert portion of the IPAT scale but was —.06 with the overt subscale. For the separate verbal anxiety scores, the total IPAT correlated somewhat better (r = .17) with the final verbal sample than with the first sample taken immediately after the subject entered the experimental room. The last sample also yielded the lowest average anxiety for the group (1.82), suggesting that anticipatory anxiety was being measured in the first two samples; whereas, the third measure contained more of the "typical" anxiety factor. This interpretation is substantiated by the fact that the correlation was much higher between the first two measures than between either of these and the third measure.

In another group of 20 boys from the same population and subjected to the same experimental procedure, but who were given 20 mg. of the minor tranquilizer, chlordiazepoxide (Librium), at the start of the experiment, overt IPAT again correlated negatively with the anxiety scores for the first verbal sample but correlated .45 and .42 respectively with the second and third samples, yielding a correlation of .36 with the average score for the three verbal samples. The covert portion of the IPAT correlated .33 and the total IPAT score correlated .39 with the average verbal anxiety score. The chlordiazepoxide seemed, therefore, to have reduced or eliminated the anticipatory anxiety in the second group of boys. That anxiety was reduced in the second group was determined by comparison with a control group (Gleser *et al.*, 1965*a*).

It would appear, then, that under conditions of obtaining verbal samples that approximate the interview situation, neither the overt nor the covert subscale of the IPAT is particularly sensitive to fluctuations in anxiety relevant to the situation in which it is obtained; in contrast, the verbal measure of anxiety is sensitive to situational effects.

16PF (Cattell and Eber)

The 16PF Test, Form A (Cattell and Eber, 1957) was administered to a sample of 40 male and 40 female chronic schizophrenic patients in a state hospital. The patients were all Caucasians of ages from 24 to 54 and had been hospitalized for from six months to 25 years since their last mental hospital admission (median, 11 years). All were on large doses of phenothiazine derivatives at the time of testing. Each patient was also seen on two or three occasions during the week of testing by a nonprofessional assistant who obtained five-minute verbal samples in the standard manner. The average scores for anxiety, hostility inward, hostility outward, ambivalent hostility, and the scale of schizophrenic alienation–personal disorganization were each correlated with the 16PF scales. The correlations are shown in Table 5.4.

Although none of the scales of the 16PF are designed to measure anxiety, Cattell has identified anxiety as a second-order factor. The scales most heavily loaded on this factor are emotional stability (C—), distrustfulness (L+), insecurity (O+), self-sentiment (Q3—), and drive tension (Q4+). The IPAT, discussed above, is made up of the items from these five scales. The only significant correlation found between the verbal anxiety scale and the 16PF scales in this sample was a coefficient of —.35 with emotional stability (C), which is in the hypothesized direction. It is interesting that for this sample, ambivalent hostility appears more closely related to the anxiety factor than does the verbal anxiety score, with correlations above .15 on four of the five PF scales mentioned above, including a correlation of —.36 with C.

TABLE 5.4

Correlations between the 16PF and Verbal Behavior Scores in a Schizophrenic Sample of Patients*

Dimension		Anxiety	Hostility inward	Hostility outward	Ambivalent hostility	Social alienation–personal disorganization
16 PF						
A	Warmth					—.12
B	Intelligence					—.23
C	Emotional stability	—.35	—.19		—.36	—.17
D	Assertiveness			—.18		
F	Enthusiasm				.17	—.22
G	Conscientious	—.15			—.21	—.33
H	Venturesome	—.19		—.28	—.22	
I	Sensitivity	—.12			—.13	
L	Distrustfulness	.16			.15	
M	Autism	.16	.20	.14		.30
N	Shrewdness	—.13		—.18	—.21	—.26
O	Insecurity			.16	.20	.13
Q1	Free-thinking	—.17			—.20	
Q2	Self-sufficiency			.21		
Q3	Self-sentiment				—.17	—.21
Q4	Drive tension		—.20			

* Underlined correlations are significant (p < .05). Correlations less than .10 are omitted.

ADJECTIVE CHECKLIST

In some of our early work on verbal content scales, we made use of a mood adjective checklist as an auxiliary measure of the intensity of immediate emotional response over a small interval of time. It was hoped that such a checklist might provide some direct indication of the validity of our verbal scales. It was recognized, however, that a checklist would tap only those emotional responses that were at the level of awareness and amenable to verbalization. The checklist used was developed in our laboratory and designed to assess anxiety-fear, hostility-anger, depression, fatigue, and active-happy. The format and content were modified slightly from one study to another, but the changes were not very crucial.

In one study, five-minute verbal samples were obtained from 24 individuals on the Cincinnati General Hospital psychiatric wards; most had symptoms of depression. The patients were also administered an adjective checklist, the Buss Hostility Inventory (Buss, 1961) and the Beck Depression Inventory (Beck et al., 1961). The verbal anxiety score correlated .21 with anxiety, .21 with hostility, .28 with depression, .34 with fatigue, and —.01 with active-happy as measured by the adjective checklist. Hostility in, as measured by the verbal sample technique, correlated .31 with anxiety, .48 with depression, and .44 with fatigue. The Beck Depression Inventory was very highly correlated with all five adjective checklist scores (.69 to .88). It therefore appeared evident that a depressive affect was being tapped regardless of the adjectives chosen to describe mood. Furthermore, verbal anxiety scores and Beck Depression Inventory scores had a correlation of only .22; whereas, hostility in and Beck Depression Inventory scores correlated .47.

A second study, in which the same battery of tests were administered to 50 patients attending a psychiatric outpatient clinic, yielded slightly clearer results. This time, anxiety as measured from the verbal sample correlated .28, .16, .39, .22, and —.34 respectively with scores of anxiety, hostility, depression, fatigue, and active-happy from the adjective checklist. The correlation between the two anxiety scores was significant at the .05 level. Again, hostility in scores correlated more highly than did verbal anxiety scores with anxiety, depression, and fatigue as measured by the adjective checklist (.42, .52, and .41 respectively). In this sample, the Beck Depression Inventory was correlated only moderately with the adjective checklist scores (.29 to .45).

Thus, while the adjective checklist provides some validation of the verbal anxiety score, the confirmation is primarily to the effect that some emotional response is being tapped; precisely what emotion is unclear. Anxiety and hostility in scores are consistently correlated in our verbal samples and not infrequently have quite similar correlations with other measures. This is in accord with the findings of others that symptoms of anxiety and depression occur together frequently and might better be encompassed by a single rating scale (cf., Spitzer, 1966; Lorr *et al.*, 1963). We have some evidence, however, to indicate that meaningful differential results are obtained with the separate anxiety and hostility inward verbal scales. So we suspect that the lack of specificity in the above cited studies was primarily due to the difficulty of obtaining specificity in the self-report on an adjective checklist of naive subjects.

Correlation between Anxiety Scores Obtained by Content Analysis and by Clinical Ratings of TAT Stories

Ten male and nine female graduate students were given six TAT cards as part of a study of the effects of the interviewer on patterns of verbal behavior. The six cards used were 6 BM, 6 GF, 2, 4, 10, and 13 MF. The stories were scaled for anxiety by two methods: (1) an experienced clinical psychologist[1] rated each story for anxiety on a four-point scale with one indicating minimal and four maximal anxiety; (2) the stories were each scored by one technician using our verbal behavior measure of anxiety. The data were then subjected to a variance-covariance analysis as shown in Table 5.5.

The principal source of variance for both measures of anxiety was the subject $\times$ card interaction plus error, that is, the variance of the subject from card to card after correcting for differences in the stimulus value of the card. For the ratings, there was no evidence of population differences among cards in stimulus value. This, however, was probably because in making the ratings of anxiety, the stories given any one card were ranked and then rated. Using the verbal behavior measurement of anxiety, variance in

---

[1] We acknowledge with appreciation the participation of Dr. Cynthia Dember in this study.

TABLE 5.5

Variance-Covariance Comparison of Clinical Judgment of Anxiety and
Verbal Behavior Measures Derived from TAT Stories

			Mean squares and products		
Source	N	Rating	Rating × verbal behavior measure	Verbal behavior measure	Correlation
Subjects	18	1.455	.097	1.063	.08
Cards	5	.724	1.312	4.252	.75
Subjects × cards	90	1.006	.207	.422	.32

			Expected values of mean squares and products		
Source	N	Rating	Rating × verbal behavior measure	Verbal behavior measure	
Subjects	18	.075	−.018	.107	
Cards	5	−.015	.058	.202	
Subjects × cards	90	1.006	.207	.422	

stimulus value of cards accounted for about 28 percent of the total variance of scores. Differences among subjects accounted for a larger proportion of variance when using the verbal behavior measure than when using the clinical rating. The generalizability of the total score on these cards to the score that would be obtained from a universe of TAT cards was estimated at .60 for the verbal behavior measure and only .31 on the basis of ratings. There was a significant agreement between the two sets of scores for a single story as told by any one person (subject × card covariance) but no agreement as to individual differences in amount of anxiety over all cards; the universe of generalization for the two methods of scoring appeared to be nonoverlapping. Thus, while there was some evidence that the two methods have common variance in distinguishing stories told by different persons in response to the same card, there was no evidence that the measures obtained by summing scores from many cards yielded similar information on individual differences in anxiety.

Anxiety as a Function of Situational Variables

Several studies made by ourselves and others indicate that the verbal measure of anxiety is sensitive to differences in the total situational context in which the subject is asked to give a verbal sample. Thus, for example, average anxiety scores are higher for subjects entering an experimental situation than for subjects who are simply being interviewed. Subtler effects have been noted, which are probably attributable to the personality and sex of the interviewer or to his status as perceived by the subject (see p. 259).

Several of the studies in which situational effects have been found involve repeated measurements on the same individual; in these, it has not always been possible to avoid confounding sequential effects with other situational effects. One consistent sequential effect we have noted, however, is that associated with giving a verbal sample for the first time. In many samples, we have noted that anxiety scores are slightly higher on the average on the first interview than on subsequent ones, provided all verbal samples are obtained under similar circumstances.

THE ANXIETY CONTENT OF DREAMS, USING THE GOTTSCHALK-GLESER ANXIETY SCALE

When subjects are presented three types of movies before going to sleep (an "exciting," a "neutral," and a "sad" movie), the content of dreams throughout the night (monitored by following REMs and EEGs) reveals significantly higher verbal behavior anxiety scores following the "exciting" movie for 10 out of 13 subjects. On the other hand, 9 of these subjects showed no increase in mood-checklist anxiety from before to after viewing the "exciting" movie, which strongly suggests that these subjects were less likely than other subjects to be able to tell about their anxiety directly (Witkin *et al.*, 1965; Witkin, 1969).

ANXIETY IN HYPNOTIZED ADOLESCENT MALES

Twelve males, 16 and 17 years old, were hypnotized in connection with a psychophysiological investigation (Gottlieb *et al.*, 1967). Anxiety and hostility scores, obtained from the verbal samples taken before and during the hypnotic state and assessed by the Gottschalk-Gleser method, were higher after these boys were put into the hypnotic state, although only the increase in anxiety level reached a convincing level of significance ($p < .025$).

ANTICIPATORY ANXIETY IN PATIENTS SCHEDULED TO RECEIVE PARTIAL OR TOTAL BODY IRRADIATION

A group of 13 patients (six males and seven females) with terminal cancer gave five-minute verbal samples before and immediately after sham and actual therapy with partial or total body radiation from radioactive cobalt (Gottschalk and Kunkel, 1966; Gottschalk *et al.*, 1969). The mean anxiety scores obtained prior to the sham and actual treatment periods were significantly higher on the average (1.76) than the average posttreatment anxiety levels (1.20) by an F test (p < .01) indicating that the situational context in which an individual speaks influences his anxiety level in the expected direction. The difference between the average postsham anxiety and postradiation anxiety was not significant.

ANXIETY LEVELS OF ACUTELY DISTURBED PATIENTS BEFORE AND AFTER BRIEF PSYCHOTHERAPY

Anxiety scores (and hostility inward scores) derived from five-minute verbal samples were significantly lower by a sign test in a group (N = 22) of acutely disturbed psychiatric patients after treatment in a brief psychotherapy clinic (Gottschalk *et al.*, 1967*b*).

Cognitive and Perceptual Correlates of Shame, Guilt, and Diffuse Anxiety

The relationship of the disposition toward the arousal of different kinds of anxiety, particularly shame and guilt, and the degree of "psychological differentiation" in patients has been explored in psychotherapeutic interviews by Witkin *et al.* (1966, 1968). Psychological differentiation has been assessed by these investigators in terms of the degree of field dependence or field independence.

Psychological differentiation has been described by Witkin (1966) as follows:

"In a field-dependent mode of perceiving, perception is dominated by the overall organization of the field; there is relative inability to perceive parts of a field as discrete. This global quality is indicative of limited differentiation. Persons whose field-dependent perception suggests limited differentiation in their experience of the world about them also show limited differentiation in their experience of body and self. Their drawings of the human body are likely to lack articulation. Just as they rely on the surrounding visual field in their perception of a stimulus object within it, so do they tend to use the social context in which they find themselves for definition of attributes of the self. We have called this a lack of developed sense of separate identity and take it as indicative of limited differentiation. Persons who perceive in field-dependent fashions are also likely to use such global defenses as massive repression and primitive denial, suggestive of limited differentiation; whereas field-independent perceivers tend to use specialized defenses, as intellectualization and isolation, suggestive of developed differentiation. Thus, viewed from the standpoint of level of differentiation, people show consistency in their psychological functioning across diverse areas of perception, body concept, sense of separate identity, and nature of defense." (See also Witkin *et al.*, 1954, 1962.)

In a recent study by Witkin *et al.* (1966, 1968), four field-dependent and four field-independent patients matched for sex and socioeconomic status were selected for psychotherapy on the basis of their being at the extremes of the differentiation dimension as determined by the hidden-figures test and a figure-drawing test evaluated for articulation of body concept. The patients were told before starting that the therapy would last no more than 20 sessions. Each of the four therapists who took part in the study was assigned a more differentiated and a less differentiated patient. The psychotherapeutic interviews were tape-recorded and transcribed, and the first two interview typescripts were sent to our content analysis research laboratory in Cincinnati for "blind" scoring of anxiety and hostility. The typescripts, scored in 500-word segments, were returned to the research division at Downstate Medical Center in Brooklyn, N.Y., for tabulating and further processing. Total anxiety, hostility, "and all subscales of these affects" were calculated, and "spurts" of these anxiety subscale scores greater than 1.0 per 500 words were counted.

The total anxiety scores for the first two psychotherapeutic interviews tended to be greater for the field-dependent than for the field-independent patients, but the differences were small. The principle difference in anxiety between the two kinds of patients was in the distribution of subcategory scores for the first and second sessions combined. Field-dependent (less differentiated) patients had significantly higher scores—by a *t*-test—on shame anxiety than field-independent (more differentiated) patients. They also had lower guilt anxiety scores than did the field-independent patients.

When the coincidental arousal of different affects during the psychotherapeutic interviews was examined by looking at spurts of affects over 1.0, elevated scores on guilt anxiety and hostility out were found to occur during the same block of time (i.e., 500-word units) and elevated shame and hostility in scores were found to occur together (ambivalent hostility scores have not been included in these calculations up to this time). Moreover, shame and guilt seemed to be almost mutually exclusive reactions in that they did not occur frequently in the same segment. In only 16.1 percent of all instances of shame and guilt spurts were these reactions found within the same 500-word unit.

The field-independent patients showed an increase in overt hostility outward and guilt anxiety from the first psychotherapeutic session to the second. The field-dependent patients, although they also showed an increase in overt hostility out, showed no associated increase in either guilt or shame anxiety from first to second psychotherapeutic session. (For additional discussion of the relationship of shame and guilt to hostility, see Chapter VI, pp. 164 ff.)

Scores on the category "diffuse" anxiety were found to be higher among field-dependent patients than field-independent patients. Also, when content items scorable as diffuse anxiety did occur, a detailed examination of the time, place, and precipitating circumstances for the diffuse anxiety verbalized by the patient revealed that field-dependent patients were consistently less articulated, less specific about these aspects of diffuse anxiety than field-independent patients. Another way to state this is that field-dependent patients showed less secondary process thinking when they were experiencing diffuse anxiety than field-independent patients.

Witkin *et al.* (1966, 1968) explained the association between proneness to shame reactions and undifferentiation or field-dependence as follows. A person experiencing shame is sensitively and often painfully aware of himself as the object of disapproval or derision of someone else. Shame is particularly connected with being seen, unexpectedly caught, or compared unfavorably with another person. Shame is a reaction in which the opinion of another, real or imagined, is of key relevance. Likewise, experimental evidence shows that undifferentiated persons are strongly other-directed and characteristically use external sources of information for definition of their attitudes, sentiments, feelings, and self-evaluations.

The association between guilt reactions and differentiation or field-independence is explained as follows (Witkin *et al.*, 1966, 1968). Guilt is aroused by violation of one's own moral standards. Guilt is an affect that involves reference to inner standards rather than immediate comparisons to standards of others, as in shame, and so guilt depends upon a self which is differentiated, more inner-directed.

DeGroot *et al.* (1967) from our research team examined the relationship between shame and guilt anxiety and psychological differentiation in a group of 40 male and 47 female undergraduate college students taking an introductory course in psychology. Using five-minute verbal samples as the source of affect scores and the Embedded Figures Test (Witkin, 1950) as a criterion of field dependence and field independence, the research team found no correlation between the latter and guilt anxiety for either sex. Furthermore, shame anxiety had a negative instead of a positive correlation ($r = -.26$, $p < .05$) with field dependence for the total sample. These findings differ from those reported by Witkin. The differences in results obtained by the studies of Witkin's group and ours may stem from the different criteria used to determine field dependence and independence, from the difference in the psychological status of the two samples of subjects or from the interpersonal interactions permitted in psychotherapy but not in the procedure for eliciting our verbal samples. Further studies are needed to clarify these issues.

Analysis of Contribution of Differentially Weighted Parts of Anxiety Scale

We have attempted to determine the efficacy of the weights given to different content categories in our anxiety scale by examining separately the validity of the differentially weighted component categories. Thus, the frequency of references to the self as anxious (a) were summed separately, as were references to others (b), references to inanimate objects (c), and denial of anxiety (d) (see Anxiety Scale, p. 23).

There are some major difficulties in determining empirical weights for these categories: (1) The extent to which each category is used may be expected to vary from sample to sample according to the type of subject. (2) No one criterion is available against which validity can be maximized; rather, we are interested in obtaining external discrimination with a variety of subjects and in relationship to many other variables. (3) The content subcategories represent, we think, different levels of awareness of anxiety —use of category (a) indicates awareness of the experience of anxiety (that is, conscious anxiety), whereas use of categories (b), (c), and (d) indicates the probable occurrence of anxiety of which the speaker is incompletely or barely aware. An appropriate independent measure for preconscious anxiety is not to be found in a measure of manifest anxiety, except to the extent to which conscious anxiety may arouse memories of old anxieties. We have not, up to this time, pursued special clinical or psychological test measures as criteria for our content categories of preconscious or signal anxiety, and this should be done. The original inclusion of these content categories in our anxiety scale, however, was based on unsystematic clinical-empirical observation that these kinds of content signalled some anxiety of which the speaker was only marginally aware. Biochemical measures of adrenergic secretion—such as elevation of plasma-free fatty acid levels in fasting subjects—may provide one index of anxiety of which the patient is not entirely aware; so may vocal qualities of a speaker's speech. Hence, we have included studies using such criterion measures of anxiety to examine the validity of these content subcategories. (4) Because the final score on anxiety is achieved by a mathematical transformation, there is no simple method by which to determine the correlation of the final weighted anxiety score with an external criterion from the interrelationships among the subcategories of anxiety and their correlations with the external variable.

The results of four studies are shown in Table 5.6. In every case, the corrected frequency of references to self as anxious (a) was highly correlated with the criterion used, and in at least two of the studies these self-references served as well as the total corrected score as an index of total anxiety. References to others being anxious (b) occurred much less frequently than category (a) and was significantly correlated with the criterion in only one of the studies; the higher correlations occurring between the frequency of use of this category and the criteria of anxiety in Studies II and IV suggest that these content items may have some pertinence to some form of subconscious anxiety. Category (c), which includes statements regarding injury, destruction, or loss of subhuman and inanimate objects, evidently was scored only rarely and made no significant contribution to overall validity. The category of denial (*d*), while scored only infrequently, was positively correlated with the criterion in all but one case and, in general, appeared to contribute some valid variance which may not be adequately represented in our present weights. Furthermore, this category appears to have some relevance to unconscious anxiety,

TABLE 5.6

Analysis of Corrected Frequency of Differentially Weighted Subcategories of the Anxiety Scale in Four Studies

	Study I*			Study II†			
	Freq./100 words		Correlation with anxiety rating	Freq./100 words		Correlation with Overall-Gorham anxiety scale	
Subcategory of anxiety scale	mean	s.d.		mean	s.d.	Type-script	Sound-script
a	1.19	1.11	.67	1.14	.85	.89	.84
b	.20	.29	—.06	.29	.61	.20	.60
c	.00	....	....	.07	.21	.09	.48
d	.11	.18	.03	.08	.08	.08	.11
Total weighted transformed score	2.01	1.09	.66	1.96	.69	.74	.84

	Study III‡				Study IV§			
	Freq./100 words		Correlation with		Freq./100 words		Correlation with	
Subcategory of anxiety scale	mean	s.d.	Av. FFA	20 m. FFA	mean	s.d.	Av. FFA	20 m. FFA
a	.40	.48	.40	.45	.46	.35	.47	.59
b	.12	.14	.15	.28	.14	.18	.47	—.11
c	.08	.16	—.16	—.10	.15	.49	.04	.20
d	.08	.12	.59	.47	.03	.07	.30	.12
Total weighted transformed score	1.17	.54	.49	.54	1.29	.43	.44	.62

* *Psychiatric patients* (N = 24). (See p. 99 for complete details.) *Anxiety criterion*—clinical ratings of patients.

† *Psychiatric patients* (N = 12). (See p. 97 for complete details.) *Anxiety criterion*—Average of 16 ratings of Overall-Gorham Anxiety Scale applied to the typescripts or typescripts plus tape recordings (soundscripts) of five-minute verbal samples.

‡ *Paid male volunteers* (N = 24). (See p. 127 for complete details.) *Anxiety criterion*—free fatty acid level. Av. FFA = average free fatty acid level. 20 m. FFA = free fatty acid level obtained 20 minutes after start of experiment.

§ *Paid male volunteers* (N = 20). (See p. 128 for complete details.) *Anxiety criterion*—free fatty acid level. Av. FFA = average free fatty acid level. 20 m. FFA = free fatty acid level obtained 20 minutes after start of experiment.

as adjudged from the correlation between its frequency of use and average free fatty acid levels in Studies III and IV (Table 5.6).

PSYCHOPHYSIOLOGICAL STUDIES

To test the validity of our measure of anxiety—and at the same time to increase our knowledge concerning relationships between a psychological state and the biochemistry of the human organism—we have pursued a number of psychobiological studies. Some of these studies have involved direct measurement of biochemical substances in the blood or urine, and some have involved indirect biochemical evaluations, in the sense that physiological and pharmacological variables indirectly reflect biochemical changes to varying extents.

The idea that catecholamines are involved in the psychophysiology of emotions is an old one. We have been interested in trying to observe changes in plasma adrenalin and noradrenalin and to determine how these relate to changes in our anxiety and hostility measures. We are aware that intracerebral and intraspinal changes in catecholamine levels may be more primary determinants of affect, mood, and behavior than levels of catecholamines circulating in the blood streams. Furthermore, under normal conditions, the blood-brain barrier does not allow the free passage of catecholamines from intracerebral loci to the blood stream. The present technical difficulties in measuring the minute levels of the catecholamines in the blood stream or in the brain, as well as the rapid modification and chemical breakdown of the catecholamines by enzymatic action in the body, have obliged our finding other ways to ascertain catecholamine levels in the body than by direct measurement.

The administration of such psychoactive drugs as the phenothiazine derivatives and the antidepressants—in double-blind, placebo studies—has been an indirect means of influencing intracerebral catecholamine levels. There is evidence that the iminodibenzyl antidepressants, such as imipramine, decrease the rate of uptake of norepinephrine in the brain or other tissues (Dengler et al., 1962; Axelrod and Glowinski, 1964; Iversen, 1965). (See fuller discussion of these matters, pp. 121 f.) Also, the anti-depressants that are monoamine oxidase inhibitors increase the level of norepinephrine in the brain (Brodie et al., 1959; Krayer, 1959; Muscholl, 1959; Shore, 1960; Zbinder et al., 1960; Gey and Pletscher, 1961; Sjoerdoma and Undenfriend, 1961; von Euler and Lishajko, 1961; Shore, 1962). The fact that neurochemical changes occur in response to psychoactive drugs has enabled us to explore the relationship of such changes to changes in the verbal behavior, and hence in the psychological responses, of human beings. Likewise, exploration of the physiological correlates of our verbal behavior measures has provided us another means of approaching the biological and the presumptive underlying biochemical substrate of affects and other psychological states.

Free fatty acid levels in fasting subjects have been found to be an extremely sensitive indicator of elevated catecholamine levels in the blood stream, particularly of primary and secondary catecholamines hydroxylated on the β carbon of the side chain. These adrenergic substances are released with stress or food deprivation and are capable of releasing free fatty acids stored in deposits of body fat for readily metabolizable fuel (Bogdonoff and Estes, 1961; Davis, 1962).

In the following sections of this book, we will describe a series of psychophysiological, psychopharmacological, and psychobiochemical studies involving the use of our content analysis scales. These studies throw light on the psychobiological correlates of our measure of anxiety.

Anxiety and Hostility in Patients with Myocardial Infarction

Miller (1965) collected five-minute verbal samples under varied interview conditions from 34 outpatients with a previous history of coronary artery disease, matched for race, age, sex, educational level, and I.Q. with 34 medical outpatients without coronary artery disease. Scores on the affects of anxiety, hostility inward, and ambivalent hostility were significantly higher for the patients with coronary artery disease than for the control patients. These differences were attributed by Miller to the patients' reactions to myocardial infarctions.

The coronary outpatients scored significantly higher on measures of death anxiety, separation anxiety, shame and diffuse anxiety, but the two groups did not differ on mutilation and guilt anxiety.

Correlations between Anxiety and Blood Pressure (with and without Hydrochlorothiazide)

In an experimental study of the pathologic psychophysiology of essential hypertension, measurements of anxiety and hostility levels of 12 hypertensive women were observed over two three-week periods; during these periods, the women received either the diuretic hydrochlorothiazide (25 to 50 mg.) or a placebo (Gottschalk *et al.*, 1964*b*). Correlations were obtained between cardiovascular changes from before to after five-minute verbal samples and psychological measures. A significant correlation (.40) was found (p < .05, one-tailed test) between anxiety scores and change in systolic blood pressure. The correlation (.24) between anxiety scores and change in diastolic blood pressure did not reach significance, as was true of the correlation (—.27) between anxiety scores and change in pulse rate. When the hypertensive patients were on hydrochlorothiazide, all correlations between the physiological measures and anxiety and hostility scores were reduced to approximately zero (see p. 169 for findings on hostility in this study).

Correlations between Anxiety Scores and Skin Temperature Changes

A group of twelve high-school boys 16 to 17 years old gave four verbal samples on each of two separate occasions while continuous measurements of skin temperature were being taken (Gottlieb *et al.*, 1967). The first five-minute verbal sample was taken prior to hypnotizing the subject, whereas the subsequent three samples were obtained while the subject was in an hypnotic state. Anxiety scores from the six verbal samples obtained under hypnosis were correlated with the decrease in skin temperature occurring during the giving of the verbal sample for each student separately, using a rank-order correlation. Ten of the 12 correlations were positive (p < .04), yielding an average intrasubject correlation of .31.

Anxiety Scores from Dreams and Inhibition of Penile Erection with Rapid Eye Movement (REM) Sleep

Karacan *et al.* (1966) studied the relationships of penile erections during episodes of rapid eye movement (REM) sleep and the anxiety scores derived from the tape-recorded dreams reported upon awakening from such periods of sleep. A statistically significant association was found between anxiety scores from such dreams and the lack of penile erections. (See pp. 139 ff. with regard to the findings of a positive correlation between dream anxiety scores and increases in free fatty acid levels during the first 15 minutes of REM sleep.)

Anxiety Scores and Electrodermal Variables

Fox *et al.* (1965) studied the relationship to anxiety of individual differences in basal skin conductance and frequency of spontaneous changes in resistance under conditions of rest and arousal in a group of delinquent boys 14 to 16 years of age. Two measures of anxiety were used, the IPAT (Cattell, 1957) administered at the beginning of the experimental session, and the average of three measures of anxiety derived from five-minute verbal samples obtained at the beginning of the session and prior to and following the period of electrodermal recording. Skin resistance was measured continuously with a Fels Dermohmeter and Esterline Angus recorder; bipalmar zinc-zinc sulfate electrodes were employed. Ten minutes of recording were taken during each of the following sequence of conditions: rest, flashing light, threat of shock, post-shock rest.

Frequency of spontaneous changes in skin resistance (600 ohms or more) during rest or arousal conditions was not correlated significantly with either verbal anxiety total score or IPAT anxiety score. In fact, many of the correlations were negative. Furthermore, no significant correlations occurred between basal conductance and either anxiety measure during rest or stimulation. Investigations by Johnson (1963), Dykman *et al.* (1963), and Katkin (1965), using the Taylor Manifest Anxiety Scale or the report of subjective experience during the experimental situation, also revealed no correlation between anxiety scores and skin resistance variables. These studies bring into question the assumption often made that the galvanic skin response is a measure of anxiety or tension.

PSYCHOPHARMACOLOGICAL STUDIES

See Chapter VI, pp. 174 ff., for details on associated changes in hostility scores with psychoactive pharmacologic agents in the studies described below.

Suppressing Effect of Amobarbital on Anxiety Scores

Eighty sophomore medical students in a double-blind psychopharmacologic study (Ross *et al.*, 1963) were asked to write (instead of speak) for five minutes about any interesting or dramatic personal life experiences they wanted to at the time. The anxiety scores on the written verbal samples obtained from students administered 65 mg. of amobarbital were significantly lower (p < .05) than anxiety levels obtained from students on either 10 mg. of dextroamphetamine or a placebo.

Acute Suppressing Effect of Chlordiazepoxide on Anxiety Levels

Forty-five male white adolescents 14 to 16 years of age incarcerated in a juvenile detention center for asocial or delinquent behavior were randomly chosen to take the minor tranquilizer chlordiazepoxide or a placebo (Gleser et al., 1965a). The day prior to that of the actual experimental procedure, each boy on the drug schedule received 10 mg. of chlordiazepoxide by mouth three times during the day, and on the following day, each of these boys was brought into an air-conditioned laboratory and was given 20 mg. of chlordiazepoxide orally. The boys on the placebo schedule were given comparable doses of an identical-appearing placebo on each of the above occasions. Neither the subject nor the experimenter knew the drug assignment. Immediately after the drug administration, each subject was asked to talk for five minutes using our standard instructions. This verbal sample, a second one obtained 40 minutes later, and a third obtained 60 minutes thereafter were tape recorded and scored for anxiety and hostility by two technicians having no knowledge of the experimental procedure or drug assignment. Results are summarized in Table 5.7.

The average scores on anxiety dropped significantly from the first to the second verbal sample and remained at the lower level

TABLE 5.7

Comparison of Mean Anxiety Scores of Groups of Boys on Chlordiazepoxide or a Placebo

Group	1st V.S.*	2nd V.S.	3rd V.S.	Prob. diff. among means
Chlordiazepoxide (N = 21)	2.61	1.85	1.78	.01
Placebo (N = 24)	2.18	2.22	2.17	n.s.
Prob. diff. between means†	<.05	<.08	......	......

* V.S. indicates verbal sample.
† Probability of difference between mean scores of boys on chlordiazepoxide and placebo on second and third verbal samples when corrected for initial values.

in the third sample for subjects on chlordiazepoxide. No such drop occurred in the placebo group. Analysis of covariance indicated that the difference between these trends in the two groups was significant. The scores on the second verbal sample for the group on the active drug were significantly lower than those for the placebo group on anxiety when these scores were corrected for initial values. The differences in initial affect scores between the two groups were not significant by a t-test. This fact implied that there was no significant residual effect of chlordiazepoxide on anxiety 12 to 18 hours after ingestion of three doses of 10 mg. in a 24-hour interval. Immediate anxiety-fear, as measured by the content analysis of speech samples, was significantly reduced within 40 minutes following oral drug administration, and this suppression of anxiety lasted for the remainder of the observation period, that is, at least two hours.

Suppressing Effect of Perphenazine on High Anxiety Levels

Twenty dermatologic patients at the Cincinnati General Hospital participated in a double-blind, placebo, crossover study in which the psychoactive drug administered was perphenazine (a phenothiazine major tranquilizer), 16 to 24 mg. by mouth per day (Gottschalk et al., 1960b). Five-minute speech samples were elicited with standard instructions and recorded on tape at approximately the same time on five successive days while the patient was receiving perphenazine and on another five days while receiving a placebo. Those patients who, when on placebo, had free anxiety indices in the upper third range of the group tended to show a decrease (or no change) in level with perphenazine, whereas patients in the middle or lower third of the range of anxiety showed no consistent direction of change with perphenazine.

Stimulating Effect of Imipramine on Anxiety Scores

An initial longitudinal study of the psychological effects of imipramine (Gottschalk et al., 1965a) on a 27-year-old Negro male with idiopathic narcolepsy, in which the active drug was alternated with a placebo, led to short-term studies on four other general medical patients who were not clinically depressed. Five-minute verbal samples, elicited with standard instructions, were obtained at frequent intervals and the typescripts of these speech samples were later scored by a technician for anxiety and hostility. The dosage range of the imipramine, administered by mouth, was 100-300 mg. per day.

A trend toward increased levels of anxiety with imipramine, as compared with the placebo, occurred in the first subject, but this difference was not statistically significant. However, anxiety scores for the next four subjects were significantly greater on the average with imipramine (1.19) than with placebo (.93). Even when on imipramine, these subjects had relatively low anxiety as measured by the verbal behavior scale.

PSYCHOBIOCHEMICAL STUDIES

Relationship of Anxiety (and Hostility) to Phases of the Menstrual Cycle

An indirect study of psychoendocrine relationships was carrier out by an investigation of the emotional changes in women accompanying different phases in the menstrual cycle (Gottschalk et al., 1962). There were five subjects, all of whom were paid volunteers. Two of the subjects were studied over a period of three menstrual cycles, two for two cycles, and one for a single cycle.

The subjects were requested to keep careful records of onset and duration of menses, to obtain basal temperatures before arising in the morning, and to keep notes on any symptoms possibly suggesting ovulation time, such as "mittelschmerz." These data were used to provide presumptive evidence for hormonal cycles. The hormonal phases classified and examined were: (1) "estrogen" phase—from the second day after the termination of menses through one day preceding ovulation time; (2) "progesterone" phase—from the second day following ovulation time through three days before the onset of menses; (3) "low hormone" phase— from one day before onset of menses through the first four days of menses.

The assessments of psychological state were made by means of the verbal sample technique. The five subjects gave five-minute verbal samples, elicited by standard instructions to talk about any interesting or dramatic personal life experiences, three to seven days per week at approximately the same time of the day.

The verbal samples were scored for anxiety, hostility directed outward, and hostility directed inward; in this section, we shall discuss only the results obtained for anxiety.

The anxiety scores for each subject obtained on days presumed to correspond to a particular phase of their menstrual cycle
were combined for all cycles to yield average anxiety scores for
"estrogen," "progesterone," and "low hormone" periods. These
were compared for each subject separately by analyses of variance.
For three women, the total anxiety score was found to be lowest
during the "low hormone" phase. This difference was significant
at the .01 level for one subject, did not quite reach significance
for another, and was minimal for another for whom data on only
two cycles were available. A further analysis, using a running
average of the combined data on the several cycles to obtain a
graphic description of the typical fluctuations in anxiety throughout the entire menstrual cycle, revealed a decrease in anxiety both
in the period of menstrual flow and around the time of ovulation
for these three women. One of the other two women also showed a
decrease in anxiety at ovulation, but not during the "low hormone"
phase.

The fifth woman, for whom only one menstrual cycle was
available, showed no significant trends.

We feel that this study was particularly valuable, not only
because of the findings that regular rhythmic variations in emotional state are correlated with the menstrual cycle in some women,
but also in demonstrating the potential usefulness of our verbal
sample technique for making repeated measurements and obtaining fluctuations that relate meaningfully to rhythmic physiological
(endocrine) processes.

More recently, Ivey and Bardwick (1968), using our content
analysis method on five-minute speech samples from a group of
college women, corroborated the finding of a dip in anxiety during ovulation and, furthermore, demonstrated an increase in anxiety premenstrually.

Relationship of Anxiety Scores and Plasma
17-Hydroxycorticosteroid Levels

Other investigators, using different samples of subjects and
different means of assessing anxiety than we, have reported a positive relationship between anxiety and urinary or plasma 17-hy-
droxycorticosteroids (Hamburg, 1962; Persky et al., 1958, 1966).

Using our verbal behavior measure of immediate affect, we
have found in natural history studies essentially no correlation
between anxiety scores and plasma 17-hydroxycorticosteroids in

28 medical inpatients or 49 chronic schizophrenic inpatients. Correlations have been found, however, between certain of our verbal hostility scores and plasma corticosteroid levels; these are described in more detail in our validation studies of the hostility scores (see pp. 181 ff.).

Relationship of Anxiety (and Hostility) to Plasma Lipids

Two recent studies of the relationships of anxiety (and hostility) to plasma-free fatty acids have established that our verbal behavior measure of anxiety is associated with the simultaneous secretion of adrenergic substances. We have found that our anxiety scores correlated significantly and positively with plasma-free fatty acids in waking subjects (Gottschalk *et al.*, 1965*b*, 1968) and in the dreams of sleeping subjects (Gottschalk *et al.*, 1966*b*). The two earlier publications reporting these investigations are reprinted below in their entirety.

STUDIES OF RELATIONSHIPS OF EMOTIONS TO PLASMA LIPIDS[2]

Abstract

A natural history study disclosed different relationships between several types of emotions and blood lipids in a group of 24 men. Findings were cross-validated in a study of a second group of 20 men. Anxiety scores had a significant positive correlation with plasma FFA in both groups, whereas three types of hostility indices had essentially zero correlation. More anxious men tended to have higher FFA levels and sharper rises in FFA than non-anxious men in reaction to venipuncture and free associating for five minutes. There was evidence for positive correlations between triglyceride levels and both anxiety and hostility inward scores, as well as for total hostility outward scores and levels of blood cholesterol. In contrast to studies where higher levels of emotional arousal have often been involved and no differential relationship has been found between blood lipid levels and the kind of emotions, plasma lipid levels in this study were found differently related to anxiety than to hostility at relatively low levels of acute arousal.

[2] From L. A. Gottschalk, J. M. Cleghorn, G. C. Gleser, and J. M. Iacono, *Psychosomatic Medicine*, 27: 102–111, 1965—with permission of the publisher.

These studies had two principal purposes. One was to explore the relationships of the magnitude of different labile emotions, such as anxiety and hostility, with variations in plasma-free fatty acids which, in the fasting individual, can serve as indirect indicators of catecholamine activity or autonomic arousal. Another purpose was to explore how levels of not only plasma-free fatty acids but also triglycerides and cholesterol—biochemical substances apparently implicated in the pathogenesis of various conditions (Friedman and Rosenman, 1959; Albrink, 1962; Sloane et al., 1962)—may relate to minor or moderate differences in levels of anxiety and hostility.

Procedure

These psychobiochemical relationships were successively examined in a natural history study of one group of 24 men and of another group of 20 men, all of whom had been fasting for 12 to 15 hours. No attempt was made experimentally to stress the men in these investigations, and differences occurring in the intensity of their emotional responses were considered to be a function of their typical personalities plus their individual reactions to the standardized data-collecting situation described below.

The first group of 24 men was comprised of ten medically healthy, nonpsychotic, psychiatric inpatients and 14 medically healthy college or medical students ranging in age from 18 to 48 years (mean age, 29.8 ± 9.4 years). Subjects were told that this was a study of the relationship of blood chemistry to emotions, that they could be quiet and relax as much as possible, and that there would be only two experimental procedures—a venipuncture and a five-minute period of talking.

Blood samples were obtained from the subjects between 8 and 10 A.M., after 12 to 15 hours of fasting. Subjects relaxed in a comfortable chair or lay supine on a stretcher, and blood was drawn from the right arm, which had been placed through an opening in a curtain so that the investigator and the blood withdrawal could not be seen by the subject. Blood was drawn through a No. 18 indwelling needle fitted with a six-inch segment of rubber tubing and a three-way stopcock allowing either withdrawal of blood or slow infusion of normal saline solution to prevent clotting. Blood samples were drawn, unobserved and undetected by the subjects, at the onset and at five-minute intervals from the twentieth to forty-fifth minutes of a one-hour observation period. About 25 minutes after the venipuncture, each subject was asked to free associate for five minutes about any personal life experiences he had ever had. The speech samples were tape recorded by the investigator and scored independently by technicians unfamiliar with the nature of the study. The following characteristics of feeling were scored by the methods of Gottschalk et al. (1961b, 1963): (1) anxiety; (2) outward hostility; (3) inward hostility; and (4) ambivalent hostility.

Plasma FFA was determined on each plasma sample by the method of Dole (1956) for the initial group of 24 subjects. For the second group of 20 subjects, the FFA determination used was that of Dole as modified by Trout et al. (1960). The latter modification improves the specificity of the FFA determination.

On the initial blood sample of each subject, serum triglyceride levels were measured by the method of Carlson[3] (1959), and serum cholesterol levels were obtained by a modification of the method of Sperry and Webb (1950).

In the cross-validation study, the group was comprised of 20 men ranging in age from 20 to 30 years (mean age, 24.25 ± 3.31), of whom four were medically healthy, nonpsychotic, psychiatric inpatients and 16 were medically healthy college or medical students. The procedures were identical in this study to those carried out with the first group of men, except that blood was drawn every five minutes throughout a 45-minute period of observation.

Results

INITIAL GROUP (24 SUBJECTS)—Table 5.8 shows the means and standard deviations for the three lipid measures and the affect scores obtained on the initial group of 24 subjects. The intercorrelations of the various measures are also shown; correlations below ± .20 are omitted from the table. In the initial group of subjects, a significant correlation is indicated between the anxiety

---

[3] The triglyceride method of Carlson was modified in the following manner: 15 ml. of plasma extract are pipetted into a screw-cap culture tube. The extract is dried under a stream of air, and 10 ml. of chloroform and 1.5 gm. of silicic acid (Biorad Laboratories, Richmond, Calif.—325 mesh) are added to the tube. The cap is securely screwed on the tube, and the sample is shaken intermittently for two hours. The extract is filtered through filter paper previously washed with chloroform and dried, and a 4-ml. sample of the filtered chloroform extract is taken through the subsequent steps of the procedure as outlined by Carlson.

TABLE 5.8

Group 1. Correlations among Lipids and Verbal Affect Measures

Measure	Mean	s.d.	Serum lipids			Immediate affect scores				
						Hostility				
						Outward				
			Triglyc-erides	Av. free fatty acids	Anxiety	Overt	Covert	Total	Inward	Ambivalent
Cholesterol, mg, % (corrected for age)	218.70	31.40	.30	.15	.14	.00	.36	.16	.05	.16
Triglycerides, mg, %	73.20	33.20	.....	.25	.54	.00	.00	.01	.31	.29
Av. free fatty acids, mEq/L	.59	.19	.....	.....	.49	−.16	.02	−.13	.25	.27
Anxiety	1.17	.54	.....	.....	.....	.11	.01	.04	.68	.77
Hostility outward										
Overt	.91	.46	.....	.....	.....	.....	.44	.89	.00	.25
Covert	.70	.49	.....	.....	.....	.....	.....	.78	−.42	.22
Total	1.16	.61	.....	.....	.....	.....	.....	.....	−.20	.25
Hostility inward	.77	.47	.....	.....	.....	.....	.....	.....	.....	.47
Ambivalent hostility	.62	.40	.....	.....	.....	.....	.....	.....	.....	.....

scores and the average free fatty acid (FFA) levels for each subject (r = .49, p = .02, two-tail test). Triglyceride levels also correlated significantly with anxiety scores (r = .54, p = .01). The correlation between average FFA and triglyceride levels was positive but not significant (r = .25).

Positive but nonsignificant correlations were found between the hostility inward and ambivalent hostility scores and FFA or triglyceride levels. Essentially zero correlations were obtained between outward hostility scores and both of these lipid measures.

No correlations of interest occurred between anxiety or hostility scores and cholesterol levels except for a low correlation (r = .36) between cholesterol levels (corrected for age) and covert hostility outwards—one of the two subscales for the outward hostility score.

Figure 5.1 shows that the more anxious subjects (above the median for anxiety in this group) had higher plasma-free fatty acid levels than did the nonanxious subjects at the onset, at 20 minutes after the venipuncture, and again about 15 minutes after they began giving a verbal sample. The anxious and nonanxious subgroups were so designated on the basis of scores derived from the verbal samples.

The maximal correlation of anxiety scores and FFA levels (Fig. 5.1) was obtained from the blood samples drawn 20 minutes after the venipuncture (r = .54; N = 23) and again 15 minutes after the verbal sample was requested (r = .47; N = 17).

These findings suggest that the rising FFA level following the venipuncture, and peaking at about 15 to 20 minutes thereafter, represents the biochemical response to the psychologic meaning of the experimental situation for the subject, including the venipuncture and the ensuing period of observation. The more anxious the subjects, the greater the rise in plasma FFA levels, and hence the greater the correlation between these two variables.

We infer that the second buildup of correlations between the total anxiety score and FFA levels—that is, the increment following a subject's five-minute talk—was related to the subject's complex psychophysiologic reaction to revealing his thoughts in response to relatively unstructured and ambiguous instructions to speak. This relative ambiguity of the verbal behavior procedure for assessing emotional contents—a feature purposely designed in the method, which, like a projective test, aims to maximize the

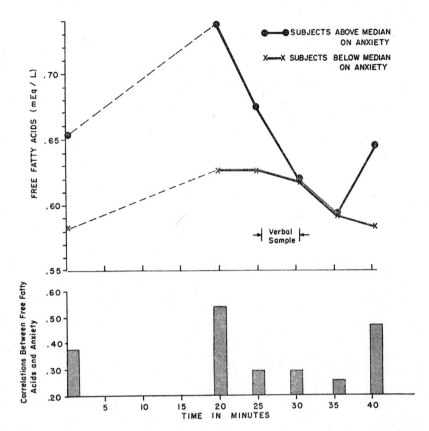

Fig. 5.1. Group 1. Variations in free fatty acids over time in anxious and nonanxious subjects.

individuality of the subject's psychological responses to the situation—tends to evoke more anxiety responses in anxious or anxiety-prone individuals.

CROSS-VALIDATION (20 SUBJECTS)—Table 5.9 shows that the scores for emotions or affects were comparable for the two groups of men except for overt hostility outward, which was significantly lower in the second group (t = 2.29, p = .05). Covert hostility out and hostility in were somewhat lower in the second group than in the first, but this difference was not significant.

The average triglyceride and cholesterol levels were lower than for the first group but not significantly so. The difference in average cholesterol between Groups 1 and 2 can be completely accounted for, in fact, by the difference in age.

TABLE 5.9

Group 2. Correlations among Lipids and Verbal Affect Measures

			Serum lipids			Immediate affect scores				
						Hostility				
						Outward			Inward	Ambivalent
Measure	Mean	s.d.	Triglyc-erides	Av. free fatty acids	Anxiety	Overt	Covert	Total		
Cholesterol, mg. % *	185.10	29.36	.30	−.13	−.24	.51	.08	.37	−.28	−.03
Triglycerides, mg. %	59.35	35.64	.....	.17	.26	−.03	−.11	−.18	.47	.07
Av. free fatty acids, mEq/L	.66	.13	.....	.....	.44	−.08	−.07	.00	.36	.04
Anxiety	1.29	.53	.....	.....	.....	.14	.00	.08	.52	.42
Hostility outward										
Overt	.64	.28	.....	.....	.....	.....	.32	.87	−.03	.47
Covert	.56	.26	.....	.....	.....	.....	.....	.72	.02	.02
Total	.81	.35	.....	.....	.....	.....	.....	.....	−.08	.33
Hostility inward	.60	.22	.....	.....	.....	.....	.....	.....	.....	.04
Ambivalent hostility	.66	.33	.....	.....	.....	.....	.....	.....	.....	.....

* Age was not partialed out for this group, since the age range was extremely limited.

The hypothesis that anxiety is correlated with average FFA level was completely substantiated in the second study ($r = .44$; $p < .025$, one-tail test). Again, no significant correlations were found between FFA level and our three hostility scores.

From the data on the second study, using a one-tail test, we could not reject the hypothesis that cholesterol level was uncorrelated with covert hostility out. For this sample, however, overt hostility out was significantly correlated with cholesterol ($p < .05$). The correlations for total hostility outward and blood cholesterol in the two groups of men were $+.16$ and $+.37$, respectively.

The triglyceride levels were significantly correlated ($r = .47$, $p < .05$) with hostility in but not with anxiety in the second study. The two studies taken together, however, would seem to indicate that there is a positive correlation between triglyceride levels and both anxiety and hostility in. Both studies indicated that triglyceride, cholesterol, and free fatty acid levels were only slightly, if at all, correlated with each other.

Figure 5.2 illustrates the FFA changes over time in the anxious and nonanxious subgroups of men in the cross-validation study. One can again see that, after the venipuncture, FFA levels rose, reached a peak in about 15 minutes, and returned toward an initial level until about the 25-minute point, when the subject spoke for five minutes. Then a second rise in FFA levels occurred, apparently through intervening neurohumoral variables, in response to emotional reactions aroused by having to speak extemporaneously and manifested in the content of the verbal communication. In Group 2, the curve for the anxious subjects remained above that of the nonanxious subjects throughout the period of observation, and as in Group 1, the more anxious subjects showed a much sharper rise in FFA level than the nonanxious ones in the first 15 minutes. Both anxious and nonanxious subjects showed a rise in FFA values after the verbal sample.

The intercorrelations observed between our measures of emotions in the present study are similar to what we have found in other samples of individuals; that is, anxiety scores were positively correlated with hostility inward, and ambivalent hostility scores and hostility outward scores were negatively correlated with hostility inward. As psychodynamic theory would predict, these intercorrelations vary with the nature of the group of people examined.

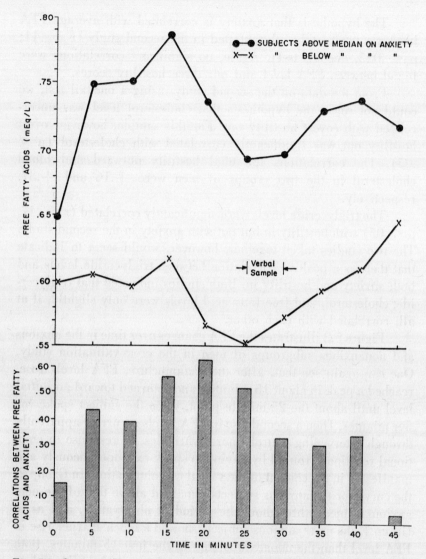

Fig. 5.2. Group 2. *Variations in free fatty acids over time in anxious and nonanxious subjects.*

Psychiatric inpatients, for example, tend to have relatively high correlations between anxiety and hostility inward scores, which simply reflects the clinical observation that anxiety and self-hate or low self-esteem are commonly seen among psychiatric patients (Gottschalk *et al.*, 1963). Among teen-age delinquent boys, a relatively high correlation has been found between anxiety scores and scores on overt hostility outwards (r = .71), reflecting the clinical association between hostile aggressive urges (hostility out scores) and anxiety based on fear of retaliation for manifesting these hostile impulses.

Discussion

This investigation illustrates psychobiochemical relationships occurring in individuals not deliberately subjected to emotional stress but exposed to a laboratory situation involving a venipuncture and a period requiring free associating for five minutes. In this type of situation, physically healthy men who had been fasting 12 to 15 hours showed a significant relationship between the magnitude of immediate anxiety and the average FFA level, but no such relationship occurred between various types of immediate hostility and average FFA.

Dole (1956) and Gordon and Cherkes (1956) noted that FFA concentrations can be elevated after parenteral administration of epinephrine to human subjects, and later other investigators (Bruce et al., 1961; Havel and Goldfien, 1960) found that parenteral norepinephrine and isoproterenol can increase FFA levels. Mueller and Horwitz (1962) found that this effect on FFA is greatest with primary and secondary catecholamines hydroxylated on the β carbon of the side chain. Our present findings suggest that our measure of immediate anxiety, but not of hostility, covaries with the secretion of certain catecholamines in the bloodstream.

Bogdonoff and Estes (1961) and Fishman et al. (1962) found, however, that various types of emotionally stressful situations are associated with elevation of FFA in human subjects, but they found no definite differential relationship between emotions and FFA elevation. We consider that our investigation reveals a differential relationship of certain emotional states to FFA elevation because we were observing relatively low levels of acute arousal of anxiety and hostility. Under these circumstances, anxiety —presumably through the mediation of the types of catecholamines outlined by Mueller and Horwitz—is associated with FFA elevation. Hostility of various kinds at relatively low levels does not turn out to have such a functional relationship with FFA elevation. At higher levels of arousal of these emotional states, such a differential relationship with FFA level in the fasting subject may not be observed because: (1) at high levels of arousal of one emotion, other emotions are often secondarily mobilized (e.g., with great anger, the emotion of fear or anxiety is often aroused as a reaction to fear of retaliation); and/or (2) the thresholds of activation of different neurohumoral mediating mechanisms may be differentially triggered by different emotional states at low levels of arousal but not at high levels.

We have evidence that the timing of the measuring of the acute emotional state is of crucial importance in trying to determine how the intensity and kind of labile emotion covaries with a labile biochemical variable such as FFA. Immediately after the termination of our cross-validation study with the second group of men, when the blood-drawing apparatus had been disconnected and the patient was sitting up, he was asked to give another five-minute verbal sample and fill out an adjective checklist. The correlation of the anxiety scores from this verbal sample and the average FFA level of each subject was +.12. In fact, this anxiety assessment had no relationship with the first three FFA determinations, and low positive correlations (a maximum correlation of .25) occurred with the last seven FFA levels in the series. The correlation of the average FFA levels and the scores on the adjective checklist for anxiety was —.14 and for hostility was —.11. Thus it appears that, in studies of the relationship of labile emotional reactions and labile biochemical variables, the synchronization point of maximal interaction should be explored before any conclusions are drawn about the nature of the relationships.

The history of psychosomatic research has been colored, if not plagued, by a variety of different procedures to measure emotions, and the results of such evaluative processes have frequently not been comparable. Some of the discrepancies may be accounted for, not only because of the complexity and intangibility of psychological processes, but also because evaluative procedures have been based on differing personality theories or because inadequate or no reliability and validity studies have been carried out on the evaluative procedure or the emotions have been assessed in dissimilar contexts or at dissimilar times.

In the development of our verbal behavior measures of emotions or affects, which are based on clinical psychoanalytic theory, we have done detailed reliability and validity tests and, in the process, have found that scores using our procedure for measuring the immediate psychological state can give quite different results in some samples of people from self-report procedures (e.g., adjective checklists), projective tests, behavioral rating scales, and even a clinical assessment. It would be pretentious, at this stage of our science, to assert that one procedure necessarily gives a truer picture of the magnitude and kind of emotional phenomena than another. It would be in order, however, to attempt to determine the constellation of biological concomitants associated with one type of measure of emotions in order to see what leads this might provide toward developing a biologically rooted concept and measure of emotional states.

In this connection, we have evidence that our verbal behavior measures of immediate anxiety, hostility out, hostility in, and ambivalent hostility have somewhat different biologic concomitants. Scores of ambivalent hostility ($r = .53$) and hostility outward ($r = .40$) were found to have significant positive correlations with plasma 17-hydroxycorticosteroids in 40 verbal samples produced by 28 patients, whereas anxiety scores had no significant correlations with plasma 17-hydroxycorticosteroids (Sholiton *et al.*, 1963; Gottschalk *et al.*, 1963). Studies of the psychological effects of psychoactive drugs indirectly reveal psychobiochemical relationships. In one study, the average anxiety score but not the average hostility outward or inward score was decreased significantly in a double-blind, placebo study using phenobarbital (Ross *et al.*, 1963). Scores on anxiety, overt hostility outward, and ambivalent hostility all dropped significantly in a group of delinquent boys 16 to 17 years old on chlordiazepoxide HCl (Gleser *et al.*, 1965a). The tranquilizer perphenazine, a phenothiazine derivative, reduced hostility outward scores in a double-blind, placebo study but did not reduce anxiety scores in a group of 20 dermatologic patients (Gottschalk, 1960). The energizer imipramine in a double-blind, placebo study in five males significantly increased scores on overt hostility outward and anxiety but produced no significant changes in the other emotional variables (Gottschalk *et al.*, 1965a).

These previous findings, in combination with the present findings involving the positive correlation of anxiety scores with plasma-free fatty acids, strongly suggest that different neuro-

humoral patterns are associated with the emotional variables measured by the verbal behavior method. We are in the process of
doing studies to delineate further these psychophysiologic relationships.

Summary

1. Two groups of fasting, medically healthy men, ranging in
age from 18 to 48, were observed consecutively over a one-hour
period between 8 and 10:00 A.M. in a relatively unstressful situation involving only two experimental procedures: a venipuncture,
and a period of free associating for five minutes. Plasma-free fatty
acids, triglycerides, and cholesterol were obtained by venipuncture
at the onset of the experimental situation. Then, through the indwelling needle, blood was drawn at approximately five-minute
intervals for free fatty acid determinations by a procedure that
prevented the subject from observing or detecting the blood drawing. About 25 minutes after the venipuncture, the subject was asked
to free associate for five minutes about any personal life experiences he had had. The speech samples were tape-recorded by the
investigator and scored independently by technicians on immediate
anxiety, hostility outward, hostility inward, and ambivalent hostility.

2. Anxiety scores were found to have a significant positive
correlation with average plasma free fatty acid levels ($r = .49$),
and this finding was completely substantiated in the second group
of men ($r = .44$). In both groups, no significant correlations were
found between plasma-free fatty acids and the three hostility
indices.

3. After the venipuncture, free fatty acid levels rose to a
peak in about 15 minutes and returned toward the initial level
until the 25-minute point, when the subject spoke for five minutes.
This was followed by a second rise in free fatty acid level. The
more anxious men—as adjudged from their verbal sample scores
—tended to have higher free fatty acid levels and sharper rises in
free fatty acids than the nonanxious men in reaction to the venipuncture and to speaking. Evidence was obtained indicating that
in studies of the relationship of labile emotional reactions and
labile biochemical variables, the synchronization point of maximal interaction should be explored before drawing conclusions
about the nature of the relationship.

4. There was some evidence for a positive correlation between triglyceride levels and both anxiety and hostility inward. The correlations for total hostility outward and blood cholesterol in the two groups of men were $+.17$ and $+.37$ respectively, which may be of interest but these are not statistically significant.

5. In both groups of men, the blood triglyceride, cholesterol, and free fatty acid levels were only slightly, if at all, correlated with one another.

6. The implications of these findings are discussed, particular attention being directed to the evidence for differential correlations of types of emotions with biochemical substances in the blood.

ANXIETY LEVELS IN DREAMS: RELATION TO CHANGES IN
PLASMA-FREE FATTY ACIDS[4]

Abstract

Blood samples for determination of plasma-free fatty acids were obtained throughout the night by means of an indwelling catheter. The first sample was drawn at the onset of rapid eye movements and a second after 15 minutes of these movements. Subjects were then awakened and asked to relate their dreams; a third sample was drawn 15 to 25 minutes later. Anxiety scores derived from 20 dreams of nine subjects had significant positive correlations with changes in free fatty acids occurring during REM sleep. No statistically significant relation was found between anxiety and the changes in free fatty acids occurring from the time just before awakening to 15 to 25 minutes later. Presumably, anxiety aroused in dreams triggers the release of catecholamines into the circulation, and these catecholamines mobilize proportional amounts of free fatty acids from body fat.

Other studies of the relation of emotions and blood lipids during the waking state revealed a significant positive correlation between low levels of arousal of anxiety, as determined from a five-minute period of free-associative speech (Gottschalk *et al.*, 1965*b*; Gottschalk *et al.*, 1968), and concentrations of free fatty acids (FFA) in plasma. No essential correlation was found in

[4] From L. A. Gottschalk, W. N. Stone, G. C. Gleser, and J. M. Iacono, *Science*, 153: 654–656, August, 1966—with permission of the publisher. We acknowledge the technical assistance of Carolyn Winget, Betty Stewart, and Terry Ishikawa and the collaboration of John M. Cleghorn in preliminary explorations in this area of study.

this study between hostility and concentrations of FFA. The positive correlation between anxiety levels and FFA raised the question whether a similar relation might occur while subjects are in a dream state. Our study was undertaken to explore such a possibility.

Nine paid volunteer male subjects, ranging in ages from 19 to 25, were asked to sleep overnight in a dream laboratory, arranged to appear as a hospital room. Subjects slept one or two nights in the laboratory but were not given preliminary periods in which to become accustomed to sleeping in this room. They were told that we were investigating sleep, dreams, and changes in body chemistry. Subjects were instructed not to eat after their evening meal at 6:00 P.M. and to report to the laboratory at 11:00 P.M. At this time, a venipuncture was performed in the left antecubital vein with a No. 18 thin-walled needle. A fixed-core stainless steel wire (diameter, 0.8 cm.) was inserted into the vein, the needle was removed, and the tip of a 122-cm. thin-walled polyethylene catheter (inside diameter, 0.18 cm.) was inserted over the wire into the vein. The wire was then removed. The catheter was attached to a three-way stopcock so that normal saline could be slowly infused to prevent clotting and the subject could move comfortably throughout the night. Blood samples were drawn through the stopcock, and since only 1.5 ml. of catheter dead space was present, the first 2 ml. of each sample was discarded to eliminate possible dilution by the saline drip. These samples could be obtained without awakening the subject.

The rapid eye movement (REM) dream state was detected by means of electrodes attached to the outer angles of the eyes, and ocular movements were recorded on a Grass polygraph, model 5, at a paper speed of 0.5 mm./sec. according to the method of Aserinsky and Kleitman (1953, 1955).

The initial sample of blood was drawn at the time of venipuncture, and samples for determination of FFA were drawn at onset of the REM state and 15 minutes afterwards. Subjects were then awakened and asked to report any dreams; all verbal responses were recorded on electronic tape. Subjects were then allowed to go back to sleep. Another sample of blood was drawn 15 to 25 minutes after this brief awakening. In all instances, the subjects had presumably resumed sleeping by this time, but no REM's were occurring. This procedure was repeated for all REM states during the night. Subjects were not permitted to sit up or eat during the experimental period.

The reports of dreams were independently analyzed and scored by two technicians for anxiety, hostility outward, hostility inward, and ambivalent hostility by the Gottschalk-Gleser method (1961, 1963). Reports having 70 or more words were the only ones used for analysis because the reliability of smaller samples has been found to be relatively poor. The two sets of scores were averaged on 20 scorable dreams occurring on 14 nights in all subjects. Concentrations of FFA were determined by the method of Dole (1956) as modified by Trout *et al.* (1960).

Figure 5.3 shows a curve of the average concentration of FFA obtained throughout the 14 nights of sleeping and dreaming of the nine subjects. A small average increase in the concentration was found to occur and reach its peak two to three hours after retiring at 11:00 P.M. Free fatty acids returned to the bedtime (five-hour, postprandial) level about five hours after going to sleep. These findings have not been previously reported, and they are important to note as a nocturnal baseline rhythm in the concentration of FFA on which is superimposed the more transient changes in FFA associated with dream anxiety.

The rank-order correlation of anxiety scores derived from 20 dreams and the associated change in FFA occurring between the onset of REM activity and 15 minutes of REM sleep was .62 (P < .01). The range of changes in FFA during the 15-minute REM periods was +14 to —11 meq./liter, which was +28 to —21 percent of the FFA level at the onset of REM periods. None

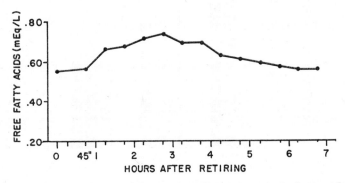

Fig. 5.3. Average free fatty acid level at half-hour intervals during sleeping and dreaming (9 males over 14 nights).

of the correlations between these specific changes in FFA and the hostility scores derived from the dreams was significant. Furthermore, there were no significant correlations between the dream anxiety or hostility scores and changes in FFA that occurred between the time just before awakening the subject to tell his dream and 15 to 25 minutes later (see Table 5.10).

TABLE 5.10

Rank-Order Correlations between Levels of Anxiety and Hostility and
Changes in Free Fatty Acids (FFA) During Sleeping and Dreaming

FFA changes	Anxiety	Hostility outward	Hostility inward	Ambivalent hostility
During first 15 minutes of REM	+.62*	+.31	−.24	+.13
From preawakening to 15 to 25 minutes later	+.11	+.02	−.37	+.27

* Significant at P < .01.

Figure 5.4 shows the average concentrations of FFA during REM sleep and 15 to 25 minutes after the interruption of REM sleep for the nine subjects over the one or two nights they slept in the laboratory. With these nine subjects, the concentration of FFA tended to increase during the first 15 minutes of REM sleep in the instance of the first and third REM periods and to decrease during the comparable interval of the second REM period. None of the variations in the average concentration of FFA during each of the

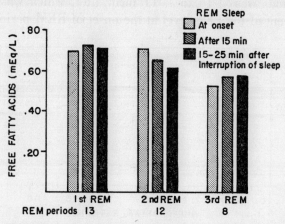

Fig. 5.4. Average free fatty acid levels during REM sleep and 15–25 minutes after the interruption of REM sleep (9 males).

REM periods and the corresponding non-REM period immediately thereafter was statistically significant.

Further analysis of our data reveals that most of our subjects reported scorable dreams (i.e., 70 words or more) after awakening from the second or third REM periods. Eight awakenings after the first REM period elicited either reports of no dreams at all (on five occasions), "feelings and thoughts" (on two occasions), or dreams with too few words (on one occasion); most of these first REM's occurred before three hours of sleep had elapsed. Four out of five of the first REM's that were followed by scorable dreams on awakening occurred three or more hours after going to sleep.

Finding of a positive correlation between magnitude of the anxiety content of dreams (using the Gottschalk-Gleser anxiety scale) and changes in FFA that occur during the first 15 minutes of REM sleep has not been previously pinpointed. This finding strongly suggests that the anxiety content of dreams is capable of triggering adrenergic discharges.

Lack of a significant correlation between anxiety scores from dreams and the changes that occur in the concentration of plasma FFA from the preawakening level to that observed 15 to 25 minutes later may be due to any one of a number of factors or combination of factors. Our previous work (Gottschalk *et al.*, 1965*b*) indicated that in waking subjects, changes in concentration of FFA reach their peak within 15 to 20 minutes after an anxiety stress, such as from a venipuncture, and then tend to return to the prestimulus level; it is likely that, for most people, any changes in FFA due to the anxiety content of the dream largely disappear 30 to 40 minutes after onset of the dream state. In addition, the gradual nocturnal rhythm that occurs in concentrations of FFA after fasting from 6:00 P.M. (Fig. 5.3) may tend to obscure other more transient changes in plasma FFA that occur during and immediately after REM sleep. Still another possibility is that shifts from REM sleep to the waking state and then to non-REM sleep may be accompanied by mild changes in either metabolic rate or the level of catecholamine secretion or both, which can affect the concentration of FFA and hence mask possible prolonged or delayed reactions to the level of anxiety in dreams.

Scott (1965) has reported two major patterns of change in FFA during REM sleep—one in which the concentration rises (Pattern II) and which occurs more frequently early in the night;

the other in which the concentration drops (Pattern I). He speculated that these changes in the concentration of FFA correspond to changes in "sympathetic tonus," but he carried out no independent measure of sympathetic nervous system arousal. Our findings with respect to the direction of changes in FFA during REM sleep (Figs. 5.3 and 5.4) correspond roughly to Scott's observations, except that a small average rise in the concentration was observed later in the night on those nights during which there was a third REM period. Our subjects probably did not have more than two or three REM periods per night because, as previously noted (Rechtschaffen and Verdone, 1964), they were not adapted to the dream laboratory before collection of data began.

Other kinds of evidence strongly suggest that arousal of anxiety associated with stimulation of the sympathetic nervous system accounts for the changes in FFA that we observed. Gottschalk *et al.* (1965*b*) found significant correlations between anxiety scores derived from verbal behavior and concentrations of FFA in two groups ($N = 24$ and 20) of fasting males. Gottlieb *et al.* (1967) found a significant correlation between anxiety scores measured by verbal behavior and decreases in skin temperature in 12 boys 16 to 17 years old. Karacan *et al.* (1966) found that the penile erections that commonly occur in male subjects during REM sleep are inhibited when dreams have high anxiety levels, measured by the Gottschalk-Gleser anxiety scale. Fisher (1965), using a clinical method of assessing anxiety, reported a similar finding. Snyder (1965, p. 382) reported "a marked correlation between REM periods and episodes of nocturnal angina." Nowlin *et al.* (1965) also found a high degree of association with nocturnal angina, and, in addition, he found a significant depression of the ST segment in the electrocardiogram after onset of REM activity. Although the patients of Nowlin *et al.* were not asked the content of dreams when they awakened with nocturnal chest pain, they were questioned for any dream recall on the morning after each study; generally, dreams that preceded an awakening with chest pain involved either strenuous physical activity or the emotions of fear or anger. We speculate that the angina occurs principally with REM dreams that have a high anxiety content, and that otherwise the angina is minimal or absent.

There is substantial evidence that epinephrine and norepinephrine (Dole, 1956; Gordon and Cherkes, 1956) can increase concentrations of FFA and that this effect on FFA is greatest with primary and secondary catecholamines hydroxylated on the β carbon of the side chain (Mueller and Horwitz, 1962). Furthermore, Bogdonoff and Estes (1961) and Fishman et al. (1962) found that emotionally stressful situations induce elevation of FFA in human subjects. These findings strongly suggest that the affect of anxiety, measurable from the dream content, leads to adrenergic stimulation and consequent transient elevation of FFA in plasma during sleep.

It has long been common knowledge to every troubled sleeper that nightmares may awaken him and that he may find himself in a state of high autonomic arousal with a great deal of associated physiological activation; but there has been no satisfactory evidence that mild to moderate emotional experiences during dreams are capable of activating physiological and biochemical activities. Our study, with the studies of Karacan and Fisher, begins to provide some of the missing evidence.

CHAPTER VI
Hostility Scales—Validation Studies

In this chapter, we shall present the evidence we have accumulated on the validity of our three hostility scales as measures of three distinct but possibly interrelated constructs. As we have indicated in Chapter V, the problem of construct validation is a complex one, especially for measures of transient psychological states, since relatively few criteria are available other than behavioral ratings and self-reports. These latter measures are, themselves, often characterized by insufficient data with respect to reliability and validity. As with our measure of anxiety, we have leaned heavily on biological variables as evidence of the arousal of hostility. We have consistently sought to explore relations between the affects we are measuring and biological variables, in the hope that such affects can be discriminated biologically as well as psychologically.

Our validation studies are grouped for convenience into psychological, psychophysiological, psychopharmacological, and psychobiochemical. These, however, do not necessarily represent the chronological order in which the studies were done. Moreover, many of the investigations reported here involved validation of other constructs, such as anxiety, social alienation—personal disorganization, and newer scales. Hence, some repetition in the description of various studies is unavoidable. Cross-references have been provided for those interested in obtaining further information on any specific study.

PSYCHOLOGICAL STUDIES

We have undertaken a number of different studies to ascertain the extent to which our constructs of three different kinds of hostility correspond to scores obtained with other measures of immediate hostility or aggressive behavior, including measures which take into consideration the direction of the hostility.

Some of the studies were undertaken at an early stage in the development of these scales and formed the basis for revision and modification of scoring categories and weights. Such revisions resulted in small changes in the size of the correlations but in no case seriously affected the general pattern of relationships. In all except the first study described below, the findings are those obtained using the latest scaling of our hostility measures and the data were processed by IBM computers.[1]

Pilot Study on Chronic Schizophrenic Patients

This investigation was a pilot study to validate our hostility directed outward scale. We compared observers' ratings of aggressive behavior to scores derived from five-minute verbal samples elicited from chronic schizophrenic patients at Longview State Hospital, Cincinnati. Ten belligerent schizophrenic patients were matched with respect to age, sex, and educational level with ten autistic, withdrawn schizophrenic patients. The mean total hostility outward scores of the belligerent group was significantly higher (p = .02) than the comparable scores derived from the verbal samples of the withdrawn schizophrenic patients.

Experimental Manipulation of Hostility Outward in Male High School Students

This was an experimental study involving 19 male high school students 15 to 16 years of age who were pledging a fraternity. The boys were scheduled to come to the research laboratory in groups of four. They were taken into a room by pairs, and then they were either complimented for their cooperative spirit or adversely criticized and mildly hazed by two of the active fraternity members who were assisting in the experiment. After about ten minutes, the boys were sent to another room where a female psychologist, who did not know which treatment they had received, obtained the verbal sample.

Only 16 boys were used for a comparison of treatment effects, since a slip-up in procedure resulted in the last three boys obtaining information from the earlier subjects as to what they might

---

[1] The initial validation studies (summarized on pp. 147–160) and the related discussion have been excerpted in part from L. A. Gottschalk, G. C. Gleser, and K. J. Springer. "Three hostility scales applicable to verbal samples," *Arch. Gen. Psychiat.*, 9: 254–279, 1963—with permission of the publisher.

expect. The average score for the eight boys who had been hazed was 1.26 on the total outward hostility scale, whereas that for the eight controls was .93. This difference, while in the predicted direction, was not significant.

Before giving the verbal sample, the boys filled out an adjective check list designed by one of us (G. C. G.) to tap current feelings of anxiety, hostility-anger, and unhappiness (Table 6.1). The scores on the hostile adjectives were correlated with the scores on the verbal measure of hostility outward. The values obtained were .38, .74, and .65 for the overt, covert, and total scales, respectively.

Ambivalent hostility also correlated .37 with the angry-hostile score on the adjective checklist, whereas the correlation with hostility inward was —.13.

TABLE 6.1

Adjective Checklist

Below is a list of words which one might use to describe how he feels. Put a *checkmark* in front of each one which *describes how you feel today*. Draw a line through those words that *definitely do not describe* how you feel. You may leave any number of words unmarked, but be sure to *read every one* and decide whether or not it is applicable to how you feel. Work quickly and do not worry about duplications or contradictions.*

(A)	1.	active	(H)	24.	furious	(H)	48.	quarrelsome
(A)	2.	adventurous	(A)	25.	gay	(H)	49.	rebellious
(T)	3.	afraid	(D)	26.	gloomy	(–T)	50.	relaxed
(A)	4.	alert	(H)	27.	grouchy	(H)	51.	resentful
(A)	5.	ambitious	(A)	28.	happy	(T)	52.	restless
(H)	6.	angry	(T)	29.	helpless	(D)	53.	sad
(T)	7.	anxious	(D)	30.	hopeless	(–T)	54.	secure
(H)	8.	annoyed	(H)	31.	impatient	(F)	55.	sluggish
(H)	9.	bitter	(H)	32.	irritable	(F)	56.	sleepy
(D)	10.	blue	(A)	33.	jolly	(T)	57.	shaky
(–T)	11.	calm	(A)	34.	joyous	(F)	58.	slow
(A)	12.	cheerful	(A)	35.	lighthearted	(D)	59.	sorrowful
(A)	13.	confident	(A)	36.	lively	(T)	60.	tense
(A)	14.	contented	(D)	37.	lonely	(T)	61.	threatened
(D)	15.	dejected	(D)	38.	moody	(F)	62.	tired
(D)	16.	despondent	(H)	39.	mean	(–H)	63.	tolerant
(H)	17.	disgusted	(D)	40.	miserable	(T)	64.	uneasy
(D)	18.	discouraged	(T)	41.	nervous	(D)	65.	unhappy
(F)	19.	dull	(T)	42.	panicky	(T)	66.	upset
(A)	20.	energetic	(A)	43.	peaceable	(D)	67.	useless
(T)	21.	fretful	(A)	44.	peppy	(F)	68.	weary
(–H)	22.	friendly	(T)	45.	on edge	(D)	69.	worthless
(T)	23.	frightened	(–H)	46.	pleasant	(T)	70.	worried
			(F)	47.	plodding			

* Scoring key: (A) = active-happy; (D) = sad-depressed; (H) = angry-hostile; (F) = fatigued; (T) = anxious-tense.

Psychiatric Inpatient Validation Study

Verbal samples were obtained in the standard manner from 19 patients (15 female and 4 male) on the psychiatric wards of the Cincinnati General Hospital in the summer of 1959. The patients were rated at the time on the Wittenborn Psychiatric Rating Scales (1955) by the psychiatrist in charge of their cases. The five-minute verbal samples were obtained by a medical student who did not see the Wittenborn ratings.

HOSTILITY DIRECTED OUTWARD

Since none of the Wittenborn scales, per se, were designed to measure aggression, the items were examined and five were chosen as describing aggressive behavior. These items were as follows: 11 (impudent to deliberately disrupts routine); 12 (expresses irritation to gross rage reactions); 14 (insistent manner of speech to shouts, sings, talks loudly); 30 (attention demanding); and 36 (belligerent and assaultive). The scores on this scale could range from 0 to 15.

The correlations between the aggression scores derived from the Wittenborn Rating Scales and scores of hostility outward, as derived from verbal samples, were .16, .30, and .31 for the overt, covert, and total scales, respectively. Although low, the correlations were all in the predicted direction.

The number of words in the sample, which again was essentially uncorrelated with the content scores, also showed a low positive correlation (.38) with the scores derived from the items of the Wittenborn Scales.

Findings of additional interest were obtained. Total hostility outward scores had low positive correlations with acute anxiety ratings (.39), conversion hysteria ratings (.31), and phobic compulsive ratings (.34) on the standard Wittenborn Psychiatric Rating Scales. Negative correlations were obtained with depressed state (—.28), paranoid condition (—.21), and the paranoid schizophrenic rating (—.42) of this scale.

HOSTILITY DIRECTED AMBIVALENTLY

Ambivalent hostility scores correlated .28 with the aggression scores derived from the Wittenborn Scales. Positive correlations were obtained with acute anxiety (.39) and phobic compulsive scores (.54) and negative correlations with the paranoid condition (—.25) and paranoid schizophrenic ratings (—.30) of the Wittenborn Scales.

HOSTILITY DIRECTED INWARD

Because it was assumed that the Wittenborn scale labeled "depressed state" does not coincide with the construct of hostility inward that we are assessing, we selected five items from the Wittenborn behavioral rating scale which we thought described some of the behavioral counterparts of hostility directed inward. These items were: 5 (delusional belief of being guilty, unworthy, evil); 18 (feelings of impending doom); 22 (signs of feelings of hopelessness); 38 (has made attempts at suicide); and 41 (shows uncertainty in making decisions). The scores on this scale could range from 0 to 15.

The correlation between the hostility inward scores derived from the Wittenborn Rating Scales and the scores derived from our hostility inward scale was .66. The correlations of our hostility inward scores with the hostility outward scores derived from the Wittenborn measure was essentially zero (—.16). Of further interest are the correlations found with relevant standard Wittenborn Rating Scales: depressed state (.35), acute anxiety (.74), conversion hysteria (.54), and phobic-compulsive (.45).

Psychiatric Inpatient Validation Study of Depressed and Nondepressed Patients

Another group of 24 inpatients (12 men and 12 women) on the psychiatric wards of the Cincinnati General Hospital gave five-minute verbal samples, elicited by the standard method. Patients selected were considered to be either definitely depressed or nondepressed. The criterion measures used were an adjective checklist (scorable for anxiety, hostility, depression, fatigue) (Gleser, 1960) (Table 6.1), the Beck depression inventory (Beck et al., 1961), and the Buss hostility measure (Buss et al., 1956; Buss, 1961). These criterion measures were alternately administered before or after the verbal sample. One research technician collected the verbal samples and criterion measures, and different technicians independently scored the verbal samples.

HOSTILITY DIRECTED OUTWARD

In this group of patients, the verbal total hostility directed outward scores correlated negatively with the depression scores on the adjective checklist (—.22) and the Beck depression inventory (—.18) and positively with the Buss assault subscale (.27) and total hostility scale (.24). These correlations were in the expected direction. A puzzling negative correlation (—.23), however, occurred between our total hostility outward scores and the hostility scale of the adjective checklist with this particular sample of patients.

AMBIVALENTLY DIRECTED HOSTILITY

The scores on this verbally derived measure showed expected low positive correlations with the Buss hostility scale, the most notable being in the subscales categorized as indirect hostility (.32), negativism (.29), and suspicion (.29). No correlation whatsoever occurred between the scores on this verbal measure and the Beck depression inventory or the adjective checklists.

HOSTILITY DIRECTED INWARD

The hostility inward scores from this group of patients showed positive correlations with the depression (.48), anxiety (.31), and hostility (.38) scales of the adjective checklist, the Beck depression inventory (.47), and the Buss negativism (.39) and suspicion (.38) subscales.

The Municipal Court Psychiatrist Clinic Validation Study

The subjects of this study were 25 persons (18 men and 7 women) referred by Cincinnati Municipal Court judges to a Municipal Psychiatric Clinic for psychiatric evaluation. The referrals had been charged with asocial acts such as petit larceny, assault and battery, disorderly conduct, habitual or public drunkenness, resisting arrest, obscene discourse, indecent exposure, and so forth. The psychologist [2] who conducted the personality assessment rated these individuals for immediate hostility. These ratings were made according to the Oken hostility scale (1960) and were based on observations of the behavior of the individuals during a

---

[2] We acknowledge the contributions of Robert Mills, Ph.D., Psychologist, Cincinnati Municipal Court, Psychiatric Clinic.

diagnostic interview. The results of this validation study are summarized in Table 6.2.

HOSTILITY DIRECTED OUTWARD

In this group of subjects, the total outward hostility scale and both subscales (overt and covert) were significantly correlated with the Oken ratings of immediate hostility (.52). The number of words spoken was also correlated with immediate hostility (.59) and was found to be relatively independent of the content scales. When the females were eliminated from the groups of subjects, the correlation of the total hostility outward scale with the immediate hostility ratings tended to increase (.64). The correlations between the Oken hostility ratings and scores from our outward hostility subscales, overt (.55) and covert (.53), also increased when only males (18) were used in the calculations.

HOSTILITY AMBIVALENTLY DIRECTE

Ambivalent hostility scores from this group of subjects had a positive correlation (.32) with the Oken ratings, and no appreciable change in correlation occurred when the women's scores were omitted from the calculations.

HOSTILITY DIRECTED INWARD

Inward hostility scores had the expected zero or negative correlation (—.18) with the Oken rating in this group of subjects, and the negative correlation increased (—.38) when it was calculated only for the 18 males in the sample.

Psychiatric Clinic Outpatient Validation Study

A definitive validation study was undertaken on 50 psychiatric outpatients comprising 20 males and 30 females with an average age of 30.7 ± 11.5 years. The subjects were new patients applying to a clinic for psychiatric treatment. Each subject gave a five-minute verbal sample, which was scored for hostility on each of our three hostility scales. The evaluative measures to which our verbal hostility scores were compared were: (1) an adjective checklist (Gleser, 1960) providing scores for hostility, depression, and fatigue (Table 6.1); (2) the Beck depression inventory (1961); (3) the Buss hostility scales (Buss *et al.*, 1956; Buss, 1961); (4) the Oken hostility rating (1960); and (5) a clinical

TABLE 6.2

Correlations among Hostility Measures with Court Clinic Subjects

	Mean	s.d.	Hostility inward	Ambivalent hostility	Hostility outward Total	Overt	Covert	Oken hostility rating Total sample	Males only (N = 18)
Number of words	595.00	167.70	−.32	.00	.28	.28	.11	.59	Not done
Hostility inward	.93	.64	.....	.08	.38	.51	−.04	−.18	−.38
Ambivalent hostility	.84	.56	.....	.....	.45	.39	.40	.32	.30
Hostility outward									
Total	1.02	.55	.....	.....	.....	.93	.68	.52	.64
Overt	.85	.51	.....	.....	.....	.....	.38	.44	.55
Covert	.60	.31	.....	.....	.....	.....	.....	.46	.53
Oken hostility rating	3.50	2.30	.....	.....	.....	.....	.....	.....	.....

depression rating scale (Table 6.3). The Oken hostility scale and the clinical depression ratings were made by one of the two psychiatrists after a one-hour diagnostic interview. Immediately after the interview, each patient was asked to give a five-minute tape-recorded talk in response to our standardized instructions. Thereupon each patient was administered the Buss hostility scales, the Beck depression inventory, and the adjective checklist. The order of administration of these latter measures was rotated every five patients so that every possible permutation occurred. The inventories and verbal samples were obtained by a psychologist (K. S.) or a research technician. (See Tables 6.4 and 6.5 for a summary of results.)

TABLE 6.3

Clinical Rating Scale for Depression

In the left-hand margin of this page, encircle one of the following letters (*a, b, c, d*) which best indicates to what extent, during the past 24 hours, each of the statements below is applicable to the person you have just examined.

> *a*—not at all
> *b*—a little
> *c*—a moderate amount
> *d*—a large amount

a b c d 1. Evidences of self-criticism, self-depreciation.

a b c d 2. Evidences of feeling of depression, grief, sadness.

a b c d 3. Evidences of suicidal ideas or other punitive, mutilating urges against oneself.

a b c d 4. Evidences of feelings of failure, lack of accomplishment or achievement.

a b c d 5. Evidences of "vegetative signs"—loss of appetite, loss of sexual interest, constipation, amenorrhea, insomnia or other sleep disturbances, lethargy.

a b c d 6. Evidences of itching, nausea, vomiting, abdominal cramps, overeating or overweight on a nonspecific etiological basis.

a b c d 7. Evidences of feelings of being criticized, depreciated, belittled by others.

a b c d 8. Evidences of feelings of persecution, by others, or of feelings others have intentionally destructive urges to self.

a b c d 9. Evidences of feeling betrayed, deserted, rejected, abandoned by others.

HOSTILITY DIRECTED OUTWARD

The highest correlations between the verbal total hostility outward scores and other affect measures occurred, in this group of subjects, with the adjective checklist hostility score (.30) and the Oken hostility rating (.36). Table 6.4 indicates that the males in the group primarily accounted for the positive correlations; using only males, the correlation of the total outward hostility scores with the hostility scores of the adjective checklist was .57

TABLE 6.4

Correlations among Various Affect Measures for a Group of Psychiatric Outpatients (N = 50)

Affect measure	Mean	s.d.	Hostility inward	Ambivalent hostility	Hostility outward Total	Overt	Covert	Adjective checklist Hostility	Depression	Fatigue	Beck inventory	Buss scales Hostility	Guilt	Lie	Oken hostility rating	Clinical depression rating
Number of words	531.1	226.6	−.19	−.09	−.05	−.19	−.06	.09	−.17	.02	−.12	.17	−.08	−.24	−.09	−.07
Verbal measure																
Hostility inward	.76	.53		.48	.13	.50	−.26	.33	.52	.41	.34	.09	.24	−.04	.00	.20
Ambivalent hostility	.68	.44			.31	.44	.06	.14	.20	.07	.37	.22	.13	−.10	.21	.16
Hostility outward																
Total	1.06	.53				.68	.79	.30	.03	.21	−.06	.06	−.16	−.06	.36	.05
Overt	.80	.42					.14	.29	.16	.16	.09	.20	.04	−.04	.28	.32
Covert	.72	.46						.16	.07	.12	−.16	−.07	−.24	−.07	.26	−.13
Adjective checklist																
Hostility	10.3	7.7							.64	.62	.32	.41	.28	−.23	.39	.35
Depression	14.2	10.3								.72	.44	.12	.32	−.06	.18	.37
Fatigue	4.8	4.0									.29	.17	.29	−.04	.19	.29
Beck depression inventory	18.9	9.1										.35	.38	−.20	−.02	.41
Buss scales																
Hostility*	31.9	11.1											.34	−.69	.27	.21
Guilt	5.7	2.4												−.33	−.01	.32
Lie	3.3	2.6													−.21	−.15
Oken hostility rating	1.9	1.5														.07
Clinical depression rating	7.8	3.9														

* Total omitting guilt.

TABLE 6.5

Comparison between Male and Female Psychiatric Outpatients in Verbal Hostility Scores, Scores on Other Measures, and Correlations between the Two

Verbal measure	Verbal hostility score (mean)		Correlation with other measures														
	Males (20)	Females (30)	Adjective checklist						Beck depression inventory		Buss scales				Oken hostility rating		Clinical depression rating	
			Hostility		Depression		Fatigue				Hostility		Guilt					
			M	F	M	F	M	F	M	F	M	F	M	F	M	F	M	F
Mean score on other measures	......	......	8.5	11.5	10.2	16.9	4.0	5.4	17.2	20.1	33.6	31.6	5.8	5.9	2.0	1.9	8.5	7.3
Number of words	535.00	528.00	.11	.08	−.15	−.19	.04	.01	−.28	−.01	.39*	.04	−.11	−.05	.36*	−.26	−.11	−.04
Hostility inward	.59	.88	.21	.32	.18	.59*	.11	.50*	.19	.36	.06	.15	.01	.31*	.13	−.07	.27	.26
Ambivalent hostility	.60	.75	.19	.07	.05	.20	−.06	.10	.06	.51*	.07	.31*	−.07	.19	.34	.10	.27	.13
Hostility outward																		
Total	1.00	1.12	.57*	.13	.13	−.09	.25	.15	−.21	−.01	.27	−.12	−.16	−.21	.50*	.25	.58*	−.27
Overt	.82	.81	.53	.14	.14	.19	.18	.17	−.13	.27	.24	.08	−.13	.09	.41*	.08	.58*	.10
Covert	.65	.77	.44*	.04	.20	−.24	.29	.02	−.16	−.19	.10	−.14	−.24	−.27	.41*	.24	.51*	−.37

* Correlations that are most strikingly different for males and females.

and with the Oken hostility rating .50. Scores on hostility outward were essentially uncorrelated with the several depression
scores in the total sample.

The lack of correlation between our hostility outward measure
and the Buss hostility scale (.06) was notable. Since the Buss
scales are intended to measure typical hostility and aggression
rather than immediate hostile affect, it was expected that only low
positive correlations might be obtained but that these correlations
might give some indication of the common factors being measured.
For the males, there were suggestive correlations between the
verbal behavior measures and the Buss scale factors classified as
assault (.32), negativism (.42), and suspicion (.22). For the
women, no positive relationships were indicated with the Buss
scales; nor were the Oken ratings found to relate to the scores
derived from the Buss scales.

An additional finding of interest in this study was the lack of
correlation between the verbal hostility scales and the lie subscale
of the Buss scale. The lie scale is essentially a measure of the
tendency to give socially acceptable responses, and it is adapted
largely from the MMPI lie scale. Persons scoring high on the
scale tend to deny behavior or feelings that are considered socially
undesirable. The lack of correlation with our hostility outward
scores gives some evidence that our hostility outward scores were
not readily influenced by conscious attempts of the person to make
himself look socially acceptable and to cover up his hostility.

AMBIVALENTLY DIRECTED HOSTILITY

With this sample of subjects, the ambivalent hostility scores
showed the highest positive correlation (.37) with the Beck depression inventory and lower positive, yet noteworthy, correlations
with the Buss hostility total scale (.22), the depression score on
the adjective checklist (.20), and the Oken hostility rating (.21).
The ambivalent hostility scores of the females accounted for most
of the correlation obtained with the Beck depression inventory
(.51) and Buss hostility scale (.31).

HOSTILITY DIRECTED INWARD

The hostility inward scores were found to correlate most
highly (.52) with the depression scores of the adjective checklist,
a fact accounted for principally by the females (.59). Some sizable

positive correlations also occurred with the adjective checklist fatigue scores for males and females (.41) and for only females (.50) and with hostility scores (.33). The inward hostility scores showed a positive correlation with the scores from the Beck depression inventory (.34), the Buss guilt subscale (.24), and the clinical depression rating (.20). Hostility inward scores showed zero or negligible correlations with the Oken and Buss hostility scales.

SUMMARY OF THE INITIAL VALIDATION STUDIES OF THE THREE HOSTILITY SCALES

The different samples of subjects used in these first six validation studies were drawn from normative, neurotic, and psychotic populations. Criterion measures included self-report and personal inventories as well as assessment procedures made by someone other than the subject. Results of comparisons made between scores from criterion measures and the hostility scores derived from verbal behavior varied, to some extent, with the sample of subjects examined. Certain typical and recurring findings appeared, however, and these pointed to the conclusion that it was statistically, as well as heuristically, valid to separate the affect of hostility into three types based on the direction of the drive or impulse.

The psychological state assessed by our measure of hostility directed outward was found similar to the assaultive and angry impulses and feelings that a person is aware of and can describe in various self-report test procedures. It is also similar to the harmful, asocial, and destructive behavior and attitudes toward objects outside oneself that an external observer can perceive or infer. The emotional phenomena measured were found dissimilar to the psychological constructs measured by the depressive scales of adjective checklists, the Beck depression inventory, and the depression and paranoid subscales of the Wittenborn system of ratings.

Our verbal behavior procedure of assessing hostility outward and the two other types of hostility tends to preclude a subject's covering up and not revealing his hostility. Although it is believed that the verbal behavior method is capable of detecting differences in awareness of hostile affect, the above-reported validation studies were not designed to substantiate this feature.

Our construct of ambivalent hostility overlaps the constructs of both hostility directed inward and hostility directed outward and the overt much more than the covert portion of the latter measure

(Table 6.2). This was demonstrated by the intercorrelations among these different hostility measures and also by the intercorrelations between ambivalent hostility scores and the various criterion measures labeled "hostility," "depression," "indirect hostility," "suspicion," "negativism," and so forth. These correlations are understandable from a clinician's point of view if one pauses to recall that the patient who feels adversely self-critical and expresses this self-criticism (such a patient would obtain a high hostility inward score) often tends to assert that he is criticizable by others (verbal behavior associated with a high ambivalent hostility score). Furthermore, it is clinically commonplace that psychiatric patients with strong consciences who overtly express their hostility outward also tend to feel they should be criticized adversely. Also, the patient is not unfamiliar who expresses his anger by complaining that others are hurting or criticizing him, thus trying to provoke a possibly sympathetic listener to feel angry at those who have wronged him.

We believe that ambivalent hostility, though it includes aspects of both outwardly and inwardly directed hostility, is different enough from either of the others to warrant discrete classification. Some evidence to justify this division is that: (1) the scores for this measure are derived from language denoting and connoting different events than the other two measures of hostility, namely, verbalizations about hostile activities directed toward oneself from forces outside oneself; (2) other investigations (see p. 83) indicate that the measure of ambivalent hostility can vary independently from hostility inward or outward.

The measure of hostility directed inward was found to be a similar construct to the psychological constructs of "depression" and "fatigue" as assessed on adjective checklists, the "depression" and "acute anxiety" scores derived from the Wittenborn rating scales, and the scores obtained from the Beck depression inventory and from our clinical depression scale (Table 6.3). It measures a psychological construct dissimilar to that measured by the Oken hostility scale and other assessment procedures designed to measure anger or outwardly directed hostility.

One of the interesting and provocative aspects of these studies is the conspicuous difference found between males and females with respect to how their verbal hostility scores correlate with other measures of verbal hostility and depression (Table 6.5). It would appear that, for males, measures of hostility outward are concordant with other measures of aggression; in general, this is not true for females. On the other hand, hostility inward scores correlate consistently higher with measures of guilt and depression for females than they do for males. In addition, males obtaining high clinical ratings of depression tend to show high hostility outward verbal scores; no such relationship occurs for women.

We suspect that these differences are culturally determined and reflect the fact that women's experience and expression of hostility in our society contrasts considerably with that of men. For example, child rearing practices encourage passivity and discourage outward aggression as adaptive mechanisms to frustration in girls while sanctioning assertiveness and some aggressive retaliation in boys. An associated phenomenon may be the higher incidence of reactive depressions in women as compared to men. These data may provide some support for the psychoanalytic hypothesis that anger or hostility toward an external object—when in conflict with some internalized standard—may become directed to the self. However, only longitudinal studies of the relationship of hostility outward, hostility inward, and depression in many types of subjects can clarify these complex psychodynamics. In exploring such psychodynamic relationships, one must continually realize that there are different kinds of depressive reactions, some revolving largely around feelings of guilt, some around feelings of shame and inadequacy, and some around separation and loss (Gottschalk, 1966). The nature and direction of hostility in these various types of depressive reactions can be quite complicated and can depend on many individual personality factors, all of which prevent drawing easy generalizations on the subject. Using our verbal behavior method in a study of the psychodynamics of depression, Gershon et al. (1968) have demonstrated just this point.

Hostility Scores and Mental Status Schedule Scores on Chronic Schizophrenic Patients: Intercorrelations, Including Predictive Capacity of the Verbal Behavior Measures

In a longitudinal study of 74 chronic schizophrenic hospitalized patients, each subject was interviewed by a psychiatrist using the standardized interview and Mental Status Schedule of Spitzer (1965, 1966) and Spitzer *et al.* (1964, 1965, 1967). In addition, each patient was seen two or three times a week by a non-professional assistant who obtained five-minute verbal samples by the standard procedure. Sixty-nine of the patients spoke enough words (100 or more) to provide reliable samples (see p. 67).

Initially, these two different types of measures—verbal behavior scores and clinical ratings (using the Mental Status Schedule)—were obtained while all 74 patients were on large doses of various tranquilizers, all phenothiazine derivatives. The Mental Status interview was repeated four weeks after a placebo had been substituted for the psychoactive drug. Final measurements were made four weeks after the second measurement period, at which time half of the patients were given daily doses of thioridazine (Mellaril) comparable to their original phenothiazine dose schedule, and the other half were maintained on the placebo (Gottschalk *et al.*, 1968).

The intercorrelations are given in Table 6.6. To be noted is the fact that overt (but not covert) hostility outward scores correlated with hostility-negativism (.37), insight deficiency (.35), and somatic preoccupation (.35). Initial overt hostility out scores also were predictive of neurotic (r = .34) and psychotic (r = .31)

TABLE 6.6

Intercorrelations of Hostility Scores and Selected Mental Status Schedule Scales (N = 69) Verbal Behavior Hostility Scores in Baseline Period (T₁*)

Mental status schedule scales		Hostility outward			Hostility inward	Ambivalent hostility
		Total	Overt	Covert		
Hostility-negativism	T₁	.33	.37	.03	.21	.10
Insight deficiency	T₁	.26	.35	−.03	.13	.26
Somatic preoccupation	T₁	.26	.35	.09	.19	.31
Neuroticism	T₁	.04	.13	−.09	.06	.16
	T₂†	.25	.34	.02	.30	.20
Psychoticism	T₁	.09	.22	−.15	.03	.24
	T₂	.26	.31	.06	.08	.26
Disorientation	T₁	−.10	.09	−.25	.04	.03
	T₂	−.15	.00	−.28	.09	−.01

* T₁ = while on phenothiazine drugs (baseline period).
† T₂ = after four weeks off phenothiazine drugs.

phenomena appearing four weeks after discontinuation of phenothiazine drug therapy. Covert hostility out scores correlated negatively with disorientation during the baseline period ($r = -.25$)
and four weeks after drug therapy was terminated ($r = -.28$).
One other interesting correlation is that between hostility in scores
and neurotic symptoms ($r = .30$) after four weeks off phenothiazine drugs. These findings encourage the possibility that such
affect scores may be used to predict response to drug withdrawal
(possible uses of social alienation–personal disorganization scores
as predictors of subsequent behavior or responses are referred to
on p. 219).

Clinical Ratings from Psychoanalytic Interviews and Hostility Outward Scores

In several studies involving the assessment of hostility, we
have applied our scaling method to verbal behavior obtained
under different circumstances than provided by our standard procedures. These studies suggest that our assumptions and methods
for quantifying psychological events can be applied to other material involving language, both spoken and written. A fuller discussion of this issue in general occurs on pp. 256 f. and 276 f. At
this point, we will review four studies, using in each language
behavior obtained under different circumstances or in different
ways than by our standard procedure. These studies all contribute
in a small way toward the validation of the hostility constructs
we are using.

Two five-minute segments of a psychoanalytic interview were
tape-recorded during the psychoanalytic session of six different
analysands. These were all sessions during which the therapist
said little or nothing. One such five-minute verbal sample was
obtained during the first and one during the last 15 minutes of
an analytic session of each patient. A poor recording, however,
prevented the transcribing of the second five-minute verbal sample
of one of the patients. Hence, a total of only 11 such verbal samples was obtained. During each psychoanalytic interview using all
clinical data available, the analyst rated on a scale of 0 to 18 what
he estimated was the relative intensity of the total immediate hostility outward of the patient during the five-minute periods the
patient's free associations were being tape-recorded. A year later,
the verbal samples were independently scored for total hostility
outward by a research technician using our total Hostility Outward

Scale. The rank-order correlation between the two sets of scores was .76.

This finding strongly suggests that a patient's verbal behavior, as it occurs in the psychoanalytic or some other type of psychotherapeutic situation, can be validly assessed to provide a measure of immediate hostility in the same way that we have evaluated the hostility levels in five-minute verbal samples elicited by our standard procedures. The findings also suggest that the affect score derived from our verbal behavior method, with all its various assumptions and statistical manipulations, is respectably similar to the quantitative assessments that the psychoanalyst makes when listening to the total context and content of the verbalizations as well as having available, as relevant information, the paralanguage and nonverbal behavioral cues from the patient.

Thematic Apperception Test (TAT), Hostility Scores, and Verbal Hostility Outward Scores

Thematic Apperception Tests on 24 individuals, comprising 12 to 14 cards in each test, were scored by a technician for hostility according to the method described by Hafner and Kaplan (1960). The same TAT protocols were also scored independently by another technician for hostility using our Hostility Outward Scale.

The rank-order correlation between the two sets of scores was .72. This finding indicates not only that the affect scores derived by the two methods are highly correlated, and hence involve overlapping constructs, but also that other material besides free associations or verbalizations during the psychotherapeutic interview may be assessed for affective content by our method.

A recent investigation of differences in the process and outcome of interaction between couples with good and poor marital adjustment (Clements, 1968; Winget *et al.*, 1969) provided us with further TAT data and a testable hypothesis regarding group differences. In this study were compared 15 couples who applied for counseling at the Marriage Counseling Service of the Hamilton County (Ohio) Court of Domestic Relations and a matching group of 15 couples who had been approved as potential parents by an adoption agency. The couples were asked to look at each of four TAT cards in turn, discuss them, and arrive together at a story to fit each picture. The cards used were 4, 6GF, 11, and 13MF, presented in random order. The couples' interactions and their final stories were tape-recorded and transcribed. The investigator made these data available to us for analysis. We hypothesized that the couples with marital problems would tell TAT stories having more hostility and poorer human relations than would the couples with good marital adjustment.

The stories for the four cards were combined for purposes of content analysis, since many of the individual stories contained too few words for reliable scoring. The groups did not differ on the average in number of words spoken. The average hostility out scores for the poorly adjusted marital group was 2.33, and that of the well-adjusted group was 1.82. The combined estimate of the standard deviation was .63. The difference in means was significant at the .05 level. (See p. 227 for comparison of these same data on the human relations scale.)

Rosenzweig Picture-Frustration Test and Verbal Hostility Scores

Eighty sophomore medical students participating in a double-blind, placebo-drug study were asked to write for five minutes about any interesting or dramatic personal life experiences (Ross et al., 1963).

Scores on hostility derived from the written verbal samples were compared to hostility scores obtained from the Rosenzweig Picture-Frustration Test (1947, 1950). Low but significantly positive correlations were found between our hostility outward and ambivalent hostility scores and the extrapunitive scores on the Rosenzweig test. The intrapunitive Rosenzweig scores were negatively correlated with these verbal hostility scores but positively correlated with our inward hostility scores.

Cognitive and Perceptual Styles and Verbal Hostility Scores Derived from Psychotherapeutic Interviews

Witkin et al. (1966, 1968) examined the relationship of hostility to shame and guilt anxiety in a series of psychotherapeutic interviews of eight patients—four who were classified as highly "differentiated" and four who were classified as "undifferentiated" on the basis of their cognitive and perceptual styles from tests developed by Witkin and his co-workers (1962). The four psychotherapists in this study each had one "differentiated" and one "undifferentiated" patient. Patients in each group were matched for sex and socioeconomic level. Regardless of patient type, a strong tendency was found for both shame and guilt anxiety scores (per 500-word units) to be associated with feelings of hostility. Within this general relation, a more specific tendency was noted: regardless of patient type, shame anxiety tended to be associated with hostile feelings directed toward the self and guilt anxiety to be associated with hostility directed outwards. The evidence for this conclusion was found in the frequency of coincidence, in 500-word units, of "spurts" of feelings [3] of shame anxiety, guilt anxiety, hostility out, and hostility in. In 500-word units where shame spurts occurred, there were hostility in spurts in 62 percent of the units and hostility out spurts in only 37 percent of the units. Conversely, guilt spurts were accompanied by hostility out spurts in 79 percent of the units and by hostility in spurts in 58 percent of the units. The consistent association between a tendency toward shame and a tendency toward hostility in was also evident with individual patients. When the weighted shame anxiety scores of the eight patients, for the first two psychotherapy sessions combined, were correlated with their hostility in scores, the resulting correlation was .84 ($p < .01$). The correlation for the percent spurts measure of shame and hostility in was equally high (.86, $p < .05$). Moreover, the relation tended to hold in individual sessions. For the first session, for example, the correlation between shame and hostility in spurts was .79 ($p < .01$); for the second session, the correlation was .71 ($p = .05$). Patients prone to strong shame reactions were also prone to strong hostility in reactions, and there was a tendency for the relation to persist. No such consistent relation was found in individual patients [4] between a tendency toward

---

[3] "Spurts" of feeling were calculated by computing the usual corrected weighted score (per 500-word units) and then obtaining the percent of 500-word units in which a weighted score of 1.0 or higher occurred.

[4] Since in our verbal behavior analysis method, the same phrase may sometimes receive multiple scores—for in everyday language, feelings of hostility toward the self and feelings of shame may at times be expressed in similar words—Witkin et al. (1966) examined the possibility that some of the linkages found between shame and hostility in might have stemmed from the fact that the same information in the typescripts of the psychotherapeutic interviews had been scored in both scales. Examination of individual scoring units in the therapy typescripts suggested that this problem of overlap in information drawn upon was not a very important factor in the relations observed. Of the 1891 clauses scored in all patient records for guilt and/or hostility out, only 6.9 percent were scored for both. Similarly, of 1178 clauses scored for shame and/or hostility in, only 17.1 percent were scored for both.

guilt and hostility out, shame and hostility out, or guilt and hostility in.

Witkin *et al.* (1966) also looked at the relationship of the degree of differentiation of the patients and the relative magnitude of hostility outwards and hostility inwards. Table 6.7 illustrates the findings.

When weighted scores were considered, undifferentiated patients did not show a consistent difference between hostility inward and hostility outward scores. For the differentiated patients, however, hostility outward scores were higher than hostility inward scores in three pairs by quite large amounts; the overall difference in mean scores was substantial. When spurt scores were considered, both groups of patients showed a tendency in the expected direction; undifferentiated patients tended to have higher hostility inward than hostility outward scores, and differentiated patients showed higher hostility outward scores. A *t*-test indicated that the differential comparison was significant for the spurts measure but not for the weighted score measure.

That feelings of hostility are accompanied by feelings of shame and guilt are findings quite consistent with common sense and clinical observation. One would expect, moreover, that there are different groups of individuals: some who are predominantly experiencing feelings of guilt; some, feelings of shame; some, separation anxiety; and some, fears of retaliation (e.g., those who experience mutilation and/or death anxiety when aroused to hos-

TABLE 6.7

Comparison of Hostility Inward and Outward in Undifferentiated (Field-Dependent) and Differentiated (Field-Independent) Psychotherapy Patients *

Weighted scores				% spurts			
Undiffer. pts. (U)		Differ. pts. (D)		Undiffer. pts. (U)		Differ. pts. (D)	
Hostility inward	Hostility outward	Hostility inward	Hostility outward	Hostility inward	Hostility outward	Hostility inward	Hostility outward
U1 1.38 → 1.86		D1 1.22 ← .94		U1 64.2 ← 61.6		D1 43.1 ← 33.8	
U2 1.70 ← 1.63		D2 .90 → 1.75		U2 88.4 ← 50.0		D2 30.5 → 68.6	
U3 1.65 → 1.80		D3 1.02 → 1.89		U3 74.9 → 77.4		D3 39.8 → 95.4	
U4 1.34 ← 1.08		D4 1.30 → 2.05		U4 71.4 ← 34.2		D4 50.0 → 70.8	
Mean 1.52 → 1.59		Mean 1.11 → 1.66		Mean 74.7 ← 55.8		Mean 40.8 → 67.2	

* From Witkin *et al.*, 1966—with permission of the authors.

tility). This is our clinical impression, and it serves as a good working hypothesis for further studies exploring the relationships between different kinds of anxiety and anger.

Cognitive and Perceptual Styles and Hostility Scores Derived from Five-Minute Verbal Samples

Like Witkin, we find in the five-minute verbal samples elicited by our standard procedure a relationship between shame and hostility in. We also find a consistent relationship between guilt and hostility out. For example, in a study of 50 psychiatric outpatients, shame anxiety and hostility inward were correlated .43, shame and hostility outward .10, and guilt and hostility outward .56. In the sample of 94 employed subjects from Kroger, shame and hostility inward correlated .43, shame and hostility outward —.09, guilt and hostility inward —.09, and guilt and hostility outward .26.

Our explanation of these findings concerning the relationship of the direction of hostility to shame and guilt are in agreement with Witkin *et al.* (1966). With shame anxiety, there is a need to correct the poor opinion of oneself in the eyes of others and to safeguard the relationship with others, and hence hostility is directed toward the self in preference to others. With hostility directed outward, an important deterrent toward acting out with physical aggression in psychotherapy patients is the internalized sense of guilt; hence, when the patient feels sufficient confidence in himself and in the therapeutic relationship to express hostility outward, he will also be likely on occasions to condemn, criticize, or abuse himself (guilt anxiety) in order to control or to temper his outspoken aggression.

There are, without question, people who characteristically experience no self-criticism when they express hostility outward— for example, some paranoid individuals or criminals—and they would usually neither seek psychotherapy nor show the hostility outward-guilt linkage.

With regard to the relationship between hostility scores and degree of cognitive differentiation, our results differ from those of Witkin, at least for a nonpatient sample. The Embedded Figure Test (Witkin, 1950) was administered to 87 male and female undergraduate college students, in an introductory psychology course at the University of Cincinnati, who also gave five-minute verbal samples during the same testing session (deGroot *et al.*, 1967). Correlations of .26 for males and .02 for females were obtained between extent of cognitive differentiation, as measured by the Embedded Figure Test, and hostility in scores obtained from the verbal samples. The correlations for hostility outward were —.14 and —.27, respectively. These correlations, while not significant, are in the *opposite* direction from those obtained by Witkin. It is likely, therefore, that the relationships he obtained are limited to differentiated and undifferentiated patients in a psychotherapeutic situation (see pp. 112 f. for further discussion).

Effect of Brief Psychotherapy on Levels of Hostility Inward and Anxiety

Patients coming to an emergency brief psychotherapy clinic (MacLeod and Tinnin, 1966) were interviewed by a research team before and immediately after psychotherapy and three to six months after termination of treatment. Part of the evaluation interviews was the obtaining of five-minute verbal samples elicited and analyzed according to our procedures. Significant decreases occurred in hostility in (p < .05) and total anxiety scores (p < .01) by a sign test; no significant changes were found after psychotherapy in hostility outward or ambivalent hostility scores (Gottschalk *et al.*, 1967). (See pp. 225 f. for further details of use of our content analysis method in the prediction and assessment of outcome with brief psychotherapy.)

PSYCHOPHYSIOLOGICAL STUDIES

Coronary Artery Disease and Hostility Scores

Sixty-eight volunteers from the Neurocardiology Research Program at the Oklahoma Medical Center participated in a study that involved giving five-minute verbal samples in response to our standard instructions (Miller, 1965). Thirty-four of the patients had a diagnosis of myocardial infarction, and a control group of 34 medical patients was judged free of coronary artery disease; the two groups of patients were matched for race, sex, education, and I.Q. The verbal samples were scored for anxiety and hostility and on a scale developed by Miller that he called "need achievement." For greater reliability of results, the average scores of two independent coders were used.

The coronary patients were found to score higher than the noncoronary patients on measures of hostility inward (p < .01) and ambivalent hostility (p < .06) but not on either overt or covert hostility outward. The coronary group also scored higher on anxiety (p < .01) and lower on need achievement (p < .05) than the noncoronary group.

Essential Hypertension and Hostility Scores

In an early study, single verbal samples were obtained from five male and five female hypertensive patients being treated at the Cincinnati General Hospital Outpatient Clinic and from five male and five female normotensives attending the Clinic for other ailments. The hypertensive patients obtained significantly higher scores (p < .05) on hostility outward as compared to the normotensives (Kaplan *et al.*, 1961).

In another study (Gottschalk *et al.*, 1964b), levels of hostility and anxiety and blood pressure and pulse rate of 12 hypertensive women (three with labile and nine with fixed hypertension) were observed over two three-week periods. During these periods, the patients were receiving 25 to 50 mg. per day of hydrochlorothiazide (an antihypertensive diuretic with no known direct action on the central nervous system) or a placebo. Measurements of the emotional variables were made from five-minute verbal samples scored by our verbal behavior analysis method.

No evidence was found in our small group of subjects that women with fixed hypertension had typically more hostility outward or were typically more anxious than women with labile hypertension. The sample of fixed hypertensives, however, had somewhat higher inward hostility scores than the labile hypertensives.

While the women were taking the placebo, significant positive correlations were obtained between their inward hostility levels and their average systolic (r = .47, p < .05) and average diastolic (r = .55, p < .01) blood pressures. Significant negative correlations were found between hostility outward levels and average systolic (r = —.50, p < .05) and average diastolic (r = —.55, p < .01) blood pressures (see Table 6.8). At the same time, positive correlations were found between hostility outward and the change in their systolic (r = .46, p ≤ .05) and diastolic (r = .50, p < .05) blood pressures from before to after a verbal sample (see Table 6.9 and Figs. 6.1 and 6.2).

TABLE 6.8
Correlations between Cardiovascular and Psychological Measures during Three Occasions in Hypertensives Taking Hydrochlorothiazide or Placebo

Psychological measures	Average systolic blood pressure*						Average diastolic blood pressure*					
	Placebo (N = 8)			Drug (N = 12)			Placebo (N = 8)			Drug (N = 12)		
	Within person	Be-tween persons	Total	Within person	Be-tween persons	Total	Within person	Be-tween persons	Total	Within person	Be-tween persons	Total
Anxiety	.12	.21	.17	.12	.05	.07	.07	.07	.07	.13	-.03	.01
Hostility outward	-.43	-.56	-.50†	.36	-.37	-.07	-.48†	-.62	-.55‡	.35	-.41	-.09
Hostility inward	.59†	.40	.47†	-.30	.14	.04	.62†	.51	.55‡	-.17	.18	.09
Ambivalent hostility	.06	.34	.23	.31	-.06	.03	.17	.55	.34	.20	-.07	.00

* Average of pre- and postverbal sample blood pressure readings.
† p < .05, two-tailed test.
‡ p < .01, two-tailed test.

TABLE 6.9

Correlations between Cardiovascular and Psychological Measures from before to after
Verbal Samples in Hypertensives Taking Hydrochlorothiazide or Placebo *

Psychological measures	Change in systolic blood pressure		Change in diastolic blood pressure		Change in pulse rate	
	Placebo	Drug	Placebo	Drug	Placebo	Drug
Anxiety	.40	—.18	.24	—.23	—.27	—.22
Hostility outward	.46†	—.20	.50†	—.13	—.09	.16
Hostility inward	.28	—.02	.06	—.15	.04	—.12
Ambivalent hostility	.34	—.05	.13	—.18	—.18	—.18

* 24 pairs of measurements were available for placebo and 36 pairs for hydro-chlorothiazide.
† p < .05, two-tailed test.

Though small but statistically significant decreases in systolic and diastolic blood pressure occurred (see Table 6.10) when these women were taking hydrochlorothiazide (p < .05, one-tail *t*-test), no significant changes occurred in hostility or anxiety levels of

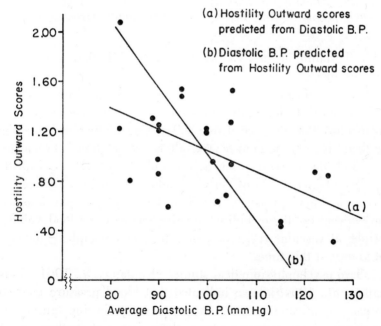

Fig. 6.1. Relationship of hostility outward scores to average diastolic blood pressures (mean of the diastolic blood pressures obtained before and after the five-minute verbal sample).

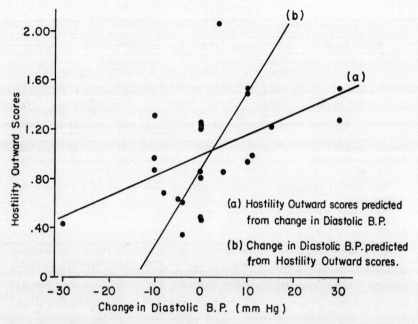

Fig. 6.2. Relationship of hostility outward scores to change in diastolic blood pressures (from before to after five-minute verbal sample).

either the labile or the fixed hypertensives while they were receiving this drug.

All significant correlations between blood pressure and anxiety and hostility levels disappeared when the women were given hydrochlorothiazide (see Table 6.9). This finding suggests that the drug, in some unknown way, alters the relation between hostility and blood pressure levels, probably by interfering with the capacity of increments of certain kinds of hostility to trigger increases in blood pressure. Whether the mediating physiological mechanisms for these findings involve changes in blood volume, peripheral vascular resistance, or some other complex factors is not known at this time.

Two psychophysiological studies (Kaplan *et al.*, 1961; Gottschalk *et al.*, 1964*b*) have indicated that blood pressure tends to increase significantly among hypertensives following talking for five minutes into a tape recorder in the presence of another person, in contrast to significant decreases of systolic and diastolic blood pressure occurring among normotensives after such an event.

TABLE 6.10

Average Blood Pressure, Change in Blood Pressure, and Pulse Rate before and after Verbal Samples in Hypertensives and Normotensives Taking Hydrochlorothiazide or Placebo

Group	Number of women	Drug					Placebo				
		Sys. B.P.	Dias. B.P.	Change in			Sys. B.P.	Dias. B.P.	Change in		
				Sys. B.P.	Dias. B.P.	Pulse rate			Sys. B.P.	Dias. B.P.	Pulse rate
Labile hypertensives	3	134.0	88.7	4.4	1.9	77.7	140.7	91.7	.0	0.5	71.4
Fixed hypertensives	5	148.0	98.7	6.6	1.3	78.4	163.5	105.3	7.4	3.9	78.0
Fixed hypertensives (no placebo)	4	162.2	102.9	10.4	4.2	81.3	......	......	......	......	......
Normotensives	2	104.4	69.2	−2.5	−0.6	84.8	110.0	73.3	−4.7	3.0	85.7

Pulse Rate and Hostility (and Anxiety) Scores[5]

Change in pulse rate after giving a five-minute verbal sample had no significant relation with hostility (or anxiety) scores derived from these verbal samples. The correlations, though not statistically convincing, are mostly in a negative direction rather than a positive one. This finding might be of interest to those investigators who assume that a positive relation is likely to occur between mildly increased hostility or anxiety and increased heart rate.

PSYCHOPHARMACOLOGICAL STUDIES

Effect of Chlordiazepoxide on Hostility Scores[6]

Forty-five male white adolescents, 14 to 16 years of age, were randomly assigned, on a double-blind basis, to receive either chlordiazepoxide (a minor tranquilizer) or a placebo (Gleser *et al.*, 1965*a*). The day prior to the experimental procedure, each boy in the drug group received three doses of 10 mg. of chlordiazepoxide by mouth. The boys in the placebo group were given comparable doses of an identical-appearing placebo on each of the above occasions. On the day of the experiment, each boy was again given a pill (chlordiazepoxide or placebo) upon entering the laboratory. Immediately after the administration of the pill, following our standard procedure, the subject was asked to talk for five minutes. About 25 minutes later, the IPAT Anxiety Scale (Cattell, 1957) was administered, and then a second verbal sample was obtained (about 40 minutes after obtaining the first verbal sample). A third verbal sample was obtained 60 minutes thereafter. The typescripts of these speech samples were scored for hostility and anxiety by two technicians who had no knowledge of the drug assignment or experimental procedure.

The results are summarized in Table 6.11. The average scores on ambivalent hostility and anxiety dropped significantly from the first to the second verbal sample and remained at the lower level in the third sample for the subjects on chlordiazepoxide. No such drop occurred in the placebo group. The group on chlordiazepoxide also evidenced a decrease in overt hostility outward which did not quite reach the .05 level of significance.

---

[5] See Table 6.9.
[6] See p. 122 for effect on anxiety scores.

TABLE 6.11

Mean Anxiety and Hostility Scores of Groups of Boys on Chlordiazepoxide or a Placebo

Treatment	Anxiety				Ambivalent hostility				Hostility inward			
	1st VS*	2nd VS	3rd VS	Prob. diff. among means	1st VS	2nd VS	3rd VS	Prob. diff. among means	1st VS	2nd VS	3rd VS	Prob. diff. among means
Chlordiazepoxide (N = 21) ..	2.61	1.85	1.78	.01	1.93	1.27	1.36	.05	.84	.62	.63	ns
Placebo (N = 24)	2.18	2.22	2.17	ns	1.79	1.68	1.63	ns	.79	.62	.86	ns
Prob. diff. between means† ..	.....	.05	.08	.....	.....	.02	ns	.....	.....	ns	ns	.....

Hostility outward

Treatment	Overt				Covert				Total			
	1st VS	2nd VS	3rd VS	Prob. diff. among means	1st VS	2nd VS	3rd VS	Prob. diff. among means	1st VS	2nd VS	3rd VS	Prob. diff. among means
Chlordiazepoxide (N = 21) ..	1.44	1.04	1.08	.06	1.14	1.35	1.04	ns	1.82	1.68	1.46	ns
Placebo (N = 24)	1.34	1.35	1.05	ns	1.26	1.36	1.15	ns	1.84	1.94	1.62	ns
Prob. diff. between means† ..	.....	.01	ns	.....	.....	ns	ns	.....	.....	ns	ns	.....

* VS indicates verbal sample.

† Probability of difference between mean scores of boys on chlordiazepoxide and placebo on second and third verbal samples when corrected for initial values.

Analysis of covariance further indicated that the difference between these trends in the two groups was significant. The scores on the second verbal sample for the group on the active drug were significantly lower than those for the placebo group on anxiety, ambivalent hostility, and overt hostility outward when these scores were corrected for initial values. None of the differences in initial affect scores between the two groups was significant at the .05 level by a t-test. This would imply that there was no significant residual effect of chlordiazepoxide at a dose level of 10 mg. three times a day, 12 to 18 hours after ingestion.[7]

The average number of words spoken in each of the three samples was examined to determine whether there was a differential trend in the amount of speech accompanying the differential changes in affect. In the chlordiazepoxide group, the averages were 442, 565, and 494 words, respectively; for the placebo group, the corresponding averages were 413, 514, and 431. An analysis of variance of the data yielded a highly significant overall trend ($F = 6.96$, $p < .0025$) and a nonsignificant interaction ($F = .13$, $p < .50$). Both groups spoke significantly more words in the second sample than in the first sample.

The IPAT Anxiety Scale did not differentiate the two groups. The average score for the subjects on chlordiazepoxide was 37.47, and that for the subjects on placebo was 38.28. The negligible difference in average score on this scale may be due to the fact that it is not sensitive enough to detect the effect of chlordiazepoxide at this dosage level without the additional control obtainable with initial values. An interesting, but as yet unexplained, finding was that there was a positive correlation between the IPAT scores and the verbal anxiety measures for the subjects on chlordiazepoxide ($r = .39$, $p = .05$) but not for the subjects given the placebo ($r = .05$).

Randall (1961) and Randall et al. (1960) have noted that chlordiazepoxide has a unique taming effect in monkeys far below the ataxic dose and that this differential response separates the compound from other tranquilizers. The lack of hypnotic effects at high doses distinguishes chlordiazepoxide from meprobamate and phenobarbital. Animals under high doses of chlordiazepoxide can be aroused by gentle prodding; they show ataxia but not true

---

[7] The difference in initial anxiety, however, had a probability of .10 of being a zero difference. Thus, it is possible that the subjects given chlordiazepoxide were somewhat more anxious initially than those given the placebo.

hypnosis. In addition, the lack of autonomic blocking effects differentiates chlordiazepoxide from chlorpromazine, which has marked effects on body temperature, blood pressure, and the autonomic nervous system.

Others have accumulated direct or indirect evidence that chlordiazepoxide can lessen fear, anxiety, or tension. For instance, Kamano and Arp (1964), studying avoidance conditioning in rats, found that these conditioning responses were more rapidly extinguished in rats given chlordiazepoxide than in controls not receiving drugs, suggesting that chlordiazepoxide lessens the fear upon which the conditioned avoidance response is based. In a double-blind, placebo study on a group of 150 male outpatients newly accepted for individual psychotherapy at V.A. mental hygiene clinics, Lorr et al. (1962) found anxiety-tension reduced at the end of the first week following administration of chlordiazepoxide as compared to a placebo group. But there was no difference in anxiety-tension scores between the drug and placebo groups by the end of four weeks. The evaluative measures used by Lorr and his colleagues were self-report and therapist rating scales developed by Lorr et al. Kelly and Gisvold (1960), in a study employing no controls and using patient reports and MMPI scores, found decreases in overt anxiety and tension in 66 psychoneurotics and psychotic patients treated with chlordiazepoxide for two to eight months. In a number of studies of children, which employed no controls and evaluated change principally by clinical observations and patient reports (Corboz, 1962; Krakowski, 1963; Leconte and Orval, 1963), chlordiazepoxide was found to reduce symptoms inferred to be associated with anxiety or fear.

The present study, using an objective method of measuring psychological variables, tended to confirm the above findings. Immediate anxiety and fear as measured by content analysis of speech samples was reduced within 40 minutes following acute drug administration and remained lowered for the remainder of the observation period (i.e., about two hours).

Two other psychological variables were also found affected by chlordiazepoxide in the present study. Overt hostility outward, a score derived from verbal references in which the speaker asserts destructive or aggressive statements directed from himself to objects in the world external to himself, was reduced following ingestion of chlordiazepoxide. Ambivalent hostility was also significantly decreased in the group. This hostility score, derived from statements that others are blaming, criticizing, or injuring the speaker, appears to be an alternate way of coping with aggressive feelings and the accompanying anxiety. Now, our subjects in this study were boys who had been recently involved in some asocial or delinquent activity for which they were being temporarily detained until their legal status had been settled by the Juvenile Court. It is not surprising that the content of their speech, in response to an open-ended instruction, should contain a relatively high frequency of assertions that other people—court, police, family—are blaming, criticizing, hurting, disapproving of one's self. The frequency of expression of such sentiments was lessened within an hour after ingesting 20 mg. of chlordiazepoxide.

The placebo and active drug groups both showed the same trend in average number of words spoken on the three verbal samples. Thus, there was no indication that chlordiazepoxide produced a sedative or euphoric effect resulting in a decrease or push of speech. The differential trend in affect scores for the two groups cannot be attributed to a difference in rate of speech.

From this study, there is no indication that the 30 mg. of chlordiazepoxide administered during the previous day had any lasting effect on the measures used in this study. No significant differences were observed in anxiety or hostility scores for the subjects given chlordiazepoxide as compared to placebo-treated controls 12 to 18 hours after ingestion of the drug. The practical application of this investigation is, perhaps, that chlordiazepoxide, at a modest dosage level, can stem for brief periods the disrupting emotions—anger, spite, and anxiety-fear—of juvenile delinquent boys. Chlordiazepoxide is considered one of the minor tranquilizers (Kapp and Gottschalk, 1962); whether one of the so-called major tranquilizers might be as broadly effective as chlordiazepoxide on these crucial emotions has not been ascertained, nor has anyone determined whether a major tranquilizer might have a longer-lasting effect at a comparable dosage level.

Effect of Perphenazine (a Phenothiazine Derivative— Major Tranquilizer) on Hostility Scores[8]

In a study utilizing a double-blind, crossover design to compare the psychological effect of the pharmacologic agent per-

---

[8] See also p. 123 for effect on anxiety scores.

phenazine and a placebo, it was found that there was a significant reduction of the median scores on outward hostility for 16 out of 20 patients during perphenazine administration as compared to the placebo (Gottschalk et al., 1960b). This group of patients was composed of both Negro and white males and females, all obtained from the dermatology wards of the Cincinnati General Hospital. The perphenazine or placebo was administered daily for a week, and five-minute verbal samples were obtained on five successive days under each treatment.

Effect of Imipramine (an Antidepressant) on Hostility Scores[9]

The effect of the antidepressive pharmacologic agent imipramine on anxiety and hostility levels of five general medical patients was assessed from verbal samples (Gottschalk et al., 1965a). The research design involved essentially a double-blind, placebo versus drug, cross-over arrangement. A pilot study was first done with one patient (J. K.) followed by a cross-validation study on the four other patients (see Fig. 6.3 and Table 6.12). A significant increase in the level of overt hostility out (p < .01)

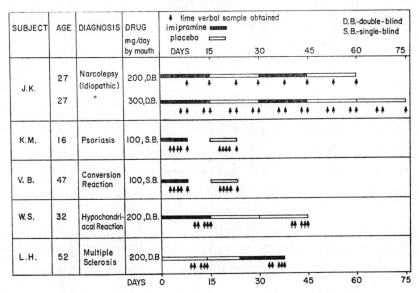

Fig. 6.3. Summary of subjects, drug dosage, and order.

[9] See also p. 123 regarding effect on anxiety scores.

TABLE 6.12

Average Affect Scores of Subject J. K. while on Imipramine and/or Placebo

Date	Number of observations Imipramine	Placebo	Hostility outward Imipramine	Placebo	Ambivalent hostility (self attacked, wronged, imposed upon) Imipramine	Placebo	Hostility inward (self-injury, self-recrimination, guilt, despair) Imipramine	Placebo	Anxiety Imipramine	Placebo
1960*	2	2	.76	.45	.35	.45	.35	.45	.98	.84
	2	2	.88	.28	.29	.28	.47	.79	1.38	1.09
1961*	4	4	.74	.45	.53	.54	.80	.50	1.40	.90
	4	3	.64	.33	.44	.27	.41	.41	.97	.51
				.65		.26		.50		1.03
Mean			.74	.46	.40	.36	.51	.53	1.18	.87
Mean difference			.28		.04		−.02		.31	
Standard error of mean difference†			.10		.08		......		.20	
P			.01		......		......		.12	
			(two-tail)						(two-tail)	

*Imipramine dosage was 200 mg./day in 1960 and 300 mg./day in 1961.
†Computed from the within treatment variance over all samples.

was found to be associated with imipramine administration (see Table 6.13). Anxiety level also tended to be elevated with imipramine (p < .025) (see Table 6.14). No significant change occurred in the scores on hostility inward or ambivalent hostility, possibly because none of the five patients was clinically depressed.

TABLE 6.13

Average Overt and Covert Hostility Outward Scores for All Subjects

Subject	Overt hostility outward		Covert hostility outward	
	Imipramine	Placebo	Imipramine	Placebo
J. K.	.47	.41	.59	.33
K. M.	.63	.49	.71	.83
V. B.	.50	.37	.83	.47
W. S.	.64	.39	.64	.71
L. H.	.66	.42	.49	.52
Mean	.58	.42	.65	.57
Mean difference	.16		.08	
Standard error of mean difference	.06		.10	
P	.01 (two-tail)		......	

PSYCHOBIOCHEMICAL STUDIES

Plasma 17-Hydroxycorticosteroid Levels and Hostility Scores

IN MALE MEDICAL PATIENTS

The hostility scales were employed as a control variable in a study of the effect of lung cancer on the plasma 17-hydroxycorticosteroid levels of patients (Sholiton, Wohl, and Werk, 1963). The study was carried out on male patients at the Cincinnati Veterans Administration Hospital. The total outward hostility score for 40 verbal samples produced by 28 patients was found to correlate .33 (p < .05) with the average of two measures of plasma 17-hydroxycorticosteroid, one obtained before and one after a period of psychological testing. The within-group correlation was .42 when data for cancer and control patients were analyzed separately using observations from one session for each subject. The covariance of total hostility out with plasma 17-hydroxycorticosteroid did not account, however, for the high level of the corti-

TABLE 6.14
Average* Affect Scores for Four Additional Subjects

Subject	Drug dose mg./day	Hostility outward		Ambivalent hostility (self attacked, wronged, imposed upon)		Hostility inward (self-injury, self-recrimination, guilt, despair)		Anxiety	
		Imipra-mine	Pla-cebo	Imipra-mine	Pla-cebo	Imipra-mine	Pla-cebo	Imipra-mine	Pla-cebo
K. M.	100	.93	.97	.69	.49	.40	.46	1.75	1.35
V. B.	100	.95	.50	.33	.40	.33	.32	.95	.71
W. S.	200	.87	.79	.45	.37	.60	.31	1.39	.95
L. H.	200	.76	.61	.30	.30	.30	.30	.66	.72
Mean	......	.88	.72	.44	.39	.41	.35	1.19	.93
Mean difference	......	.16		.05		.06		.26	
Standard error of mean differences†	......	.115		.075		.075		.125	
P	......	.10 (one-tail)		......		......		.025 (one-tail)	

* Average of five observations per drug period.
† Computed from the combined error and interaction sum of squares obtained by a two-way analysis of variance with five measures per cell.

costeroid in the group of patients with lung cancer as compared to the control group. A correlation of .32 was found between the average 17-hydroxycorticosteroid and hostility inward scale as it was then coded. These data were brought up to date and re-examined after the last revision of our hostility scales. With our present method of weighting and scoring categories, a correlation of .40 was obtained between hostility outward levels and the average 17-hydroxycorticosteroid level over all samples. The correlation was somewhat higher with the corticosteroid level obtained after the psychological testing session (.47) than with that obtained before testing (.31). Furthermore, with our present method of weighting and scoring, ambivalent hostility scores correlated .53 and hostility inward scores correlated —.14 with the mean plasma hydroxycorticosteroid levels (themata comprising these two scores were all coded as hostility in, in the previously reported data of this study).

IN CHRONIC SCHIZOPHRENIC PATIENTS

Blood was drawn sometime between 8:00 A.M. and 9:00 A.M. from 49 chronic schizophrenic patients who were receiving placebo in connection with a phenothiazine withdrawal study; the blood was used to obtain plasma 17-hydroxycorticosteroid determinations (Gottschalk, Cleghorn, and Gleser, 1964c). That same morning, verbal samples were obtained from each patient by the standard procedure. Additional verbal samples had been obtained two to five days prior to this time. The affect scores for the two verbal samples were averaged, and correlations were computed between these scores and the 17-hydroxycorticosteroid values for males and females separately. Two of the biochemical measures were discarded prior to this computation because of hemolyzation resulting in unusually low values. Several other determinations showed traces of hemolyzation but were included since they fell within normal limits. The results are shown in Table 6.15.

None of the correlations obtained in the schizophrenic sample between 17-hydroxycorticosteroid levels and affect scores was significantly different from zero, although there was some similarity in the patterning of correlations to those obtained on the medical patients. Further studies are needed to determine whether the attenuation of correlations in chronic schizophrenic patients is a direct result of the schizophrenic process itself, a product of long-

TABLE 6.15

Plasma 17-Hydroxycorticosteroids (HOCS) and Affect Scores in Chronic
Schizophrenic Patients

	Females (26)			Males (21)		
	Mean	s.d.	Correlation with 17-HOCS	Mean	s.d.	Correlation with 17-HOCS
Anxiety	1.58	.73	−.11	1.80	.88	.08
Hostility inward	.76	.40	−.20	.96	.66	.26
Ambivalent hostility	.80	.50	.04	.92	.61	.18
Hostility outward	1.11	.58	.16	1.17	.52	.14
17-hydroxycorticosteroid (meq.)	14.18	5.16	......	14.72	4.77	......

term institutionalization, or an artifact due to sampling or to the
difficulty in obtaining representative affect measures on such patients as the result of decreased verbalization and idiosyncratic
thought processes.

The complexity of factors involved in mobilization of the
pituitary adrenocortical axis has been well documented. Studies
of the relationship of the arousal by emotional stress of corticosteroid secretion in parents of fatally ill children (Wolff et al.,
1964), in schizophrenic reactions (Sachar et al., 1963), and in
Rhesus monkeys (Mason et al., 1966a) indicate that complex factors are involved in determining whether or not endocrine reactions
occur to stressful situations. Investigators report that various psychological defenses can block the stress-induced increased production of corticosteroids, whether the stress comes from outside or
within the individual. Possibly the defense mechanisms involved
in chronic schizophrenia also interfere with the relationship between
affect and mobilization of 17-hydroxycorticosteroids.

Along another line, Silverman (1964) and Silverman et al.
(1965), in studying effects of institutionalization in general, have
recently observed narrowing of perceptual and cognitive respon-
sivity in chronic as compared to acute schizophrenics in mental
hospitals, in prisoners as compared to nonprisoners, and in long-
term as compared to early term prisoners in penal institutions.
The explanation they offer—the "cognitive filtering hypothesis"—
holds that the narrowing of perceptual and cognitive categories
allows individuals to minimize their awareness of external or
internal threats so that they may selectively cope with disturbing

stimuli. Such a mechanism may tend to reduce the relationship of hostile affects to plasma 17-hydroxycorticosteroids as noted in our sample of chronic, institutionalized schizophrenics as compared to short-term hospitalized subjects.

Menstrual Cycle Phases and Hostility (and Anxiety) Scores

An investigation was made of the variations in magnitude of anxiety and hostility occurring during phases of the menstrual cycle (Gottschalk *et al.*, 1962). Five women gave five-minute samples of speech at approximately the same time of day for periods ranging from $1\frac{1}{2}$ to 3 months. The number of verbal samples given by each woman ranged from 30 to 60. Two of the women spoke into a tape recorder in the presence of a female research technician who elicited the verbal samples by reading standardized instructions. The other three women spoke about anything that came to their mind, that is "free associated," into the tape recorder without anyone else being present. Menstrual cycle phases were noted by keeping records of the onset and duration of menses and of body basal temperature before arising each morning. Four of the five women showed statistically significant rhythmical changes in the magnitude of at least one of the affects—hostility outward, hostility inward, or anxiety—during the sexual cycle. The changes in these affects were not similar among the women; these individual variations were considered related to individual differences in psychosexual development and conflicts. There was a significant tendency in this small group of women for the levels of "tension" measured—specifically, anxiety and the summation of hostility inward and ambivalent hostility—to decrease transiently around the time of ovulation, and this observation was presumed related to some undetermined hormonal change. A decrease in the level of anxiety around the time of ovulation, using the Gottschalk-Gleser content analysis method of measuring psychological states, has recently been confirmed by Ivey and Bardwick (1968).

Plasma Lipids and Hostility Scores

See pp. 126 ff., section on plasma lipids and anxiety scores, for complete details of these studies.

CHAPTER VII
Social Alienation–Personal Disorganization Scale—Validation Studies

Our content analysis scale of social alienation–personal disorganization, unlike most of our affect scales, aims to measure a psychological state which fluctuates relatively slowly and which is manifested to a considerable extent in observable behavioral variations. For these reasons, validation of the scale followed a somewhat different pattern than did that of the previously discussed scales. In particular, more reliance was placed on modifying content category weights on the basis of empirical findings.

The succession of studies which has led to our presently weighted scoring categories will be presented chronologically together with the intermediary scoring systems. The scale, at present, contains several categories for scoring content which are given a zero weight in the total score (see Chapter II, Schedule 2.5). We have kept these content items because we find that they help to delineate the boundaries of the categories, which might otherwise become fuzzy so that themata which are scored in these categories, when they are available, would tend to be placed into other closely related categories by a scorer if such categories were removed. In other words, it is often necessary for reliable content coding to specify what is being excluded in order to clarify what is being included in a content category.

LONGITUDINAL STUDIES: MEASURING INTRAINDIVIDUAL VARIATIONS OVER TIME IN DEGREE OF SOCIAL ALIENATION–PERSONAL DISORGANIZATION

The initial study of content analysis of the speech of schizophrenic patients (Gottschalk *et al.*, 1958a) had the following aims:

(*a*) To analyze the verbal productions of a group of schizophrenics over a period of time according to certain a priori cate-

186

gories (structural, emotive, and informative) which were believed to have relevance to the schizophrenic pattern of relating to the environment.

(*b*) To test whether the frequency of occurrence of themata in these categories was quantitatively related to the degree of personal disorganization, social alienation, and isolation of the patients.

(*c*) To modify the categories used for analyses and their weighting according to the empirical objective evidence of their value in distinguishing the degree of personal and social disorganization of schizophrenic patients and revalidate.

Procedure

Eight chronic male schizophrenic patients ranging in age from 27 to 41 were used as subjects, five for the experimental sample and three for cross validation. The subjects were picked from the psychiatric wards of the Veterans Administration Hospital, Cincinnati, Ohio. During the period they were observed for this study, the only medication they received was reserpine for short periods (up to four weeks) and occasional barbiturates. None of the patients received any other type of somatic therapy.

METHOD OF ELICITING VERBAL SAMPLES

The subjects were asked by their individual psychiatrists to speak at approximately weekly intervals for three minutes on any topic they chose. The specific instructions they were given, at the time their first verbal sample was obtained, were as follows:

> While you are here in the hospital, and getting treatment, there are certain examinations that I will be doing every week. I'd like to explain one of these. I would like you to pick up this "telephone" and talk into it for three minutes. It doesn't matter what you say; anything that comes into your mind. The important thing is to say everything that comes into your mind. I will tell you when three minutes are up. You probably wonder where this "phone" goes to. It goes to a dictating machine so that one of our secretaries can type up what you say. In this way we will have a weekly record which will be kept confidential in your hospital chart. Do you have any questions?

After all the patient's questions about the procedure were answered, the recording session was started. The patient spoke into a telephone in the presence of his psychiatrist and his speech was recorded on a tape recorder located elsewhere in the building. The psychiatrist was advised not to reply to any questions the patient might ask once the three-minute recording was started. The spoken material was transcribed by a secretary, and the typescripts of these three-minute samples of speech were analyzed according to schemata of categories that will be described later.

The eight patients were given the same instructions each time another verbal sample was sought except that explanatory information given the first time was omitted. The instructions repeated on recording sessions after the first one read essentially:

> I would like you to pick up this telephone and talk into it for three minutes. It doesn't matter what you say; anything that comes into your mind. The important thing is to say everything that comes into your mind. I will tell you when three minutes are up.

For varying reasons not relevant to this study, these patients remained in the hospital for different lengths of time, so that a different number of verbal samples was obtained from each patient.

THE CRITERIA FOR EVALUATING PSYCHOSOCIAL ALIENATION AND PERSONAL DISORGANIZATION

Two psychiatrists from the Veterans Administration Hospital, Cincinnati, Ohio, independently rated each patient on a ten-point scale along three continua: (1) interpersonal relations; (2) intrapsychic phenomena (mental status); and (3) personal habit patterns. The ratings were anchored by descriptions of behavior, but as can be seen from the rating scales (Table 7.1), we could not avoid having the psychiatrists make discriminations between such comparatives as rare, occasional, moderate, frequent, and so forth.

The psychiatrists who were using these rating scales were instructed to give a rating that most accurately typified the patient over a specified span of time. The time span covered a period of six days, including the three days preceding and the two days following the day on which the verbal sample was obtained. The psychiatrists had access to all data charted in the patient's daily record, including interview notes or other material by attending psychiatrists and other physicians, nurses' notes, and comments by

TABLE 7.1

Psychiatric Rating Scales Used to Assess Severity of Psychosocial Disorganization

Ratings	Behavioral patterns

A. Interpersonal relations

10   Out of contact with others, uncommunicative.

8   (*a*)   Belligerent, aggressive, physically destructive.
     (*b*)   Brief attempts to relate with others, but usually withdrawn, asocial.

6   (*a*)   Hostile, periodically aggressive, but not physically attacking others. Acting out of physical aggression controllable by verbal limit-setting of others.
     (*b*)   Avoidance of relationships with others, but some participation when others initiate relationship.

4   (*a*)   High frequency of aggressive relations with others, but some autonomous control against hurting others. Some "group" acceptance.
     (*b*)   Avoidance of relationships with others, but some self-initiated participation with others.

2   (*a*)   Some mastery of aggressive impulses towards others.
     (*b*)   Self-initiated participation with others associated with occasional withdrawal and avoidance.

0   Interpersonal relations congenial, constructive, and without notable tension and/or anxiety.

B. Intrapsychic phenomena (mental status)

10   (*a*)   Openly hallucinating and delusional. Almost constant projection.
     (*b*)   Severe depression interfering with all activities. Severe psychomotor retardation. Marked excitement. Constant motor activity.
     (*c*)   Thought processes fragmented. Obsessive doubt.
     (*d*)   Associations entirely irrelevant. Constant blocking.

8   (*a*)   Hallucinations and delusions occasionally and temporarily suppressed.
     (*b*)   Occasional brief periods of being less depressed or excited.
     (*c*)   Beginning organization of thought processes, although minor stress produces fragmentation. Much doubt persistently verbalized.
     (*d*)   Associations impoverished, but showing some relevance. Flight of ideas.

6   (*a*)   Occasional verbalization of hallucinatory or delusional material. Ideas of reference. Obsessions, phobias.
     (*b*)   Moderate depression, despondent. Moderate sustained euphoria.
     (*c*)   Thought processes organized, but loosely. Constant rationalization.
     (*d*)   Association organized, but circumstantial. Brief associations, but little spontaneity.

4   (*a*)   Rare evidence of hallucinations and delusions. Hypochondriasis.
     (*b*)   Mild constant depressive or euphoric mood. No vegetative signs.
     (*c*)   Very shallow thought processes.
     (*d*)   Circumstantiality less marked. Associations brief, with some spontaneity.

2   (*a*)   Frequent use of projection or introjection without major break in reality.
     (*b*)   Occasionally mildly depressed or euphoric, although mood generally appropriate.
     (*c*)   Thought processes somewhat shallow.
     (*d*)   Associations show only occasional circumstantiality or conciseness. Spontaneity frequent.

TABLE 7.1 (contd.)

Ratings	Behavioral patterns

0 (*a*) Rare use of projection or introjection.
  (*b*) Mood shows appropriate fluctuation without persistent tone.
  (*c*) Thought processes normally variable.
  (*d*) Associations spontaneous, relevant, and without circumstantiality or conciseness.

C. Personal habit patterns

10 (*a*) Incontinent of urine and faeces with smearing. Bizarre.
  (*b*) Refusal to eat or drink. Tube feeding a necessity. Omniphagic, rapid weight gain or loss.
  (*c*) Inability to sleep or awaken.
  (*d*) Sexually assaultive. Homosexually assaultive. Open masturbation.

8 (*a*) Incontinent of urine and faeces.
  (*b*) Refusal of food and drink with frequency, but tube feeding not required. Gluttinous. Moderate weight gain or loss.
  (*c*) Moderate insomnia. Somnolent. A large amount of time in sleep both day and night.
  (*d*) Enjoying homosexual activity. Actively soliciting sexually. Masturbating but generally under some concealment.

6 (*a*) Occasional incontinence. Slovenly. Able to take care of personal appearance only with direct supervision. Meticulous.
  (*b*) Refuses to eat with infrequency. Usually anorectic. Constant over-eating. Slow weight gain or loss.
  (*c*) Sleeping with difficulty. Lethargic. Daytime sleeping interferes to a degree with necessary ward activities.
  (*d*) Rare overt homosexual act. Passive participation. Frequent suggestive remarks to opposite sex.

4 (*a*) No incontinence. Interest in own personal appearance, but generally unkempt. Meticulous at times.
  (*b*) Anorectic but eats each meal. Some over-eating.
  (*c*) Persistent but mild sleep disturbance.
  (*d*) Moderate anxiety in sexually provoking situation.

2 (*a*) Spontaneous interest in own appearance. Some exaggeration of neatness and orderliness.
  (*b*) Mild anorexia or increased appetite not present consistently.
  (*c*) Occasional mild sleep disturbance. Restlessness.
  (*d*) Impulses generally under control, but mild discomfort in stressful sexual situation.

0 (*a*) Personal appearance appropriate.
  (*b*) Appetite normal. Weight constant.
  (*c*) Sleep pattern normal.
  (*d*) Able to participate in activities with both sexes without overt conflict.

social workers and occupational and recreational therapists. Sometimes, when the patients happened to be in their care, the raters had additional, unrecorded information about them.

It is worthwhile mentioning at this point—because it tends to happen in spite of the most careful efforts to avoid the problem—the occurrence of a subtle but important discrepancy in the rating orientation of the two psychiatric judges, discovered only after the results of our first experiment were being discussed and plans for the cross-validation study were being made. One psychiatrist consistently tended to arrive at a rating by determining the average or typical behavior of the patient; the other psychiatrist tended to give a rating in line with the worst descriptive feature of the patient over the six-day time span. We decided that for the cross validation, the two psychiatrists should base their final judgments on the worst feature occurring over the six-day time span, not only to improve consensus of the judges, but also to give more weight to maladjustment and psychopathologic factors, for this was the principal focus in selecting categories of relevance in the analysis of speech patterns.

The subtle difference in the approach of the two psychiatrists to the task of rating the patients will be shown later not to have had much discernible effect on the reliability of quantifying relative degree of emotional sickness within a patient, that is, intraindividual differences. It is possible, however, that this difference in approach by the raters was one of the factors resulting in a low correlation between them in rating relative degrees of sickness among patients, that is, interindividual differences.

The ratings by the two psychiatrists on each criterion scale were tabulated separately. After reliability coefficients were computed, the ratings of the two psychiatrists were combined, and these were arranged, for each patient, in the order from the lowest score (least sick) to the highest score (sickest). These rank orders were then compared to the rank orders obtained by the analysis of the three-minute verbal samples.

VERBAL SCALE OF SOCIAL ALIENATION—PERSONAL DISORGANIZATION

The scale of social alienation—personal disorganization used in scoring the verbal samples has been described previously (see Chapter II). In this first study, our category weightings were slightly different than those we are presently using (see note, p. 44).

Each category was assigned a weighting, plus or minus one, or plus or minus a half. A minus weighting was assigned to the category when the item was considered to indicate personal malfunctioning and/or social alienation. A plus weighting was assigned to an item when it was thought to imply personal and/or social integration and well-being. Categories signifying evidence of the schizophrenic syndrome are now, in our present scale (see Schedule 2.5, p. 42), given positive weights.

Results: Part 1

The scores on each verbal sample were tabulated and counted; the total minus scores were subtracted from the plus scores, and a raw score obtained. To make allowance for differences in word output per three-minute verbal sample, the raw scores for each sample were divided by the total number of words spoken in the sample and multiplied by 100 to give a corrected score for each verbal sample.

In Part 1, the verbal samples were all scored by one of the investigators and no check of the reliability of scoring was made. In cross validating, however, a check was made of the reliability of the revised system of scoring. A total of 41 different verbal samples produced by three of the patients was coded independently by two different individuals, and a Pearson product-moment correlation was obtained between the two sets of scores. The correlation coefficients for the individual patient were .77, .82, and .89, with an overall correlation of .87.

The ratings of the two psychiatrists were correlated to determine the reliability of this method. The product-moment correlations between raters for each subject and for each of the three scales used, as well as for the ratings obtained when the three scales were combined with equal weighting, are shown in Table 7.2.[1] It can be seen that there was respectable correlation between the scoring of the two raters for the first three subjects and for the fifth subject (although the total number of time periods he was assessed amounted to only five), but the coefficient was lowest with subject 4. Examination of the standard deviation of ratings on subject 4 reveals, as compared to those on other subjects, that this patient varied little in his degree of disorganization over 15 periods of observation; he fluctuated within a narrow range. Such a restriction of range in general has the effect of attenuating the correlation

---

[1] The ratings of each psychiatrist on each criterion scale was transposed to a mean of 5 and a standard deviation of 2 on the total sample before combining them into a composite score in order to give equal weighting to each criterion factor. This also resulted in giving equal weight to each psychiatrist's ratings when these were combined to be used as the criterion for the experimental assessment procedure.

TABLE 7.2

Pearson Product Movement Correlations between Ratings of Two Psychiatrists Made at Various Times on Each of Five Individuals

Patient	Number of samples	Correlations between psychiatrists on criterion scales				Composite scale mean		Standard deviation	
		Mental status	Inter-personal relations	Personal habits	Composite ratings	Psychiatrist		Psychiatrist	
						#1	#2	#1	#2
1	21	.95	.38	.09	.66	8.47	11.57	3.51	3.44
2	20	.42	.65	.24*	.71	9.60	16.88	3.88	3.92
3	15	.88	.89	.68	.94	12.59	13.53	4.09	4.96
4	15	.27	.17	.37	.54	9.91	8.93	1.06	1.57
5	5	.75	indeterminate	.50	.66	15.58	14.00	3.21	1.10
Total	76	.43	.42	.48	.59	......	......	......	......

* Based on only 13 ratings.

between two variables and probably explains the low correlations obtained for this subject.

The raters showed fairly good agreement on judgments made within individuals, but they showed practically no agreement as to the relative degree of personal and social disorganization of different individuals, with the exception of ratings on "personal habits." Thus, for the composite rating, the average correlation within individuals was .80, while between individuals, it was only .22. This lack of correlation over individuals tended to lower the reproducibility of ratings over all samples and made it unlikely that we would be able to predict, by means of the verbal analysis data, the interindividual differences as adjudged by the set of criteria.

The principal criterion to be used for the verbal analysis was the combined composite ratings for each individual. The reliability of the combined ratings was found to range from .80 to .97. The reliabilities (within individuals) were all sufficiently high to warrant their use in validating the scores on the experimental verbal material.

Table 7.3 presents the rank-order correlations obtained for each subject by use of the two methods of assessment. Those correlations marked with an asterisk reach a convincing level of statistical significance. The correlations between the two different methods as applied to subject 5 appear to be high, but because only five periods were assessed with this subject, only the correla-

TABLE 7.3

Spearman Rank-Order Correlations of Combined Psychiatric Ratings (for Each of Five Individuals) with Original and Revised Verbal Analysis Scores

		Rank order correlations with criterion scales							
	Number of samples	Mental status		Inter-personal relations		Personal habits		Composite scale	
Patient		orig.	rev.	orig.	rev.	orig.	rev.	orig.	rev.
1	21	.85‡	.86	.29	.36	.41*	.51	.62†	.71
2	18	.80‡	.87	.76‡	.77	.66†	.84	.81‡	.88
3	15	.71†	.80	.64†	.75	.67†	.75	.70†	.77
4	15	.35	.33	.30	.54	.30	.56	.35	.67
5	5	.98*	.88	.45	.65	.66	.77	.80	.90

* Significant at .05 level (one-tailed hypothesis).
† Significant at .01 level (one-tailed hypothesis).
‡ Significant at .001 level (one-tailed hypothesis).

tion with mental status is high enough to satisfy a 5 percent level of confidence. The correlations are high enough, however, to encourage belief that in this subject, as well as the first three subjects, the method of analysis of speech patterns to assess severity of schizophrenic illness is valid. None of the correlations for subject 4 reach a satisfying level of statistical significance, but this is not surprising; as previously discussed, the spread of criterion ratings and their reliability for this subject were low.

The overall results gave strong support to the theory that counting the frequency of occurrence of certain typical features in the verbal communications of a schizophrenic person provides a quantitative estimate of the relative severity of his disorder from one time to another. The experimental method of assessing severity of schizophrenic disorder from time to time within an individual correlated well with the standard method of evaluation. The results, however, though very encouraging from the viewpoint of the experimental method's giving valid results in distinguishing changes within a patient, did not appear to give very satisfactory results toward comparing the severity of disorder between different schizophrenic patients.

We next sought to improve the validity of our experimental method by doing an item analysis. The verbal samples were divided into three groups according to the degree of disorganization and alienation noted by the rating psychiatrists. A careful check was then made to determine which items in the verbal samples tended to differentiate these three groups. Items which were found not to have any notable bearing on relative extent of personality disorganization were eliminated. Also, it was found possible to combine several categories, because they were of about equal validity and required no differential weighting. Finally, we found that, in several instances, our a priori weights applied to each category were not accurate. In most instances, we merely had to change a score from a number (-1) indicating features highly characteristic of schizophrenic disorder to less characteristic features ($-\frac{1}{2}$) or vice versa. In rare instances, we had to reverse our weighting completely, that is from a negative score (indicative of sick behavior) to a positive score (indicative of well behavior). An example of such a reversal was the category of references to weather, as bad, unpleasant, dangerous. Our tentative assumption had been that such references by a schizophrenic reflected his inner turmoil and despair of satisfying object relations (and that this should be weighted on the sick side) and that references to good, pleasant weather reflected a more satisfying relationship with external reality (and thus should be weighted on the well side). In our sample of subjects under the experimental conditions, we found that any references by the patient to bad weather, as well as references to good weather, were probably more indicative of sociableness and readiness to follow cultural convention than of withdrawal and despair. Frequent repetitions about poor weather within a three-minute time span of talk still appeared to represent foreboding preoccupation with poor interpersonal relationships. So, until we obtained more evidence to lead us to another opinion, we decided to score the first two references per three-minute verbal sample as healthy and any references thereafter as unhealthy.

The revised system of coding and tallying peculiar and healthy aspects of the speech patterns of schizophrenic patients is given in detail in Schedule 2.5, original scoring (pp. 42 ff.).

The verbal samples were recoded in terms of this revision. The new scores obtained were then compared to the combined ratings of the two psychiatrists. Table 7.3 shows that with these revisions better rank-order correlations between the standard method of assessment (criterion) and the experimental (revised) method were obtained for all subjects. The rank-order correlation over individuals did not differ significantly from zero.

That the separate groups of categories of the verbal behavior method of assessment (after revision) were all contributing to the correlation with the composite psychiatric ratings is indicated in Table 7.4. Each group of categories is high for at least one of the

TABLE 7.4

Rank-Order Correlations of Major Categories of Verbal Analysis with Composite Psychiatric Ratings after Rescoring

	Major categories of verbal analysis after revision				
Patient	Inter-personal	Orienta-tion	Self	References to food, sleep, weather	Blocking, repetition, bizarre remarks
1	.23	.60	.67	.37	.38
2	.64	−.08	.42	.65	.56
3	.20	.10	.74	did not occur	.42
4	−.21	.21	.42	.11	.62
5	.88	.80	.70	.72	.80

five patients. No group of categories, however, yielded the highest correlation consistently for all individuals. Thus, while it appears that the categories we were using are appropriate in differentiating schizophrenic speech, a particular individual tends to show only some of these manifestations to any great extent.

Results: Part 2—Cross-Validation

Three new patients served as subjects for the cross-validation study. The same two psychiatrists assessed the severity of the patient's disorder as described in Part 1 (Table 7.1). This time, however, the different bias of the raters in evaluating the first five patients was corrected, and each rater made his judgments on the same basis; that is, they now tended to give a score on each scale that was in line with the sickest manifestations occurring during the six-day period of observation instead of trying to arrive at an approximate average.

The three-minute verbal samples of each subject were assessed this time according to the revised schemata. Table 7.5 indicates that the overall correlation between the ratings of patients 6, 7, and 8 by the two psychiatrists was .93 and that the highest concordance between the two psychiatrists was reached on the rating scales of mental status (.94) and interpersonal relations (.91).

Table 7.6 shows that significant correlations were obtained between the verbal analysis scores (revised system) on patients 6, 7, and 8 and the criterion ratings. The highest correlation (.80) occurred with patient 8. A glance at Table 7.5 shows that the mean ratings by the psychiatrists on this patient were the highest, that is, this patient was the sickest, and the variability of this particular patient was far greater than either of the other two patients. With the first five patients, we also found that the experimental method of assessment was more highly correlated with the criterion when a patient showed a relatively wide range of variability from time to time in the characteristics being measured.

A further investigation was made to determine to what extent our positively and negatively weighted items in the verbal samples separately accounted for the significant correlations obtained. For each patient in this experiment, it was found that both types of items correlated with the composite-criterion ratings, the negative scores showing the higher correlations. In every case, however, the sum of the positive and negative scores yielded a higher correla-

TABLE 7.5

Product-Moment Correlations between Ratings of Patients (6, 7, and 8) by Two Psychiatrists

Patient	Number of samples	Correlations between psychiatrists on criterion scales				Composite scale mean		Standard deviation	
		Mental status	Inter-personal relations	Personal habits	Composite scale	Psychiatrist		Psychiatrist	
						#1	#2	#1	#2
6	11	.77	.42	.11	.58	6.45	6.77	.92	1.56
7	15	.88	.45	.32	.73	5.66	5.37	1.48	1.02
8	14	.96	.96	.35	.98	7.72	8.36	4.01	4.64
Total	40	.94	.91	.33	.93	......	......	......	......

TABLE 7.6

Correlations of Verbal Analysis Scores (Revised System)
with Combined Clinical Psychiatric Ratings

Patient	Number of samples	Rank-order correlations with criterion scales			
		Mental status	Inter-personal relations	Personal habits	Total
6	11	.61*	.64*	.25	.58*
7	15	.25	.62†	—.04	.44*
8	14	.40	.81‡	.73†	.80‡

* Significant at .05 level (one-tailed hypothesis).
† Significant at .01 level (one-tailed hypothesis).
‡ Significant at .001 level (one-tailed hypothesis).

tion than either type of score alone. These findings support the assumption that positive and negative indicators may be added to give a more accurate estimate of the level of functioning of an individual.

Discussion and Conclusion

In terms of the criterion used, it was concluded that the counting and scoring of certain speech patterns of the schizophrenic patient constituted a valid method of providing a quantitative estimate of intraindividual variations in the degree of schizophrenic disturbance. But our verbal analysis method did not provide satisfactory information about interindividual differences in degree of schizophrenic disturbance for the eight patients we had examined. Our principal explanation for this finding was that our total sample was too small to give us adequate information on interindividual differences. We believed it likely that item weightings could be found which would enable such differentiation to be made, but with only five individuals available for item analysis, it was not possible to determine adequate weighting of items for this purpose. A study of single verbal samples obtained from a large group of schizophrenic patients, in which we compared scores on these samples to the same composite criterion we have used in our longitudinal experiments just reported, we felt, would give us a better idea of the item weightings necessary to obtain differentiations among individuals. We next undertook this type of investigation.

CROSS-SECTIONAL STUDIES: MEASURING INTERINDIVIDUAL
DIFFERENCES IN DEGREE OF SOCIAL ALIENATION–
PERSONAL DISORGANIZATION

This investigation was specifically designed to determine
whether our verbal behavior index of relative severity of the
schizophrenic syndrome, with or without modifications in the
weighting of the various verbal categories, might be valid in assessing differences, cross-sectionally, among schizophrenic patients in
the relative severity of disorganization and alienation (Gottschalk
et al., 1961*a*). That is, we wanted to find out whether our method
of measurement was capable of discriminating interindividual differences as well as intraindividual variations.

Procedure

We first undertook a pilot study, using 14 schizophrenic patients (seven males and seven females) from the psychiatric wards
of the Cincinnati General Hospital. Five-minute verbal samples
were elicited by employing our standardized instructions (see
Chapter II). The verbal samples were recorded on a tape recorder
(in full view of the patient) and transcribed by a secretary. Another investigator independently rated the severity of the schizophrenic illness, as adjudged from clinical observations of the
patient on the day the patient gave the experimental verbal sample;
these evaluations were made in terms of the same three scales used
in the longitudinal study—pp. 189 f. (Gottschalk *et al.*, 1958a). The
14 verbal samples were scored (by the investigator who originally
elicited the speech) according to the verbal behavior analysis
schedule and weightings arrived at from the previous investigation
(see Chapter II, Schedule 2.5, "original weights"). The rank-order
correlation of the verbal behavior measure and the clinical criterion
measure was .55, significant beyond the .05 level (one-tail test).
This encouraging concordance led us to undertake a more extensive
and definitive investigation.

A five-minute verbal sample elicited in the standard manner
was obtained from each of 152 patients, 28 males and 124 females,
from Longview State Hospital. Clinical ratings were again made on
the three ten-point scales (interpersonal, intrapsychic, personal
habits) described in the longitudinal study above (Table 7.1), and
the sum of these ratings constituted the criterion measure in the
present study. The ratings were written down just before the verbal

sample was obtained, the judgments being based on direct clinical observations and notes from nurses and attendants over a two- to three-day time span preceding the giving the verbal sample. Once the ratings were written down, they were not changed, regardless of what the patient did when he was presented with the instructions to speak. The verbal samples were, again, recorded on a tape recorder in full view and transcribed. The typed speech samples were scored by one investigator and checked by another according to the schizophrenic disorganization and social alienation scales of the previous study (Gottschalk *et al.*, 1958*a*; see Chapter II, Schedule 2.5). Three new thematic items were also coded because they were considered to have possible relevance to the schizophrenic syndrome, but tentative weights were not initially assigned to them, nor were they included in the total score.

Our total sample of schizophrenic patients was randomly split into two groups of equal size for purposes of cross-validation.

Since shorter verbal samples supply less information and consequently are less reliable representatives of an individual than longer ones, we decided that only samples of 45 words or more would be included in the validation study. Those persons speaking fewer than 45 words were classified as "reticent." There were 39 such individuals, and these patients were split between the two subgroups.

All the relevant vital statistics of each patient, such as age, sex, type of schizophrenia, duration of illness, the criterion measure of severity of schizophrenic syndrome, and breakdowns of the percentage frequency of occurrence of each category of thematic reference, were entered on IBM cards for processing. Means, standard deviation, and Pearson product-moment correlations among the verbal categories and criterion ratings were obtained separately for each subsample by means of the IBM 650 digital computer.

Results

In Table 7.7 are provided some background data on the total group with regard to race, sex, age, education, and diagnostic categories. It may be noted that the majority of the schizophrenic patients were white females, and as a group these were significantly older than any of the other subgroups classified by race and sex. No significant differences were found in average education or

TABLE 7.7

Background Data for the Total Sample of Schizophrenic Patients

Subgroup	N	Diagnosis						Age (in years)		Education (in years)		Rating		Correlations	
		Undiff. schiz.	Simple schiz.	Catatonic schiz.	Hebephrenic schiz.	Paranoid schiz.	Schizo-affective	Mean	s.d.	Mean	s.d.	Mean	s.d.	Educ. by rating	Age by rating
White females	101	39	7	3	10	39	3	48.3	13.4	9.1	2.7	15.7	8.5	−.06	.18
Negro females	23	4	1	1	2	13	2	40.5	9.6	7.9	3.2	15.5	9.8	−.28	.45*
White males	22	11	1	1	4	5	0	38.4	11.2	8.9	2.9	13.0	7.7	−.32	.26
Negro males	6	3	0	1	0	2	0	36.3	9.9	8.3	3.0	17.3	6.7	−.12	.41
Total	152	57	9	6	16	59	5	42.2	13.2	8.8	2.9	15.3	8.5	−.14	.23*

* Significant at .05 level.

psychiatric rating (i.e., severity of schizophrenic syndrome) for subgroups classified by race and sex. Age and severity of the schizophrenic syndrome were found to be correlated to a small but significant degree, probably reflecting the fact that among our patients there was a nucleus of older patients who had remained ill for a long period of time or even regressed despite all attempts at treatment (the great majority of patients were on some type of psychoactive medication).

The composition of the two subsamples is shown in Table 7.8. The two samples did not differ significantly with regard to distribution of race, sex, age, education, or psychiatric rating. They did differ somewhat, however, in distribution of diagnostic categories, with a significantly greater proportion of undifferentiated schizophrenics in Subgroup I and a greater proportion of paranoid schizophrenics in Subgroup II.

Using only those verbal samples containing 45 words or more, the complete matrix of intercorrelations among the three criterion scales and the percentage frequency scores derived in each speech category were obtained for each subgroup separately. A portion of these results is shown in Table 7.9. For both groups, the total verbal behavior score predicted each of the criterion rating scales and the combined criterion rating at or beyond the .001 level of significance. The correlation with the total criterion rating was .53 in Subgroup I and .60 in Subgroup II. It thus appeared well established that our verbal behavior scale could validly discriminate differences in severity of illness between individuals as well as within an individual.

A detailed scrutiny of Table 7.9 reveals that certain categories were much more highly and consistently related to the criterion measure than others. In particular, mumbled and inaudible phrases (IIIA1), illogical or bizarre remarks (IIIA3) and repetitions of phrases or clauses (IIIB2) were consistently positively correlated with the criterion ratings, while the category for references to people helping, being friendly to others or self, and self being friendly to others (IC1, 2, 3) was very significantly negatively correlated with ratings in both samples. On the other hand, such categories as references to food as pleasant or unpleasant (IID1 and IID2), references to weather (IIE1 and IIE2), to sleep (IIF1, IIF2) abrupt shifts of thought (IIIA2), and repetition of single words (IIIB1) were not found contributory to the

TABLE 7.8

Composition of Each Subgroup of Schizophrenic Patients

Subgroups	N	Undiff.	Simple	Cata-tonic	Hebe-phrenic	Para-noid	Schizo-affec-tive	Age Mean	Age s.d.	Education Mean	Education s.d.	Rating Mean	Rating s.d.
Subgroup I													
White females	50	24	5	2	4	14	1	49.4	14.1	9.2	3.2	15.9	8.8
Negro females	13	2	1	1	2	5	2	39.6	7.0	8.8	3.6	16.8	9.0
White males	8	6	0	0	1	1	0	43.1	10.2	8.6	3.6	12.4	6.4
Negro males	5	3	0	1	0	1	0	34.0	9.2	9.2	2.8	18.8	6.4
Total	76	35	6	4	7	21	3	46.1	13.4	9.0	3.3	15.8	8.6
Reticent	20	11	2	4	1	2	0	49.2	15.0	8.2	3.0	21.0	7.8
Nonreticent	56	24	4	0	6	19	3	45.0	12.7	9.4	3.3	14.0	8.1
Subgroup II													
White females	51	15	2	1	6	25	2	47.2	12.6	9.0	2.2	15.5	7.9
Negro females	10	2	0	0	0	8	0	41.6	12.0	6.9	2.4	13.8	10.5
White males	14	5	1	1	3	4	0	35.6	10.8	9.0	2.3	13.4	8.3
Negro males	1	0	0	0	0	1	0	48.0	.0	4.0	.0	10.0	.0
Total	76	22	3	2	9	38	2	44.2	12.9	8.6	2.4	15.0	8.4
Reticent	19	4	1	0	6	8	0	46.3	10.1	7.9	2.7	22.0	6.7
Nonreticent	57	18	2	2	3	30	2	43.6	13.6	8.9	2.3	12.4	7.7

predictions in either sample. (References to weather and to sleep occurred so infrequently in this cross-sectional study that they were not included in the correlational analysis.)

It was, therefore, decided to attempt to refine the weighting of categories in the verbal scale by making weights more nearly proportional to the independent contribution of each category to overall prediction. This involved taking into account the standard deviation of category scores and their intercorrelations as well as their validities. Those items which made no contribution to prediction in either sample were given zero weight, as were two items regarding orientation and attempts at orientation (IIA2, IIA3), which, although apparently possessing some validity, were found difficult to score unless other data were available by which to judge the correctness of the statements made. Weights were assigned to two of the three new categories: questions directed to the interviewer (IVA); and religious and biblical references (V). In general, new weights were chosen to increase the correlation with the combined criterion rating in Subgroup I, but certain restrictions were imposed in assigning these weights with the hope of also increasing the stability of the correlation from one subgroup to another, rather than seeking to maximize the correlation in any one subgroup. The new weights developed from patients in Subgroup I were cross-validated on Subgroup II. The final language category weights (with slight revisions based on subsequent comparative studies reported below) are shown in Schedule 2.5 as "modified weightings."

The verbal behavior scores resulting when the "modified" weights were used correlated .58 in Subgroup I and .68 in Subgroup II with the total criterion measure, yielding an overall correlation for the total group of schizophrenic patients of .63. A more detailed analysis of the correlations is given in Table 7.10. All correlations in both subgroups were increased slightly by the revision, and for the total group of schizophrenic patients, each of the rating scales was predicted with about equal efficiency.[2]

---

[2] The equation for predicting our total clinical rating from the verbal scores is $R = .7V + 9.7$, where R = total clinical rating and V = verbal behavior score. It should be noted that the modified weightings are arranged so that plus weightings signify the more severe schizophrenic syndrome, in contrast to the original weightings, in which pluses signify the more healthy responses. The distribution of scores obtained with the modified weights is somewhat skewed to the right and possibly could profit by a mathematical transformation to obtain a more symmetrical distribution.

TABLE 7.9

Correlations among the Three Criterion Measures and between Them and the Speech Categories for Subgroups I and II

Criterion measures	Interpersonal relations		Intrapsychic phenomena		Personal habit patterns		Total rating		Mean		Standard deviation	
	I	II	I	II	I	II	I	II	I	II	I	II
Interpersonal relations	.....	.....	.79	.65	.66	.51	.92	.84	5.70	4.88	2.86	2.87
Intrapsychic phenomena	.79	.65	.....	.....	.59	.67	.92	.92	5.43	5.00	3.75	3.53
Personal habit patterns	.66	.51	.59	.67	.....	.....	.81	.82	2.88	2.56	2.48	2.53
Total ratings	.92	.84	.92	.92	.81	.82	.....	.....	14.00	12.44	8.11	7.72
Speech categories												
IA	.09	.00	.11	−.03§	−.15§	−.19§	.04	−.08§	.32	.27	.70	.44
IB	.04	.08	.08	.04	.16	−.04§	.10	.04	.50	.36	1.00	.78
IC1,2,3	−.30†	−.45‡	−.29*	−.35†	−.39†	−.27*	−.36†	−.41†	1.00	1.20	.86	1.10
ID1	.14	.01	.11	−.14§	.19	−.12§	.16	−.08§	.64	.86	.81	1.42
ID2	−.03	−.31*	.01	−.42†	.05§	−.34†	.01	−.42†	.28	.41	.61	.53
IIA1	.11	.19	.27*	.24†	.20	.15	.22*	.23*	.09	.06	.37	.34
IIA2	−.16	−.14	−.04	.07§	.31*	−.14	−.17	−.07	.08	.06	.20	.15
IIA3	.28*	.15	.25*	.15	.22	.11	.28*	.16	.31	.16	.48	.37

IIB1	.02	.13	.07	.08	.13	.02	.08	.09	1.44	1.48	1.74	1.49
IIB2	−.11	−.07	−.16	−.05	−.28*	−.18	−.20	−.11	.16	.08	.26	.19
IIB3	−.23*	−.20	−.20	−.13	−.04	−.12	−.19	−.17	.70	.85	1.06	1.05
IIB4	.07	.37†	−.01	.31*	.02	.38†	.03	.40†	1.52	1.54	1.92	2.45
IIB5	−.07§	.19	.03	.35†	−.14§	.19	−.05§	.29*	.47	.41	.56	.79
IIC	.03	−.01	.20	.00	.19	−.04**	.16	−.01	.13	.08	.22	.17
IID1	.00	−.15§	−.06§	−.18§	.03	−.20§	−.02§	−.20§	.07	.02	.28	.09
IID2	.08§	−.03	−.04	.07§	.09§	.21§	.04§	.09§	.20	.07	.73	.24
IIIA1	.29*	.33†	.33†	.51‡	.36†	.35†	.36†	.47‡	1.17	.98	2.14	2.10
IIIA2	.04	−.09§	.03	.17	.08	.03	.05	.05	.55	.26	.57	.35
IIIA3	.30*	.25	.40†	.42†	.32†	.38†	.39†	.41†	.82	.31	1.06	.61
IIIB1	−.06§	−.01	−.14§	.18	.14	−.08§	−.04§	.06	1.27	.81	1.40	.94
IIIB2	.15	.31*	−.03§	.38†	.33†	.46‡	.14	.44‡	1.71	1.77	1.80	1.82
IVA	.08	.30*	.05	.45‡	.26*	.34†	.13	.43‡	.66	.63	1.44	1.00
IVB	−.08§	.08	−.10§	.31*	−.01	.16	−.08§	.23*	.61	.60	.89	.95
V	.06	.02	.08	.25*	−.15§	.06	.01	.14	.29	.19	.90	.69
Total	.45‡	.53‡	.43‡	.58‡	.59‡	.44‡	.53‡	.60‡	7.19	6.44	4.76	6.05

* Significant at .05 level.
† Significant at .01 level.
‡ Significant at .001 level.
§ Reversal from direction of expected correlation.

TABLE 7.10

Correlations of the Revised Verbal Behavior Index Criterion Scales
(Using the "Modified Weightings" Given in Schedule 2.5, p. 42)

Criterion scales	Subgroup I	Subgroup II	Total
Interpersonal	.48	.56	.53
Mental status	.45	.64	9.54
Personal habits	.60	.54	.57
Total	.58	.68	.63
Verbal behavior index			
Mean	5.96	4.06	5.00
s.d.	6.21	7.20	6.79

Reticent Patients

As noted previously, 39 of the 152 subjects spoke less than 45 words in the five-minute period and consequently were not used in the analysis of verbal productions. Sixteen of these were completely mute, and the others spoke from five to 44 words. An examination of the diagnoses of this group revealed a greater proportion of simple, catatonic, and hebephrenic patients and a smaller proportion of paranoid schizophrenic patients than in the non-reticent group. When we divided the total group into those who spoke less than 100 words (58 persons) and those who spoke 100 or more words (94 persons), the trend for paranoid schizophrenic patients to speak more words under our experimental conditions than other schizophrenic types still persisted and was significant beyond the .01 level.

The reticent group as a whole was rated as much sicker by the psychiatrist. They had an average rating on our clinical rating scale of 21.5 as compared to 13.2 for the nonreticent group, a difference significant beyond the .001 level. For the 16 who did not speak at all, the average rating was 25.4 (highest possible rating 30); whereas, for the remaining 23, the average was 18.8. It seems reasonable to conclude, therefore, that a schizophrenic who speaks less than 45 words under the circumstances of this verbal test, and particularly one who is completely mute, is extremely deviant in a pathological direction with respect to our clinical ratings of severity of the schizophrenic syndrome.

An examination of the productions of those who were reticent but not mute, however, revealed one exception to this conclusion. There were four patients in Subgroup I and two in Subgroup II who simply made a statement to the effect that they had nothing to talk about and then said no more for the entire period. From the psychiatrist's ratings, it would appear that such patients are not necessarily very sick; in fact, their average rating was 9.0, the ratings ranging from 2 to 22. The statement made by the one rated as 2 was, "I don't know anything to talk about." That made by the one rated 22 was, "Yeah, but I don't know anything I could say."

We have extrapolated the regression equation for predicting the verbal score on social alienation–personal disorganization from clinical ratings to obtain an estimated score for those individuals who are either mute or reticent in response to the standardized instructions. The formula is as follows:

$$V = .54R - 2.13$$

Using 25.4(R) as the average clinical rating for mute patients, the estimated verbal score is 11.6(V). For patients not mute but who spoke less than 45 words, the clinical rating is 18.8 and the estimated score is 8.0.

Discussion

This study provided evidence that the severity of the schizophrenic illness can be quantitatively assessed at any one time in different schizophrenic patients by a weighted scoring of certain speech categories in five-minute samples of speech elicited with standardized instructions. The study also indicated that in those instances where the schizophrenic patient responded with silence or relatively few words under the conditions of the verbal test used here, an approximate score of severity could be arrived at which was highly predictive of his total behavior. Only when the patient made the statement that he had nothing to talk about and then said nothing more was it uncertain whether the patient was very sick or relatively well. Only six of our total group of 152 patients fell into this classification, and this did not provide a large enough number of persons to examine for a more definitive interpretation.

Other investigators have examined the problem of lack of responsiveness or cooperation of some schizophrenic patients to diagnostic testing procedures and have raised the pertinent question whether these uncooperative patients are a population that are qualitatively different from the testable population of schizophrenics. It is not surprising that clinical psychologists have found varying percentages of untestability among schizophrenics, depending on the testing conditions and tasks. Zubin *et al.* (1953), for example, noted that 25 percent of the chronic schizophrenics used in the Columbia-Greystone project were untestable on more than one-third of a test battery including cognitive (I.Q.), perceptual, and motor tasks. Mednick and Lindsley (1958), studying a very chronic sample of patients (median length of hospitalization: 16 years), reported that 55 percent were untestable on a test battery consisting of the Wechsler-Bellevue and the Rorschach. Wilensky and Solomon (1960) reported 27 percent of a group of 101 chronic male schizophrenics (median length of hospitalization: 10 years) were untestable when a Rorschach and an abbreviated Wechsler-Bellevue were administered. The latter investigators also noted that the untestable group had the poorest mental health ratings, particularly those who were "confused," that is, who seemed willing but unable to produce scorable records, as compared to those who "refused," that is, who appeared able but unwilling to perform.

Although 26 percent (39 of our 152 patients) spoke less than 45 words in the five-minute period (and we did not score these specific verbal samples because we had set this level of production as an arbitrary cut-off point) we would not label this group of 39 patients as "untestable." The primary purpose of administering the verbal behavior test that we have been describing herein was to assess the relative severity of the schizophrenic symptom-complex, and we have been able to demonstrate that a validated index of severity was actually provided by a patient's speaking less than 45 words or not speaking at all. As far as we now know, poor predictive capacity regarding clinical psychotic behavior of our schizophrenic verbal measure, and hence in a sense "untestability," occurred only in 4 percent of the population we have specifically described above, who said that they have nothing to talk about and then said no more.

We have provided, in Schedule 2.5, two sets of weights—the "original" weights of the longitudinal study and the "modified" weights presently used. We had some tentative suggestions as to which set of weights might be best to use for different types of clinical psychiatric research problems. The "modified" weights were thought to be superior in cross-sectional studies where information was desired as to the relative severity of the schizophrenic syndrome on the day of testing as adjudged from a single five-minute verbal sample. If a more general index of the severity of illness were required, which ignored daily fluctuations, our experience with other indices of behavior derived from verbal samples led us to believe that a mean or median score should be obtained from several verbal samples. We have noted, however, that when patients are requested to talk at daily or even weekly intervals in response to the instructions used in deriving this measure of severity of symptom complex, they tended to use more content categories (for example, references to weather, sleep, food, etc.) in subsequent verbalizations than they did when given the instructions for the first time. In this language behavior, they resembled the communication activity of the patients used in our longitudinal study on whom the "original" weights were developed. It was considered possible, therefore, that the original (nonzero) weightings for these items would result in more accurate discrimination whenever repetitive measures of severity were to be made.

We checked back and tried recalculating the schizophrenic severity indices on the last three patients of our longitudinal study using the "modified" weights arrived at from the present cross-sectional study. For the three patients, the revised scores were as highly correlated with the criterion measure as were the scores based on the original weights (see Table 7.11). Thus, it was tentatively decided that the "modified" weights were applicable not only to cross-sectional studies, but also to longitudinal ones. If so, they would have the advantage of greater simplicity, since fewer items needed to be scored. However, further studies were needed using the present instructions for eliciting verbal productions, before definite conclusions could be drawn.

An additional question in which we were interested was whether this verbal behavior scoring system of schizophrenic speech might be, in fact, dealing with speech habits and symbolic activities not unique to the person with a schizophrenic syndrome but to varying extents ubiquitous in mankind. That is, the aspects of language behavior on which we were concentrating our attention in these studies of schizophrenic speech patterns were not all pathognomonic for the schizophrenic syndrome. We were quite aware that other mentally and physically ill people (and also functioning and healthy, communicative people) tend to withdraw

TABLE 7.11

Comparisons of Correlations Obtained by Using Original Weights‡ (On Last Three
Patients Followed Longitudinally) with Correlations Obtained by Using Modified
Weights Derived from Present Cross-Sectional Study

| | | Rank-order correlations with criterion scales | |
Patient	Number of samples	Using original item weighting	Using modified item weighting
6	11	.58*	.65*
7	15	.44*	.48*
8	14	.80†	.88†

* Significant at .05 level (one-tailed test).
† Significant at .001 level (one-tailed test).
‡ For weights, see Schedule 2.5, p. 42.

and become disorganized to various degrees at times. It was apparent that people who were not schizophrenic fluctuated in the
intensity of their feelings of alienation and closeness, in their
coherency and articulateness. Perhaps only some of the speech
categories we were scoring here were diagnostic of the schizophrenic syndrome, and other verbal behavior items we were scoring might occur secondarily in reaction to any illness, medical as
well as psychiatric. To answer these questions fully, we carried out
further studies in which the verbal scores from our group of
schizophrenic patients were compared to other hospitalized patients, psychiatric but nonschizophrenic, medical and surgical, and
nonhospitalized "normals."

COMPARISONS OF SCORES FROM THE SOCIAL ALIENATION–
PERSONAL DISORGANIZATION SCALE OBTAINED FROM
ACUTE AND CHRONIC SCHIZOPHRENICS, PATIENTS WITH
BRAIN SYNDROMES, PSYCHIATRIC OUTPATIENTS,
GENERAL MEDICAL PATIENTS, AND "NORMAL" INDIVIDUALS [3]

The distribution of scores obtained when our "schizophrenic"
scale was applied to the verbal communications of a group of
acute (N = 29) and chronic (N = 113) schizophrenics and several groups of nonschizophrenic (N = 152) individuals is indicated in Table 4.11. The study not only yielded normative data
for the several populations of subjects studied but also provided
evidence of the validity of this method in differentiating known
schizophrenics from other subjects (Gottschalk and Gleser, 1964a).

-----
[3] For a fuller presentation of this study, see Chap. IV, pp. 84 ff.

The scale was found to be capable of discriminating the speech samples of schizophrenic patients from those of well subjects, medically ill patients, and, to a lesser extent, patients with other psychiatric illnesses. Brain-damaged patients, however, were found to obtain total scores which were distributed similarly to the scores of schizophrenics.

Some subcategories of content were found, particularly those pertaining to interpersonal relations and disorientation, which did tend to distinguish the brain-damaged subjects from schizophrenics. A similar type of differentiation was noted in an unpublished study of verbal behavior scores obtained on interview material from six persons given psychotomimetic drugs and six schizophrenic patients.[4] All the interpersonal categories on our schizophrenic scale (including self and others—friendly, helpful, loving [IC]; and others—well, achieving, adequate [ID2]) were used more frequently by the schizophrenics, whereas disorientation scores were higher for the subjects on psychotomimetic drugs. Such items could be weighted to obtain a scale for differentiating between schizophrenic and brain-damaged patients. This possibility was explored further and has led to the development of a scale of *Cognitive and Intellectual Impairment* (Gottschalk and Kunkel, 1966; Gottschalk *et al.*, 1969) which is described in Chapter VIII.

A comparison of the frequency of use of certain other content categories among the several samples of subjects revealed a few minor modifications in weighting that appeared warranted. After making these changes in weights, we recalculated the correlation obtained in our schizophrenic validation study (1961a) between the scaled scores derived from 113 verbal samples obtained from patients at Longview State Hospital and the clinical ratings of psychiatrists. The new correlation for the total sample was .63, which was the same as previously obtained, indicating that the slight revision in scoring and weighting did not adversely affect the predictive power of the schizophrenic scale to measure the relative severity of the schizophrenic syndrome within a population of known schizophrenic patients.

This study of comparative score distributions demonstrated

---

[4] These interview transcripts were obtained by Leo Hollister, M.D., and his collaborators at the V. A. Hospital, Palo Alto, Calif., as part of a large study on drug-induced psychoses. We wish to express our gratitude for his permitting us to make use of the data.

that, in addition to its other uses, our verbal behavior measure of the schizophrenic syndrome was of potential value as an initial screening instrument to sort out schizophrenics from non-schizophrenics; different cut-off scores might be used, depending on the purpose of and precision required in such a screening procedure.

Many of the distinguishing characteristics of schizophrenic speech which we have used to some extent in our schizophrenic scale have been pointed out elsewhere. Schizophrenic verbal communications have been found difficult to understand or unintelligible (Bleuler, 1911). Self-contradictions and euphemisms have been said to be common. Frequent self-references and impersonal constructions have been found to occur frequently (White, 1949; Mittenecker, 1951; Lorenz and Cobb, 1954; Mirin, 1955; Bellak and Benedict, 1958). Schizophrenic language has been described as concretistic and as revealing a confusion of the word symbol with the symbolized object (Arieti, 1948, 1950, 1954; Bellak and Benedict, 1958; Sullivan, 1962). These authors also have provided excellent reviews and discussions of these and other peculiarities of schizophrenic language.

We have wondered, however, whether the unusual content and structural aspects of schizophrenic language are mainly a matter of degree, with similar characteristics occurring, but less frequently, in nonschizophrenics. One can readily observe that other people who are mentally and physically ill, and also people who are healthy and functioning well, tend transiently at times to withdraw socially or become cognitively disorganized. Perhaps the difference between nonschizophrenics and people whom we label schizophrenic is not simply in their feelings of social withdrawal and alienation and in their inarticulateness or incoherence, but in the degree and continuity of such characteristics.

In this connection, the present study did not locate any content or form aspects of speech which were pathognomonic of schizophrenia. Rather, it found that the speech categories we have selected in the social alienation–personal disorganization scale were distributed throughout all the groups of people we examined and that abnormal characteristics tended to occur more frequently among sicker individuals and, most frequently, among schizophrenic or brain-damaged patients. This finding tends to support a relativistic concept of the occurrence of the schizophrenic phenomenon among human beings. However, a final conclusion on the basis of this study alone would be premature. Both our verbal behavior method and the statistical procedures we have used, based as they are on quantitative data and assumptions, provide us primarily with quantitative differences between groups. Hence, this investigation could not give an unbiased and critical answer to a relativistic versus a discrete and discontinuous concept of the schizophrenic syndrome.

COMPARISONS OF SCORES FROM THE SOCIAL ALIENATION–
PERSONAL DISORGANIZATION SCALE WITH MEASURES
DERIVED FROM THE MENTAL STATUS SCHEDULE OF
SPITZER ET AL. AND THE CATTELL 16PF SCALE

One additional study, incorporating both longitudinal and cross-sectional data, has given further evidence of the validity of the social alienation–personal disorganization scale by determining its relationship to other measures of personality and adjustment.

The schizophrenic patients selected for this study, 35 males and 39 females, were all diagnosed as chronic schizophrenics. They had been hospitalized from six months to 25 years on the present admission, with a median of 11 years. Those hospitalized for the shortest periods had had one to four previous admissions. All patients had been on one of the phenothiazine drugs continually for at least six months. They were considered to be functioning sufficiently well within the hospital setting to cooperate with testing and interviewing procedures. Patients were all Caucasian and in the age range from 24 to 54.

Each patient was seen by a psychiatrist or third-year psychiatric resident, who administered a standardized interview from which he filled out the Mental Status Schedule (Spitzer, 1965; Spitzer *et al.*, 1964, 1965, 1967). The 16PF test, Form A (Cattell and Eber, 1957), was administered by a psychologist and assistant to groups of 6 to 12 patients at any one session. Directions were read aloud and repeated when necessary to make sure that each patient knew what he was to do. In addition, individual attention was given to each person at some point while he was answering the test to make sure he was recording answers correctly, and in some cases, items were read to him if he was having difficulty reading or understanding. By this means, complete test results were obtained on 35 females and 34 males or 69 of the 74 patients. In addition to the above data, each patient was seen on two or three occasions over the interval of a week by a nonprofessional assistant, who obtained taped verbal samples from each patient by asking him to speak for five minutes about any interesting or dramatic life experiences. The verbal material was scored independently by two technicians on the anxiety, hostility, and social alienation–personal disorganization (schizophrenic) scales we have developed.

The Mental Status Schedule contains a set of 248 items describing symptoms or behavior to which the psychiatrist responds true or false on the basis of a structured interview. The authors of this schedule have collected data on over 2,000 patients throughout the United States and at the time of our study were in the process of determining subscales by means of factor analysis. In particular, a verimax rotation of the first three principal component factors yielded subscores for neuroticism (feelings and concerns), psychoticism (delusions, hallucinations, grandiosity), and disorientation (confusion, retardation).[5] In addition, they had derived some 42 subscales on more specific and circumscribed symptom clusters.

The 16PF test claims to measure "functionally unitary and psychologically significant dimensions" (Cattell and Eber, 1957) as determined by factor analytic and construct validation methods. Standardization tables (1964) provide norms for males and females in the general population based on a substantial number of cases.

Table 7.12 shows the correlations involving the average "schizophrenic" scores of three five-minute verbal samples obtained from each patient during the week when both the Mental Status Schedule and the 16PF were administered to the patients. Our social alienation–personal disorganization scores showed significant positive correlations with the factors from the Mental Status Schedule labeled *delusions-hallucinations* ($r = .41$) and *confusion-retardation* ($r = .43$). Among the 16PF scores, our social alienation–personal disorganization scores showed a significant positive correlation with *autism* ($r = .30$) and a significant negative correlation with *conscientiousness* ($r = -.39$), *shrewdness* ($r = -.30$), and *self-sentiment* ($r = -.32$).

Elsewhere, we have reported evidence from this study that

---

[5] Personal communication from the authors.

TABLE 7.12

Selected Correlations between the Verbal Scale of Social Alienation–Personal Disorganization, the 16PF Scales, and the Mental Status Schedule (N = 69) *

Scales	Social alienation–personal disorgani-zation	Mental status factor scales		
		Feelings-concerns	Delusions-hallucina-tions	Confusion-retarda-tion
Verbal scale				
Social alienation–personal disorganization	......	.19	.41	.43
16PF scales				
C Emotional stability	—.17	—.47	—.29	—.34
F Enthusiasm	—.16	—.27	......	......
G Conscientiousness	—.39	—.35	—.30	—.26
H Venturesome	—.10	—.32	—.12	......
M Autism	.30	.12	.24	......
N Shrewdness	—.30	......	—.24	—.11
O Insecurity	......	.39	.19	......
Q₃ Self-sentiment	—.32	—.41	—.22	—.35
Q₄ Drive tension	......	.41	.11	.18
Mental status subscales				
Delusions-hallucinations	.31	.38	.80	......
Disorientation	.35	......	.17	.77
Apathy-retardation	.31	.32	......	.85
Silly disorganization	.38	......	.37	.22
Somatic preoccupation	.35	.18	.44	.15
Elated excitement	.36	.16	.52	.29

* Significant correlations (p < .05) are underlined.

the average rate of change in social alienation–personal disorganization scores during the first four weeks of this investigation correlated very significantly with certain combined factor scores from the Mental Status Schedule and the 16PF Scale (Gleser *et al.*, 1968; Gottschalk *et al.*, 1968). This finding provided further support that the social alienation–personal disorganization scale is a useful and valid measure of change over time of the schizophrenic syndrome. Along this line, Flegel (1967) has reported that, in following eight schizophrenics during the course of their psychosis, the Gottschalk-Gleser social alienation–personal disorganization scores followed more faithfully his own clinical evaluations and those derived from the Brief Psychiatric Rating Scale

(Overall and Gorham, 1962) of the changing state of the patients than the ratings derived from the Wittenborn Rating Scale (1955).

EFFECTS OF LSD-25 AND A PLACEBO ON THE SOCIAL ALIENATION–PERSONAL DISORGANIZATION SCORES OF A GROUP OF COLLEGE STUDENT VOLUNTEERS [6]

Twenty-seven male college students from the University of Michigan at Ann Arbor participated as paid volunteers in a double-blind, placebo-drug study in which they were told some of them might receive the psychotomimetic, lysergic acid diethyla-mide-25. Before receiving the drug, each student free-associated in a darkened room for 15 minutes and his speech was tape-recorded.[7] Then 18 of the students were given 0.5 microgram of LSD-25 per kilogram of body weight in a glass of water; the other nine were simply given a glass of water (placebo group). One hour later the students were again requested to free-associate into the microphone of a tape recorder for 15 minutes. A significant increase ($p < .05$) was found on the verbal "schizophrenic" scale between predrug–LSD-25 condition and also between predrug–placebo condition. A significant increase was also found on cognitive and intellectual impairment scores of students on LSD-25 as compared to predrug levels ($p < .01$) although the increase was not significantly greater than that obtained by the group of subjects on placebo (see Table 8.4 and discussion on p. 234).

The findings with the psychotomimetic drug, LSD-25, using our content analysis scales—measuring, on the one hand, the severity of the schizophrenic syndrome, and, on the other, the relative magnitude of cognitive and intellectual impairment—support the clinical hypothesis that LSD-25 does not produce a schizophrenic psychosis anymore than does a placebo. Our findings, indeed, suggest what most clinicians now assert, namely, that LSD-25 promotes cognitive impairment and induces a toxic mental disorder rather than a functional one. Also, our findings make clear that the increase in cognitive impairment scores with LSD-25 was independent of changes in anxiety or hostility, for these latter psychological variables actually showed a decrease (see Table 8.5).

---

[6] See pp. 228 f., Chap. VIII, *The Cognitive and Intellectual Impairment Scale*, for further details of this study.

[7] We acknowledge with appreciation the loan of these speech samples from Zegans *et al.* (1967), who obtained them in connection with another study.

PREDICTION OF OUTCOME IN A BRIEF PSYCHOTHERAPY
CLINIC USING THE SOCIAL ALIENATION–PERSONAL
DISORGANIZATON SCALE [8]

Five-minute verbal samples were obtained on two groups of psychiatric outpatients before being seen for treatment in an emergency brief psychotherapy clinic. The first group of patients (Group I) was requested to write ten-minute verbal samples in response to the standard instructions, and the second group (Group II) was requested to speak the usual five-minute period (Gottschalk et al., 1967b). Scores on the social alienation–personal disorganization scale (as well as the anxiety scale and human relations scale) were obtained as possible predictors of outcome after psychotherapy, using a standardized interview (the Psychiatric Morbidity Scale—PMS) as one of the criteria of personality and emotional change. The "schizophrenic" scale turned out to be a predictor of outcome in the sense that it tended to designate those individuals who had not improved following psychotherapy. The rank-order correlation between the pretreatment social alienation–personal disorganization scores and the posttreatment psychiatric morbidity scores (PMS) in Group I ($N = 10$) was .54 and in Group II ($N = 22$) was .39 ($p < .05$, one-tail test). The pre- and posttreatment social alienation–personal disorganization scores in Group II were highly correlated ($r = .63$, $p < .01$). Also, a t-test revealed no significant change in average score from pre- to posttreatment.

Findings were understood to signify that brief psychotherapy of the type provided in this clinic did not tend to modify schizoid character traits, although there was ample evidence (see p. 168) that acute symptoms of anxiety and depression were alleviated. Hence, verbal behavior indices of the relative magnitude of these schizoid character traits and attitudes can be used as one of the predictors of treatment outcome in such a psychotherapy clinic.

---

[8] See p. 284, Chap. X, for a fuller discussion of this study.

CHAPTER VIII
Additional Psychological Measures Derived from the Content of Speech

This chapter will describe a set of scales, applicable to the content analysis of speech, which are in relatively early stages of development. Some of the scales have gone through preliminary trials of reliability and validity (e.g., the Human Relations Scale, the Cognitive and Intellectual Impairment Scale, and the Achievement Strivings Scale). Some have not yet been used in any study that might provide evidence toward validity (Hope Scale, Dependency Strivings and Dependency Frustration Scale, Health-Sickness Scale). Some of the scales are simple frequency scales in which the categories of relevant content have identical weights. Some scales contain categories which have differential weights. The theoretical assumptions behind these scales have been outlined in Chapter II (pp. 5 ff.).

THE HUMAN RELATIONS SCALE

Purpose

Except for clinical evaluation, no systematic instrument is available which provides a quantitative estimate of an individual's degree of interest in and his capacity for constructive, mutually productive, or satisfying human relationships. Yet the clinician commonly finds himself making appraisals of the so-called object relatedness of his patients. Some clinicians use the schema and continuum of the traditional psychoanalytic levels of psychosexual development, referring to oral, anal, phallic, and genital styles of relating to objects. Other clinicians use a more general formulation of the dimension of object relatedness, speaking of the degree of collaborative versus adversary attitudes one reveals in human relationships.

The impetus for developing a scale of human relations has

stemmed from the clinical impression that the relative magnitude of such a capacity or need has often seemed to be an important factor in how well a patient responds to brief psychotherapy, or how successfully a person is advancing in a career involving mutual collaboration and dependence on other people, or even how successfully one learns at school from other people. These and other clinical impressions have made it seem worthwhile to try to develop a scale that could be applied to the content of speech so that these clinical leads could, first of all, be followed up and tested. If favorable results ensued, useful applications of such a scale might then be pursued.

Selection of Verbal Categories and Assignment of Weights

The usual problem in selecting content items and the associated weights for any such scale involves trying to determine the clues that the clinician uses to make inferences about a psychological and behavioral gradient of this kind. One of us proceeded in just this way to attempt to locate the lexical communications that provide some bits of information suggesting, on a probability basis, that the dimension of coldness–warmth in human relations was being either denoted or alluded to in speech in a positive or negative way (Gottschalk, 1968). The result of this first attempt was the accumulation of a set of content items and associated weights (positive or negative) which roughly followed the progression of the psychoanalytic levels of psychosexual development (Freud, 1915–16; Abraham, 1916, 1924), positive weights (attached to content units per clause) implying a liking of people and negative weights implying a disliking.

One departure from using a strictly psychoanalytic *psychosexual development model* in assigning these weights, on a clinical impressionistic basis, was to upgrade oral-dependent and oral-receptive references and to attach a positive weight to such statements because of the likelihood that they suggest that the speaker maintains hope that human relations will provide relief, help, and sustenance. That is, it was assumed that the occurrence of oral-dependent themes in the language behavior of an individual was associated with the likelihood that the individual had some quantum of oral optimism, rather than pessimism, and that such an object orientation presaged continuing behaviors and attitudes of an approach, rather than a withdrawal, from human object relationships. This does not exclude the possibility that, in small samples of speech, oral- dependent references pertaining to the self or others might sometimes be communicating dislike or disinterest in people and, hence, in such instances, would yield misleading results.

This is a typical problem that occurs in assigning standard weights to the probable meaning and significance of brief statements. Even the interviewing clinician, who has access to considerably more data from a patient that may have bearing on this psychodynamic relationship, may have difficulty ascertaining how much the expressed attitudes or actual behavior of a patient signifies like or dislike of people. In the usual clinical diagnostic and psychotherapeutic situation, the clinician can maintain a "wait-and-see" attitude; in fact, a definitive conclusion as to the degree of positive or negative relationship is rarely required. In the type of content analysis procedure that is being developed here, however, where high reliability, validity, and predictive capacity are sought, it is necessary to make some probability estimate of the significance and implications of even brief utterances to the momentary magnitude of a certain psychological dimension. Such estimates are implied by the prescribed weights attached to each content category within a certain scale and in turn provide a score (including zero) for every clause in a sample of speech. In those scales where positive and negative weights are used, contiguous or widely separated statements are frequently assigned weights that cancel out or contradict previous weights; one is, in effect, simply presenting a summation of the various weights in the final indices derived from each verbal sample (details are discussed in Chapter II).

To return, then, to the selection of content items and their associated weights in the Human Relations Scale, a positive weight was assigned to statements implying oral dependence because such verbalizations were considered to imply a predominance of propensities to relate constructively and collaboratively with other people. For a similar reason, verbal statements suggesting a preoccupation with competitive and aggressively rivalrous attitudes or activities were also, initially, assigned a positive weight on the basis of the working hypothesis that competition with people involved a type of human relationship requiring not only human contact of varying degrees of involvement but a relationship also prescribed or fostered by our Western culture. Such hostile themes were assigned a negative weight, however, after a pilot study exploring pretreatment human relations scores as predictors in the outcome of psychotherapy (see initial validation studies below). A further refinement of weights was undertaken after all the data on brief psychotherapy became available, using as a criterion the final outcome corrected for initial scores on a psychiatric morbidity scale. In addition, since the Human Relations Scale was believed to measure a factor similar to the needs for affiliation and nurturance as measured by the Edwards Personal Preference Scale, data from a small study involving these measures were used in determining the revised weights. The verbal content categories and associated weights for the Human Relations Scale, as presently revised, are presented in Schedule 8.1.

SCHEDULE 8.1

Human Relations Scale (Revision 4-7-67)

Score each clause of the verbal sample with one of the code symbols preceding the following thematic categories whenever the content of the clause denotes similar or equivalent content to any of these thematic categories. Many clauses may not contain themes that are similar to these categories and hence can be left unscored.

Scoring weights are given in the left-hand margin beside each category. Total words of the verbal sample should be counted and used as a correction factor to arrive at a final score. Where it is possible to score a clause under two different categories, choose scoring which is weighted minus rather than plus and give the lowest rating toward the negative pole, i.e., give priority to pathology. Give only one score per clause.

Weights   Content Categories and Scoring Symbols

A1. References to giving to, supporting, helping or protecting others.

+2   *a.* Self to others—specific.
+1   *a'.* Self to others—references in which the giving etc. is inferential or the object is unspecified.
+1   *b.* Others giving to others or others receiving from and being taken care of by others.

A2. References to warm, loving, congenial human relations or human relations in which a desire to be closer is expressed. The reference should be specific rather than inferred. Do not score such key words as marriage or friends in this category unless there is additional evidence of congeniality. Rather, score in B2, below.

+2   *a.* Involving self or self and others.
+1   *b.* Involving others.

A3. Concern for other people; references to missing others when they are away. References should be to specific others only.

+1   *a.* Self about others.
+1   *b.* Others about self.
+½   *c.* Others about others.

SCHEDULE 8.1 (contd.)

Weights   Content Categories and Scoring Symbols

A4. Praise or approval of others, indicating more than neutral relations (see B2, below) but not conveying as much positive feeling or warmth as A2, above.

+1   *a.* Self to others.
+1   *b.* Others to self.
+½   *c.* Others to others.

B1. References to manipulative relationships with other human beings. The reference should involve demanding someone do something largely in the service of one's own needs (exploitive) or deliberately making someone feel shame or guilt, e.g., by putting emphasis on how one is made to suffer.

−½   *a.* Self manipulating others.
−1   *b.* Others manipulating self.
−½   *c.* Others manipulating others.

B2. Neutral: nonevaluative references to any kinds of human relations which specify the person(s) interacted with, but which do not specify the nature of the deeper involvement and which are not classified elsewhere. All references to self and others (e.g., we drove, we reached, we thought, etc.) not scorable elsewhere are coded B2*a.*

+¼   *a.* Self or self and others.
+¼   b. Others.

−½   B3. Neutral: nonevaluative references to any kinds of human relations, which are generalized, ambiguous as to person(s) interacted with and impersonal.

C1. Expulsive: references to competitive, hostile, depreciating, and smearing attitudes, impulses, actions.

−½   *a.* Self to others.
−1   *b.* Others to self.
−½   *c.* Others to others.

C2. Retentive: references to withholding affection, interest, approval or attention from people; references to disapproval.

−1   *a.* Self from others.
−1   *b.* Others from self.
−½   *c.* Others from others.

C3. Distancing: references in which people are alienated, drawn apart, kept at a distance from one another.

−1   *a.* Focus on self.
−½   *b.* Focus on others.

D1. Optimism: references to self receiving from, getting from, being taken care of by other people in gratifying and positive ways; interest in other people based on what they can do for oneself; asking others for help; emphasis on the self as the recipient of nurturance and sustenance.

+2   *a.* Self receiving from others.

D2. Pessimism: references to frustration in being taken care of or to poor or inadequate protection, support or care.

−½   *a.* Self.
−½   *b.* Others.

SCHEDULE 8.1 (contd.)

Weights   Content Categories and Scoring Symbols

D3. Separation: any reference to separation, loss, death, not scored elsewhere.
−1   *a.* Self.
−½   *b.* Others.

D4. References to eating or to food in connection with others.
+½   (1) Positive valence.
              a. Self.
              b. Others.

+½   (2) Neutral valence.
              a. Self.
              b. Others.

          (3) Negative valence.
−1   *a.* Self.
−½   *b.* Others.

0   D5. References to difficulty talking, to not knowing what to say, to being
          at a loss for words with interviewer or others.

      D6. Direct interaction with interviewer.
+½   *a.* Asking questions of interviewer when standardized verbal sample
              instructions have been used.
+½   *b.* Other direct references: "you know," or statements addressing in-
              terviewer directly by name or as "you."

−2   E1. References to lack of humans or subhumans in the environment. The
          references must contain evidence of lack of interest in or need for hu-
          man or subhuman objects.

−1   E2. References to eating, food, drinking, meals, etc. out of the context of
          other people. Code both self and others.

−1   E3. References to bathing alone (no other people in view) or to undiffer-
          entiated or amorphous substances or surroundings involving no dis-
          cernible human beings.

Initial Validation Studies

HUMAN RELATIONS SCORES AS PREDICTORS OF OUTCOME
WITH PSYCHOTHERAPY

Initial empirical studies employing the Human Relations Scale
tended to corroborate the assignment of positive weights to the
occurrence of oral-dependent content items but not to verbal content conveying aggressive and rivalrous themes. This first test of
the Human Relations Scale involved the use of human relations
scores derived from pretreatment ten-minute written verbal samples as predictors of the outcome with therapy in an emergency,
brief psychotherapy clinic where acutely disturbed psychiatric
patients could be seen within 24 hours for a maximum of six treat-

ment sessions (Gottschalk *et al.*, 1967*b*). On the basis of the pilot study, which involved only ten patients, the content items and their associated weights were revised to improve the correlation of pretreatment human relations scores with outcome measures, the scores from this first revision showing a positive correlation ($r = +.38$) with the amount of personality change following termination of psychotherapy.

The scale derived from the pilot study was used in a second validation study involving a new group of 22 patients attending the brief psychotherapy clinic. This time, a correlation of $+.51$ ($p < .01$, two-tail test) was obtained between pretreatment human relations scores (derived from spoken, five-minute verbal samples) and the amount of symptomatic improvement occurring with psychotherapy, as measured by pre- and posttreatment difference scores on a Psychiatric Morbidity Scale. Since some relationship also existed between the human relations score and the pretreatment psychiatric morbidity score, a second criterion score was obtained consisting of the posttreatment psychiatric morbidity score corrected (by covariance) for the pretreatment score. The corrected posttreatment scores correlated —.45 with the human relations scores derived from the pretreatment verbal sample (note that the negative correlation here is due to the fact that we are now dealing with residual *morbidity* rather than improvement).

One additional correlation from this study which is relevant at this point is that between the scores on human relations and the scores on social alienation–personal disorganization (see Chapter VII). The latter scale, as the name implies, contains a component pertaining to tendencies to withdraw from interpersonal relationships. For this reason, it might be expected that scores on the scale would be negatively correlated with scores on human relations. However, for both scales to be maximally useful, it would be preferable that the overlap be minimal. The correlation obtained between the two scales on this sample was —.64 (Gottschalk *et al.*, 1967), which was somewhat higher than might be desired.

After the content categories were refined and the weights modified on the basis of the findings on this sample, the resulting human relations scores correlated —.66 with the psychiatric outcome measure. Furthermore, the correlation between the scores from the Human Relations Scale and the Scale of Social Alienation–Personal Disorganization dropped to —.37. These results, of course, now need to be revalidated on a new sample.

CORRELATIONS OF HUMAN RELATIONS SCORES AND SCORES
ON AFFILIATION, NURTURANCE, AND SUCCORANCE FROM
THE EDWARDS PERSONAL PREFERENCE SCHEDULE

A group of 22 medical inpatients, 16 males and 6 females, filled out the Edwards Personal Preference Schedule (1954) and gave one five-minute verbal sample under standard instructions. The group consisted of ten coronary infarction patients, five coronary insufficiency patients, and seven patients with lung disease. They ranged in age from 31 to 61.

The correlations between scores in the preliminary version of the Human Relations Scale obtained from the verbal sample and the affiliation, nurturance, and succorance scales of the Edwards Schedule were .25, .16, and .10, respectively. After the current revision (Schedule 8.1) of the Human Relations Scale, these correlations increased to .36, .53, and .36, respectively. The mean score for human relations was 2.11 and the standard deviation was 1.07.

Further Studies on the Human Relations Scale

Verbal samples were obtained using standard instructions from 75 male and 54 female freshmen entering college during orientation sessions. These samples were scored on the revised Human Relations Scale as well as on the four affect scales. Scholastic Aptitude Test scores and first- and second-quarter grade point averages were made available to us. The human relations scores were not correlated significantly with SAT scores or with grade-point averages for either the male or female sample. The means, standard deviations, and intercorrelations among the verbal scores are shown in Table 8.1. The average human relations score for females (1.40) was very significantly higher than that for males (.94). Furthermore, it appeared that human relations scores for females were negatively correlated with the affect scores; whereas, only hostility outward obtained a negative correlation (nonsignificant) for males.

The Human Relations Scale was applied recently to TAT data obtained in connection with a study of the interaction process between couples with good and poor marital adjustment (Clements, 1968). In this study, 15 couples who applied for counseling at a marriage counseling service were compared with a matching group of 15 couples who had been approved as potential parents

TABLE 8.1

Means, Standard Deviations,* and Intercorrelations among Five Verbal Content Scales for Male and Female Entering College Freshmen

Scales	Mean	Anxiety	Hostility outward	Hostility inward	Ambivalent hostility	Human relations
Males (N = 75)						
Anxiety	1.21	(.60)	.26	.65	.54	.10
Hostility outward	.91	......	(.43)	−.01	.29	−.19
Hostility inward	.65	......	......	(.41)	.33	.17
Ambivalent hostility	.53	......	......	......	(.31)	−.05
Human relations	.94	......	......	......	......	(.81)
Females (N = 54)						
Anxiety	1.32	(.63)	.58	.73	.70	−.28
Hostility outward	.84	......	(.39)	.49	.68	−.41
Hostility inward	.75	......	......	(.41)	.48	−.33
Ambivalent hostility	.57	......	......	......	(.34)	−.33
Human relations	1.40	......	......	......	......	(.95)

* Standard deviations are presented in parentheses as diagonal entries in the matrix.

by an adoption agency. The couples were asked to make up stories jointly to four TAT cards. We hypothesized that the stories of the couples with poor marital adjustment would obtain lower average scores for human relations than would those from couples with good marital adjustment. This hypothesis was substantiated at the .01 level of significance. The average score for the poorly adjusted couples was −1.43 while that for the well-adjusted couples was .60 (Winget et al., 1968). These results are highly encouraging for the potential usefulness of this new scale. (See p. 164 for further details of this study.)

A preliminary investigation of scoring reliability was carried out using a verbal sample from each of 16 male and 16 female students selected at random from the total group. Two coders independently scored each verbal sample on the Human Relations Scale. A correlation of .85 was obtained between the two sets of scores.

THE COGNITIVE AND INTELLECTUAL IMPAIRMENT SCALE

Purpose

Another scale on which we have done some preliminary work is one we have called the Cognitive and Intellectual Impairment

Scale. The scale was developed empirically from a comparative study of verbal samples from various populations using the content categories for Social Alienation–Personal Disorganization (see Chapter VII). In this study, we noted that although brain-damaged patients obtained a score distribution on the total scale which was very similar to that of chronic schizophrenia, there were some categories on which they differed considerably. For example, references to interpersonal relationships were used more frequently by the schizophrenics; whereas verbal statements indicating disorientation occurred more often in the speech of brain-damaged patients. These data suggested that it might be possible to develop a scale of cognitive and intellectual impairment that could be applied to short samples of speech. It was hoped that such a scale would be capable of measuring *transient and reversible changes in cognitive and intellectual function as well as irreversible changes, all due principally to brain dysfunction and minimally to transient emotional changes in the individual.* The usefulness of such a psychological measure, if it could be developed, in basic and applied psychological and psychiatric research is obvious.

Initial Validation Studies

SELECTION OF THE VERBAL CATEGORIES AND ASSOCIATED WEIGHTS
FOR THE COGNITIVE AND INTELLECTUAL IMPAIRMENT SCALE

From the data obtained on the comparative frequency of response to the content categories of the Social Alienation–Personal Disorganization Scale given by groups of schizophrenic patients, other psychiatric patients, brain-damaged patients, general medical patients, and normal subjects (see Tables 4.10 and 4.11, pp. 88 f.), those categories were selected which were used most frequently or most rarely by brain-damaged patients. The categories were weighted initially to maximize the difference between the average score of the brain-damaged patients relative to each of the other groups (Gottschalk and Kunkel, 1966). The weights were later modified on the basis of the correlation of frequency scores for each category with the Halstead (1947) and Trail Making (Reitan, 1958) tests on a sample of 20 patients. These modified weights, which we still consider to be tentative, are given in Schedule 8.2.

The mean content analysis scores on the cognitive impairment

SCHEDULE 8.2

Cognitive and Intellectual Impairment Scale

Weights	Content Categories and Scoring Symbols
	I. Interpersonal References (including fauna and flora).
	B. To unfriendly, hostile, destructive thoughts, feelings, or actions.
—½	1. Self unfriendly to others.
	C. To congenial and constructive thoughts, feelings, or actions.
—½	1. Others helping, being friendly toward others.
—½	2. Self helping, being friendly toward others.
—½	3. Others helping, being friendly toward self.

II. Intrapersonal References.

Weights	
+3	A. To disorientation-orientation, past, present or future (do not include all references to time, place, or person, but only those in which it is reasonably clear the subject is trying to orient himself or is expressing disorientation with respect to these; also, do not score more than one item per clause under this category).
	B. To self.
—½	1. Injured, ailing, deprived, malfunctioning, getting worse, bad, dangerous, low value or worth, strange.
+¼	3. Intact, satisfied, healthy, well.
+1	5. To being controlled, feeling controlled, wanting control, asking for control or permission, being obliged or having to do, think or experience something.
+1	C. Denial of feelings, attitudes, or mental state of the self.
	D. To food.
—1	2. Good or neutral.

III. Miscellaneous.

Weights	
	A. Signs of disorganization.
+1	2. Incomplete sentences, clauses, phrases; blocking.
	B. Repetition of ideas in sequence.
+1	2. Phrases, clauses (separated only by a phrase or clause).
+½	IV. A. Questions Directed to the Interviewer.

scale for the various diagnostic groups described in Tables 4.10 and 4.11 are listed in Table 8.2. The means indicate a plausible ordering of the groups with respect to cognitive impairment, if it can be assumed that a portion of long hospitalized chronic schizophrenics are, indeed, likely to have some brain damage.

CORRELATIONS OF COGNITIVE IMPAIRMENT SCORES WITH SCORES FROM THE HALSTEAD AND TRAIL MAKING TESTS

Five-minute verbal samples were obtained, using standard instructions, from a group of 20 subjects, male and female, ranging in age from 42 to 84. The Halstead Battery (1947) and the

TABLE 8.2

Mean Scores on the Cognitive Impairment Scale for Various
Diagnostic Groups

Group	N	Average score
Brain syndrome	18	2.72
Chronic schizophrenics	113	2.12
Acute schizophrenics	29	1.24
General medical	48	.79
Psychiatric (non-schizophrenic)	26	.66
Normal employed	60	.47

Trail Making Test (1958) were administered to the subjects.[1] Sixteen of the subjects were terminal cancer patients, and the other four were patients with miscellaneous ailments at a nearby Veterans Administration hospital. The verbal cognitive impairment scores from the initial interview were correlated with the scores from the Halstead and the Trail Making tests. An earlier set of weights for the content items on our Cognitive Impairment Scale yielded correlations of .33 and —.37, respectively. While neither of these correlations was significantly different from zero at the .05 level, they did indicate some possible validity.

The revised weights finally selected (see Schedule 8.2) resulted in a substantial increase in the correlation of the verbal cognitive impairment scores with the Halstead Battery ($r = .55$) and with the Trail Making Test ($r = —.48$). The average score for this group on the revised scale was 1.21 with a standard deviation of 2.05. The eight subjects showing the most severe brain damage on the basis of both tests had an average score of 2.90.

CHANGES IN COGNITIVE IMPAIRMENT SCORES COMPARED TO
CLINICAL CHANGES OBSERVED IN PATIENTS WITH ACUTE
OR CHRONIC BRAIN SYNDROMES

To test further the validity of the Cognitive Impairment Scale, verbal samples were obtained from 17 male patients at a Veterans Administration hospital, ranging in age from 23 to 83, who demonstrated an acute or chronic brain syndrome from a clinical examination. Whenever possible, those patients with acute brain syndrome were tested again when the symptoms had subsided. Altogether, 27 observations were available for analysis.

[1] We gratefully acknowledge the assistance of Phyllis Moenster, M.A., in administering these tests.

The average score obtained when the patients were rated as *moderately to severely impaired* clinically was 1.71, as compared to an average of 1.36 when they were rated as *mildly impaired* and 1.14 when *no clinical impairment* was evidenced.

The stability of the revised Cognitive Impairment Scale over a short interval of time was examined in 12 male Veterans Administration patients from each of whom two verbal samples had been obtained in a two- to four-week interval. The intraclass correlation between the two sets of scores was .70. From this data, the standard error of measurement over occasions was estimated to be .57.

LYSERGIC ACID DIETHYLAMIDE (LSD-25), DITRAN (JB-329), AND PSILOCYBIN: COGNITIVE IMPAIRMENT IN NORMAL SUBJECTS ON PSYCHOTOMIMETIC DRUGS AS COMPARED TO COGNITIVE IMPAIRMENT IN MATCHED SCHIZOPHRENIC PATIENTS

Six male nonpsychiatric patients at the Veterans Administration Hospital at Palo Alto, Calif., were administered psychotomimetic drugs. The six patients were give a standardized interview, along with six male schizophrenic patients. The typescripts of the interviews [2] were scored blindly on the content analysis scale of cognitive and intellectual impairment. Table 8.3 gives the comparative content analysis scores, on the Cognitive and Intellectual Impairment Scale, derived from the psychiatric interviews.

In this small sample of subjects, the effect of psychotomimetic drugs on the dimension of cognitive and intellectual impairment was to produce more signs of cognitive impairment in the speech of normals receiving such drugs than occurs naturally and without such drugs in the verbal behavior of schizophrenic patients. The difference between the mean cognitive impairment scores of the two groups was significant at the .05 level by a one-tail t-test and at the .07 level by a Mann Whitney U Test. Noteworthy is the fact that the psychotomimetic drugs Ditran and Psilocybin were associated with higher cognitive impairment scores than with LSD-25, and there is some suggestion the degree of cognitive impairment may be related to dosage.

---

[2] We acknowledge with appreciation the loan of the typescripts of these interviews from Leo E. Hollister, M.D., V. A. Hospital, Palo Alto, Calif.

TABLE 8.3

Cognitive and Intellectual Impairment Scores Obtained from Content Analysis of
Standardized Interviews of Schizophrenic Patients and "Normal" Subjects
on Psychotomimetic Drugs

Cognitive and intellectual impairment scores		
Drug dose	Subjects on psychotomimetic drugs	Schizophrenic patients (not on psychotomimetic drugs)
	Score	Score
"Ditran" (JB-329)—286 mcg/K	8.97	5.26
"Ditran" (JB-329)—187 mcg/K	6.90	2.75
Psilocybin—159 mcg/K	5.65	2.22
Psilocybin—140 mcg/K	5.18	1.01
LSD-25—1 mcg/K	3.72	—.57
LSD-25—1 mcg/K	—.58	—.43
Mean scores	4.97	1.71
Standard error of mean difference	1.60	
t	2.04	
P	<.05 (one-tail)	

LYSERGIC ACID DIETHYLAMIDE (LSD-25) AND PLACEBO: COMPARISON
EFFECTS WITH RESPECT TO COGNITIVE IMPAIRMENT AND SOCIAL
ALIENATION—PERSONAL DISORGANIZATION

Twenty-seven male college students from the University of
Michigan at Ann Arbor participated as paid volunteers in a
double-blind, placebo-drug study in which they were told some of
them might receive the psychotomimetic, lysergic acid diethyla-
mide-25. Before receiving the drug, each student free-associated
in a darkened room for 15 minutes and his speech was tape-
recorded.[3] Then 18 of the students were given 0.5 microgram of
LSD-25 per kilogram of body weight in a glass of water, and the
other 9 students were simply given a glass of water as a placebo;
one hour later, the students were again requested to free associate
into the microphone of a tape recorder for 15 minutes.

A significant increase was found on the cognitive and intellectual impairment scores of students on LSD-25 as compared to
similar scores during predrug periods (p < .01), but the increase

---

[3] We acknowledge with appreciation the loan of these speech samples from Zegans
et al. (1967), who obtained them in connection with another study.

in cognitive impairment was not significant in comparison to the increase obtained from the placebo group of subjects (see Table 8.4).

TABLE 8.4

Significances of Differences of Mean Cognitive Impairment Scores Obtained from LSD Group and Placebo Group of Young Males

Group	Drug condition Without	Drug condition With	Within-group mean difference		P level*
LSD (N = 18)					
Mean	.83	1.65		.82	
s.d.	.74	1.36	s.e.	.30	.01
Placebo (N = 9)					
Mean	.83	1.15		.32	
s.d.	.57	.96	s.e.	.31	n.s.
Difference between groups					
Mean	.00	.50		.50	......
Standard error (s.e.)	.28	.51	s.e.	.43	......
P level	n.s.	n.s.		n.s.	......

* Based on a one-tail *t*-test.

When the free associations of the students were coded on our content scale of social alienation–personal disorganization, both the LSD and placebo groups of subjects showed significant increases (p < .05) in social alienation–personal disorganization scores while on LSD-25 or on placebo as compared to similar scores during the predrug period. Presumably, the direct encouragement to free-associate plus the knowledge that LSD-25 might be administered enhanced the production of content scorable on our Social Alienation–Personal Disorganization Scale whether or not the subject received the psychotomimetic LSD-25. The significant increase in cognitive impairment scores of those subjects receiving LSD-25 (and not in those receiving the placebo) cannot, in this study, be attributed with certainty to cerebrotoxic effects of LSD-25, for the effect of suggestion or some other psychological factor cannot be clearly ruled out. To mitigate the argument that psychological factors accounted for the increase in cognitive impairment scores after ingestion of LSD-25 is the fact that there were no differences between mean scores of anxiety or mean hostility out scores of subjects receiving LSD-25 as compared to those not given this drug, when predrug scores (initial values) were taken into account, although the decrease for the placebo group was significant. Both the LSD group and placebo group of subjects had higher anxiety and hostility out scores, on the average, before drug or placebo was given than during the postdrug or placebo period (see Table 8.5).

TABLE 8.5

Scores on Selected Verbal Content Scales Before and After LSD-25 or a Placebo

	Mean scores			
	LSD (N = 19)		Controls (N = 9)	
	Mean	s.d.	Mean	s.d.
Anxiety scale				
Predrug	1.79	.63	1.48	.63
Postdrug	1.50	.87	1.01	.48
Difference	−.29	.82	−.47*	.45
Hostility outward scale				
Predrug	1.42	.51	1.24	.46
Postdrug	1.27	.35	1.14	.59
Difference	−.15	.43	−.10	.31
"Schizophrenic" scale				
Predrug	2.84	4.86	2.61	2.65
Postdrug	5.71	4.95	3.89	3.37
Difference	2.87†	5.75	1.28†	1.29

* $p < .01$
† $p < .05$

The findings are in line with what most clinicians now assert, namely, that LSD-25 promotes cognitive impairment and that it induces a toxic mental disorder rather than a functional one. These impressions are corroborated by the experimental studies of Amarel and Cheek (1965), who reported that the predictability of speech was reduced by the administration of LSD-25. These investigators used the Cloze procedure (Taylor, 1956), which involves the deletion of every nth word in a verbal passage, after which raters are asked to fill in each missing word with one that seems best to fit the remaining text. The number of correctly guessed words thus forms a measure of the predictability of a given verbal sample. Among other things, the Cloze procedure is considered to be a measure of cognitive function, for it has been found to differentiate the speech of aphasics from that of normal subjects (Fillenbaum and Jones, 1962).

These are preliminary studies of the Cognitive and Intellectual Impairment Scale. More validation studies will be carried out which will include further content item evaluation and revision of the tentative weights. This scale has been applied in one study

(Gottschalk *et al.*, 1969) exploring the effect of total or half-body irradiation on intellectual functioning, and it has provided suggestive evidence of temporary impairment of such functioning immediately after exposure to radiation.

ACHIEVEMENT STRIVINGS SCALE

Purpose

Scales of achievement strivings and achievement frustration, as well as scales of dependency strivings and dependency frustration, were developed in conjunction with an exploratory psychophysiological investigation on patients with acute myocardial infarction and with coronary insufficiency. The purpose of the scales was to provide a means to assess both the transient swings and typical levels of motivation toward achievement and dependency and also the relative magnitude of reactions of frustrations in each of these drives. It had been suggested, for instance, in work done by Friedman and Rosenman (1959, 1960) that patients with coronary artery disease are characteristically driven to achieve under the pressure of time and that individuals with such traits also have comparatively high levels of plasma and urinary 17-hydroxycorticosteroids. We speculated that the achievement strivings and achievement frustrations of coronary heart disease patients might be relatively high. Because the achievement drives of these individuals might be either inherently elevated or increased on the basis of the psychological mechanism of reaction formation, no prior hypothesis could be generated as to what the relative dependency strivings or frustrations of such patients might be.

To accomplish some headway in the study of the psychophysiology of coronary artery disease was only the immediate impetus toward formulating content guidelines for such scales. We were certain that there were a large number of other basic and clinical research projects that might be pursued if good measures of these types could be fashioned. Our work on these scales has not progressed much beyond the preliminary stages.

Selection of Content Categories and Associated Weights for Achievement Strivings Scale

The initial tentative content categories for the Achievement Strivings Scale were formulated by both of us, and these content items and their associated weights have undergone many revisions. In spite of these many revisions, we have not been able to find content categories which can cover achievement strivings and accomplishments relevant to all possible fields of endeavor. First of all, vocational and avocational strivings may be differentially pertinent, depending on the achievement goal. Furthermore, one person's vocation may be another person's avocation, and a person with high motivation for short-term goals may have poor motivation for long-term goals. These factors can hamper not only reliability but also validity of any global scale. Hence, we believe it may be necessary to specify the achievement goals of the subjects studied to assess the meaning of any findings obtained using such a measure of "achievement."

Our current set of content categories are listed in Schedule 8.3.

Preliminary Studies Using the Achievement Strivings Scale

In these preliminary studies, we used content categories pertaining to achievement strivings and not those involving achievement frustrations. The categories were broken down into typically *vocational* (Categories I and II, below) and *avocational* (Categories V and VI) pursuits. Also, the scores obtained for each verbal sample were based on simple frequency counts, that is, each pertinent achievement content category occurring was given a weight of $+1$. The category of "Deterrents" (IV) was given a weight of -1.

COMPARISONS OF ACHIEVEMENT STRIVINGS SCORES (AND DEPENDENCY) IN HEALTHY SUBJECTS AND MEDICAL INPATIENTS

Three groups of ten patients each were chosen from three inpatient groups at a private general hospital in Cincinnati, Ohio. The patients in these three groups had, in common, complaints centering around precordial pain or pain involving the chest and shortness of breath. One group was comprised of patients with acute myocardial infarction, another of patients with coronary insufficiency, and the third group consisted of patients without cardiac disease. A fourth group of 15 individuals was composed of nonpatients, that is, subjects not medically nor psychiatrically ill. All groups were matched for age, sex, and educational level.

Five-minute verbal samples from each of these groups were elicited by standard instructions. These verbal samples were

SCHEDULE 8.3

Achievement Strivings Scale

Score all codable clauses. Distinguish between references to the self or others by adding the following notation: (*a*) self or self and others; (*b*) others.

I. Vocational, occupational, educational references, including naming and identification.

II. Other constructive activities where emphasis is on work or labor rather than play. Emphasis may be in form of overcoming hardships, obstacles, problems, toward reaching a goal. Exclude all sports and entertainment activities.

   A. Domestic activities: moving; buying or selling major items; decorating, painting, cleaning, cooking, doing chores.

   B. Activities that require some effort or perseverance to carry out or activities done with speed or accuracy, activities involving trying new experiences as in eating new food or travelling to new places (score no more than three in succession of references to travelling to new places). Score references to learning new information or habits, needing to satisfy curiosity, or attempting to unlearn undesirable attitudes or behavior.

III. References to commitment or sense of obligation to responsible or constructive social and personal behavior; to obligation to perform well or succeed in a task; to commitment to a task and to carrying it out or completing it. References to inculcation by others or self of sense of responsibility for one's actions or for welfare of others; responsibility for leadership; evidence of positive superego or ego ideal; evidence of high standards or standards that are hard to live up to (score these even when reference is to fears of not achieving, e.g., "I felt terrible about doing so badly on the test").

IV. Deterrents

   A. External dangers or problems or fear of loss of control or limit setting on part of others. References to lack of control by others; references to errors or misjudgments by others that might injure the self.

   B. Internal obstacles: references to difficulties in setting limits on oneself or problems in disciplining the self; references to errors or misjudgments by self that might harm the self.

   C. Interpersonal: arguments or troubles getting along with others; problems in interpersonal relations, such as inability to make friends.

V. Sports (note that some sports, such as swimming, may be A, B, or C, depending on context).

   A. Spectator.

   B. Team or organized.

   C. Solitary or small group.

VI. Entertainment.

   A. Spectator.

   B. Amateur.

   C. Professional.

scored by one technician for achievement strivings and dependency strivings. The results are summarized in Table 8.6 (Gottschalk *et al.*, 1964c).

The results of this study show that more important than the

TABLE 8.6

Comparative Achievement Strivings and Dependency Strivings in Two Groups of
Cardiovascular Inpatients, a Control Group of Noncardiac Inpatients, and a
Group of Healthy Employed Individuals

Group	N	Achievement strivings (refs/100 words)			Dependency strivings (refs/100 words)
		Voca-tional	Avoca-tional	Total	
Healthy employed individuals ..	15	2.32	2.32	4.64	.98
Hospitalized medical patients ..	30	1.48	.96	2.44	1.58
Acute myocardial infarction patients	10	1.80	.26	2.06	1.72
Coronary insufficiency patients	10	.96	1.10	2.06	1.46
Noncardiac patients	10	1.68	1.51	3.19	1.56

nature of one's illness, that is, cardiac versus noncardiac, in deter-mining content of speech is whether or not one is severely enough ill to be hospitalized. The group of nonhospitalized, gainfully employed individuals showed significantly higher mean scores for total achievement strivings (p < .05) than the mean scores for all three groups of hospitalized patients. On the other hand, the mean dependency strivings score for all three hospitalized groups was significantly higher (p < .05) than the mean dependency scores for the nonhospitalized, healthy group of individuals. These findings suggest that the context in which an individual talks for five minutes "about any interesting or dramatic personal life ex-periences," that is, whether or not he is hospitalized and whether or not he qualifies by reason of sickness for the role of a patient, influences to what extent he thinks about and hence talks about achievement and dependency strivings.

Comparing the content of speech of the different kinds of patients, we found that there was a trend for the patients with myocardial infarctions to have the highest scores for the *vocational component* of the Achievement Strivings Scale and the lowest scores for the *avocational component* of this scale. The former finding, though not significant, was in the direction previously noted by Friedman and Rosenman. That the achievement strivings of our sample of cardiac patients were not more marked can be attributed, in part, to their very sick status at the time five-minute verbal sam-ples were obtained from them. No verbal sample was obtained from these three groups of medical patients until they had been in the hospital for at least one week, so that the potentially precarious status of their health could be somewhat stabilized. Even at this point of their hospital course, the patients were under the protective wing of their private physician, who typically discouraged the patients' efforts to be independent or active and sanctioned or enforced their dependency. Furthermore, these medical patients were typically under mild sedatives and tranquilizers, which may have further dampened their usual achievement strivings and enhanced their dependency needs.

EFFECT OF A SUBJECT'S MENTAL SET OR EXPECTATION ON THE EFFECT OF THE PSYCHOACTIVE DRUG AMPHETAMINE

A study was carried out on 108 college students to explore the influence of the mental set or doctor's attitude on the patient's response to psychoactive medication. The subjects wrote ten-minute verbal samples before and 45 to 60 minutes after ingesting 10 mg. of racemic amphetamine sulphate or 10 mg. of secobarbital or a placebo after reading one of three cards suggesting what effect to expect from the drug they took. The "amphetamine" set was: "This drug will probably make you feel more peppy and energetic and cheerful." The "secobarbital" set was: "This drug will probably make you feel less anxious and more relaxed, and it might even make you feel a bit sleepy." The noncommittal (placebo) set was: "It is not known exactly what effect this drug will have on you as an individual." Subjects were randomly assigned to one of the nine combinations of drugs and mental sets.

Mean achievement strivings derived from verbal samples were significantly higher with the "amphetamine" set ($p < .005$) and with amphetamine drug ($p < .025$). The drug-set interaction was not significant (Gottschalk *et al.*, 1968). The capacity of mental set to influence these content categories of speed emphasizes the importance of the context in which speech is elicited, and suggests the need to differentiate between achievement fantasy and achievement realization.

Further Studies Using the Achievement Strivings Scale

Two pilot studies have been undertaken in an effort to determine whether verbal content categories regarding achievement strivings and achievement frustration can be weighted to yield a prediction of scholastic success for college students. In the first study five-minute verbal samples were obtained from 47 female and 40 male college students who were enrolled in introductory psychology courses. These students were for the most part sophomores or juniors in Arts and Sciences, Education, Business Administration, Fine Arts, and Engineering. On the basis of a comparison of verbal samples of ten students obtaining the highest grade point average for the quarter and the ten obtaining the lowest grades, our previous categories for vocational and avocational references were elaborated and refined, and a category was added referring to achievement frustration, that is, *Deterrents*. Tentative weights were selected which tended to maximize the correlation of the total score with grade point average for both the male and female groups, although it was noted that some categories were predictive for only one or the other sex.

For the second study, verbal samples were obtained from 75 male and 54 female new college freshmen who subsequently remained at the University for at least one quarter. The verbal samples were scored for achievement strivings, and the resulting total scores were correlated with first- and second-quarter grade point averages and aptitude test scores separately for males and females. The resulting correlations were disappointingly low. Only the correlation of achievement strivings scores with second-quarter grades for males was significantly different from zero.

Frequency scores per hundred words for each subcategory were recorded separately and correlated with first quarter grade point averages.[4] These are shown in Table 8.7. It is evident from the data that correlations differ considerably according to the sex of the subjects. Thus, it is unlikely that the same weights would be predictive of scholastic achievement for both sexes. Also, very likely, different weights would be optimal according to the college in which the student is enrolled. Thus, engaging in sports might be positively related to success for a student majoring in Physical Education but negatively related to success for a student in Engineering or Liberal Arts. Also, there is, undoubtedly, a difference in the standards for grading in different colleges which may attenuate results. We, therefore, plan, in doing further work on this scale, to combine the data from these two pilot studies and regroup it on the basis of the college being attended.

---

[4] The data were processed on an IBM 7040.

TABLE 8.7

Means and Standard Deviations of Scores on Achievement Strivings and Achievement Frustration Categories and Correlations with First-Quarter Grade-Point Averages for Freshmen Male and Female College Students

Content category	Males (N = 75)			Females (N = 54)		
	Mean	s.d.	Correlation with GPA	Mean	s.d.	Correlation with GPA
I*a*. Vocational—self	.94	.83	—.04	.83	.67	—.10
b. Vocational—others	.40	.45	.20	.36	.40	—.15
II*Aa*. Domestic—self	.01	.05	.04	.02	.08	—.09
b. Domestic—others	.01	.03	.18	.00	.00	......
II*Ba*. Other activities—self ...	.33	.48	.12	.39	.48	—.01
b. Other activities—others .	.04	.15	—.09	.05	.13	.00
III*a*. Task commitment—self .	.11	.24	—.22	.12	.23	.06
b. Task commitment—others	.03	.07	.03	.02	.07	.20
IV. Deterrents						
A. External dangers	.07	.14	—.35	.06	.20	—.15
B. Internal obstacles	.07	.17	—.37	.03	.08	—.18
C. Interpersonal difficulties	.05	.14	.05	.08	.14	—.03
V. Sports						
A*a*. Spectator—self	.04	.17	—.04	.03	.09	.23
b. Spectator—others	.04	.27	.04	.00	.02	.12
B*a*. Team—self	.19	.67	—.18	.00	.02	.29
b. Team—others	.39	1.13	.04	.02	.09	.16
C*a*. Solitary—self	.13	.30	—.11	.13	.31	—.05
b. Solitary—others	.03	.11	—.11	.02	.10	.08
VI. Entertainment						
A*a*. Spectator—self	.00	.02	—.01	.03	.08	.03
b. Spectator—others ...	.00	.02	—.08	.01	.03	.00
B*a*. Amateur—self	.11	.44	—.03	.24	.54	.24
b. Amateur—others	.02	.10	—.04	.08	.25	.07
C*b*. Professional—other ..	.00	.00	......	.00	.02	—.23

DEPENDENCY AND DEPENDENCY FRUSTRATON SCALES

Purpose

Excessive dependency needs on others and the frustration of either appropriate or inordinate dependency needs have been psychodynamic areas of recurring practical and theoretical interest to clinicians. These psychodynamic areas have also been of considerable interest to the researcher, but he has found it difficult to define and measure these psychological relationships.

A number of psychiatric and psychosomatic theories prevail, generated by clinical observation, which involve the concept of excessive oral dependency drives or of dependency frustration. For example, individuals subject to manic-depressive psychosis have been considered to be plagued by unsatisfiable dependency needs (Abraham, 1916, 1924; Freud, 1917; Fenichel, 1945; Jacobson, 1953). Patients with peptic ulcer have been described as having either high, covert, frustrated dependency needs due to intrapsychic conflicts with their pride and their need to present themselves as self-sufficient and independent (Alexander, 1934, 1947) or as having high, overt, frustrated dependency needs due to such external factors as poverty or loss of emotional support (Kapp et al., 1947). Weiner et al. (1957) have obtained supportive evidence for this peptic ulcer psychophysiological hypothesis, but claim that both a physiological predisposition, manifested by a high gastric acidity, and a high level of dependency are necessary in the psychophysiology of peptic ulcer. A content analysis method applicable to verbal behavior could be used to test further these psychological theories about such illness. Our verbal behavior scales of dependency strivings and frustrated dependency strivings may be a contribution toward a content analysis method of measuring dependency and its frustration.

Content Categories

Schedules 8.4 and 8.5 give the content categories for the Dependency Strivings and Frustrated Dependency Strivings Scales.

SCHEDULE 8.4

Scale of Dependency Strivings

Types of Reference about Dependency Strivings

A. Statements referring to having, getting, wanting or needing help, support, protection, care, approval, love, doctoring, and divine assistance.
B. References to oral activities, food, etc. Includes any oral activity, such as chewing gum, eating, smoking, drinking, swallowing, sucking, and biting.
C. Denial of dependency strivings.

Person Involved in Dependency Strivings

Include possessions of self or others as extension of person involved in dependency strivings.
1. Self or self and others.
2. Others or unspecified.

Time of Occurrence of Strivings

a. Past.
b. Present.
c. Future or unspecified.

SCHEDULE 8.5

Scale of Frustrated Dependency Strivings

Types of Reference about Frustrated Dependency Strivings

A. References to self being frustrated in having, getting, wanting, or needing help, support, protection, care, approval, love, doctoring, and divine assistance.

B. References to oral frustrations. Includes any oral-gastric frustrations, e.g., difficulties or delays in getting food, water, or other objects to relieve oral tension. Need to resort to scraps or waste products for food, hunger, thirst, food deprivation, dry throat, difficulty in obtaining food, empty stomach, being out of cigarettes, difficulty in swallowing, etc.

C. Denial of oral frustration.

D. References to others being frustrated in wanting help, support, protection from speaker.

Person Involved in Frustrated Dependency Strivings

1. Self or self and others.
2. Others or unspecified.

Time of Occurrence of Frustrated Dependency Strivings

a. Past.
b. Present.
c. Future or unspecified.

Preliminary Studies

No validation studies have yet been carried out using these two scales. An exploratory study with coronary artery disease inpatients and normal controls has been described briefly in a preceding section (Table 8.6, p. 239) dealing with our Achievement Strivings Scale. Dependency strivings, as defined operationally by the scale items (all weighted $+1$), were found to be significantly higher in the five-minute verbal samples of medically ill hospitalized individuals than in those from healthy employed people.

The Dependency and Dependency Frustration Scales need item analysis, reliability, and validity studies before their usefulness to behavioral and psychiatric research can be gauged.

HEALTH-SICKNESS SCALE

Purpose

This is a content analysis scale aiming to measure the dimension of illness, physical or mental. It was developed originally to follow the course of patients with metastatic cancer who received total or partial body radiation with the cobalt bomb (Gottschalk and Kunkel, 1966; Gottschalk *et al.*, 1969). Its many possible uses have not been explored.

Content Categories in the Health-Sickness Scale

The verbal content items in this scale, given in Schedule 8.6, are very few at this stage of the scale's development. There is one set of statements classified as designating subjective feelings of health (and weighted +1) and another category of statements presumably indicating feelings of sickness (and weighted —1). Whether the negatively and positively weighted content items can be added meaningfully, that is, to give a score that relates to a definable and useful health-sickness dimension, has yet to be determined. At the present time, we are assuming only that the health-sickness construct evaluated by our present content items relates to a subjective or feeling state and may not necessarily coincide with either a biological indicator of degree of medical illness or some other measure of severity of mental illness (for example, when an individual is falsely denying the presence of illness).

SCHEDULE 8.6

Health-Sickness Scale

Weights	Content Categories and Coding Symbols
+1	HS 1. References to feelings of well-being, health, being symptom-free (physical or mental). *a.* Others. *b.* Self.
—1	HS 2. References to feelings of poor health, having symptoms, pain, suffering (physical or mental). *a.* Others. *b.* Self.

Exploratory Studies with the Health-Sickness Scale

No reliability studies have been carried out as yet using this scale.

1. A preliminary validation study has been done, comparing health-sickness scores derived from verbal samples of four groups, each of 20 individuals, matched for sex, age, and education. The four groups were: (1) gainfully employed individuals, (2) patients on a psychiatric ward, (3) patients on a medical ward, and (4) acutely and severely ill psychiatric outpatients. Results were as given in Table 8.8.

TABLE 8.8

Comparative Scores on Health-Sickness Scale

Group	N	"Health" statements (total no.)		"Sickness" statements (total no.)		Corrected* "sickness" scores (av.)		Combined and corrected* scores (av.)	
		M	F	M	F	M	F	M	F
Gainfully employed	20	0	1	4	4	—.07	—.17	—.07	—.14
Psychiatric inpatients ..	20	11	23	45	26	—.78	—.63	—.61	—.16
Acutely ill psychiatric outpatients	20	10	4	36	84	—.54	—1.66	—.38	—1.35
Medical inpatients	20	12	16	78	60	—1.57	—1.41	—1.08	—1.21

* Corrected for number of words per verbal sample.

The findings suggested that though statements of ill health are more frequent among samples of people who are likely to be considered sick by the medical profession, statements of good health are also likely to be more common among such people; actually, more preoccupation with the total health-sickness spectrum typified patient samples in comparison to a nonpatient sample. Statements of good health in groups of patients may be the result of the social-cultural context of "sick" individuals, which in our society promotes communications of this sort; such verbalizations may be the expressions of the denial of illness or anxiety about death; in some instances, such talk may be associated with the pharmacological effects of analgesics, sedatives, or tranquilizers. At the present time, it appears that in cross-sectional (extensive design) studies, the weights on negative and positive content items need not be added together to arrive at health-sickness scores to make pertinent discriminations; whereas, in longitudinal (intensive design) studies, the use of both negative and positive content items may prove useful in ascertaining the effects on this subjective state of various external factors. In any event, further studies are needed to obtain more information on matters of this sort.

2. In another preliminary study, health-sickness scores were derived from a five-minute verbal sample obtained from ten cancer patients three days after they had been exposed to partial or total body radiation. The patients were distinguished on the basis of whether the physician in charge of their treatment considered them

well enough to return home or not. The six patients allowed to return home were found to have higher health-sickness scores (p < .07 by a Mann Whitney test) than the four who were required to remain in the hospital. An item analysis indicated that this difference was due to positively weighted content, which differentiated the group at the .03 level.

Furthermore, the correlation of health-sickness scores derived from a five-minute verbal sample obtained on admission to a general hospital of 16 terminal cancer patients and the duration of their survival in days, following partial or total body radiation, was found to be —.31.

Much further study needs to be done with this Health-Sickness Scale, in addition to reliability and validity studies. Not only does the dimension require clarification at the level of a definition of the construct, but also differentiation of the severity of illness, across illnesses of all kinds, may not be possible on the same scale unless one concedes that the dimension we are using is a strictly psychological one that may not necessarily be congruent with behavioral or physiological criteria of illness.

HOPE SCALE

Purpose

This scale was devised to measure the intensity of the optimism that a favorable outcome was likely to occur, not only in one's personal earthly activities, but also in cosmic phenomena and even in spiritual or imaginary events. A favorable outcome was intended to denote one which might lead to human survival, the preservation or enhancement of health, the welfare or constructive achievement of the self or any part of mankind. Hope might also involve the fruitful survival, growth, and development of fauna and flora; the creative products of people; or positive memories, thoughts, or emotions about people or things.

Content Categories of the Hope Scale

The development and use of this scale is at an early phase. The content categories could probably be enlarged upon or further refined to advantage, not only from the viewpoint of increasing reliability of scoring but of more clearly crystallizing our construct of hope.

The content categories of the Hope Scale and their associated weights are given in Schedule 8.7.

Weights		Content Categories and Coding Symbols
+1	H 1.	References to self or others getting or receiving help, advice, support, sustenance, confidence, esteem (*a*) from others; (*b*) from self.
+1	H 2.	References to feelings of optimism about the present or future (*a*) others; (*b*) self.
+1	H 3.	References to being or wanting to be or seeking to be the recipient of good fortune, good luck, God's favor or blessing (*a*) others; (*b*) self.
+1	H 4.	References to any kinds of hopes that lead to a constructive outcome, to survival, to longevity, to smooth-going interpersonal relationships (this category can be scored only if the word "hope" or "wish" or a close synonym is used).
−1	H 5.	References to not being or not wanting to be or not seeking to be the recipient of good fortune, good luck, God's favor or blessing.
−1	H 6.	References to self or others not getting or receiving help, advice, support, sustenance, confidence, esteem (*a*) from others; (*b*) from self.
−1	H 7.	References to feelings of hopelessness, losing hope, despair, lack of confidence, lack of ambition, lack of interest; feelings of pessimism, discouragement (*a*) others; (*b*) self.

Preliminary Studies Using the Hope Scale

In clinical medicine and psychiatry, the observation is frequently made that the patient's will or hope to survive or improve or to get well is often an important contributing factor in the favorable course of an illness. Such a hypothesis is at work in the style of a physician's patient care when he encourages the patient's hope for survival or when he covers up medical information that might discourage the patient's hopeful mood.

We intend to experiment with and test the use of this scale in the near future in selected psychiatric and medical conditions in which hope (of a good outcome) has been thought to have a favorable influence on the outcome.

Thus far, no reliability studies have been completed with the Hope Scale.

It has been tried in a study of the effects on patients with metastatic cancers of various kinds of total or partial body radiation with the cobalt bomb at the Cincinnati General Hospital. In a group of 16 patients, a correlation of $+.38$ was obtained between hope scores obtained from the first five-minute verbal sample given by the patients in response to our standard instructions and the duration of survival of the patients, in days, after receiving the actual body irradiation (Gottschalk and Kunkel, 1966). Also, the third-day post-radiation five-minute verbal sample average hope scores of 11 cancer patients who returned home that day ($+5.42$) were compared by a Mann Whitney U Test to the comparable hope scores of the patients obliged to remain in the hospital ($+1.9$). The hope scores of these two small groups of patients differed significantly at the .01 level.

The Hope Scale will require further content item analysis, reliability, and validity studies before it can be of general use in research.

CHAPTER IX

Investigations Dealing with Specific Problems or Facets of Our Verbal Behavior Content Analysis Procedure

COMPARISONS BETWEEN ANXIETY SCORE OBTAINED USING TYPESCRIPTS AND THAT USING TYPESCRIPTS PLUS SOUND RECORDINGS OF SPEECH SAMPLES [1]

The estimation of the magnitude of the construct called anxiety is at best an approximation, whatever the measurement procedure might be. This is particularly so when anxiety is defined as some kind of transient, subjective, inner state which can be communicated directly or indirectly by various speech cues and/or other behavioral or physiological signs. One invariably encounters a considerable lack of precision associated with making such assessments of transient anxiety, particularly since judgments by different people differentially emphasize the importance of the various cues.

In an attempt to improve the reliability and validity with which transient anxiety can be measured, we have developed a method using content analysis of brief samples of verbal material. Our method makes use of the typescript only, without reference to the sound of the speaker's voice or to his movements, gestures, or facial expressions. Studies reported in the preceding chapters strongly suggest that when we measure anxiety using only lexical data, a meaningful psychological state can be discerned which is concomitant to relevant biological variables and which is different from other psychological states, such as hostility, elation, and so forth. But the question still remains in these studies whether a more valid estimate of anxiety could be obtained by listening to the tape recordings of the speaker's voice.

[1] Excerpted in part from L. A. Gottschalk and E. C. Frank, "Estimating the magnitude of anxiety from speech," *Behav. Sci.*, 12: 289–295, July, 1967.

Increasing interest in verbal behavior analysis has focussed attention on the relative contribution of lexical and paralanguage [2] factors (Trager, 1958, 1966) in the expression and communication of quantitative differences of affects in speech. A number of investigators (Starkweather, 1956a, 1956b; Dittmann and Wynne, 1961; Ostwald, 1963) have expressed the viewpoint that vocal variables are likely to be especially sensitive indicators of emotionality in man; some hold them possibly more indicative than the content of his speech. Although this is an intuitively appealing position, rigorous supportive evidence for any point of view on this matter is blocked by methodological problems besetting the investigator who seeks to explore the problem. One of the major difficulties is the inadequate reliability with which independent assessment of the paralanguage components of vocalization can be made. Another major problem is finding suitable criteria of the specified emotional variable on which to base a determination of the validity of the paralanguage variables.

An excellent review of the literature on paralanguage studies has been done by Kramer (1963); he enumerates some of the methodological problems involved in investigations of the nonverbal properties of speech.

Procedure

The study reported here (Gottschalk and Frank, 1967a) was undertaken as an attempt to obtain some answer to the plaguing question of the relative importance of lexical and paralanguage variables in the assessment of anxiety from speech samples. A set of twelve five-minute tape recordings of speech obtained under our standard instructions was selected from a large pool of such samples on the basis that they covered a wide range of anxiety as ascertained by our verbal content method for deriving anxiety

---

[2] Paralanguage phenomena, classified by linguists separately from linguistic phenomena and from all vocal properties of speech (Trager, 1958, 1966; Dittmann and Wynne, 1961), have been grouped as follows: 1. *Vocalizations* include (a) vocal characterizers, such as laughing, crying, and voice breaking: (b) vocal segregates, which are sounds other than words that have communicative value, such as "um-hmm"; (c) vocal qualifiers, which are the extra increases or decreases in loudness, pitch, or duration beyond what are needed to convey the linguistic phenomena of juncture, stress, and pitch patterns. 2. *Voice quality* includes tempo, rhythm, precision of articulation, register range, rasp and openness, nasality, breathiness, and resonance. 3. *Voice set* refers to current physiological characteristics of the speaker, such as fatigue, immaturity, and the like.

scores. Sixteen raters (eleven psychiatric residents and five graduate psychologists) participated in the study as judges. The judges were asked to rate the magnitude of anxiety in the speech samples following the anxiety rating scale of the Overall and Gorham Brief Psychiatric Rating Scale (1962). The raters first read the typescripts of the verbal samples and rated the intensity of anxiety; then, at least a month later, they rated the magnitude of anxiety after listening to the tape recordings of the speech samples and reading the typescripts.

Separate analyses of variance were computed on the ratings of the verbal samples by the sixteen judges, using the anxiety scale of the Overall and Gorham Psychiatric Rating Scale, when the typescript was the only source of information and when both the typescript and sound recording were made available. Reliability or generalizability estimates for a single rating and for the average of 16 ratings were obtained from the appropriate mean squares and variance estimates (Cronbach *et al.*, 1963). The reliability of ratings by a single rater was calculated by the application of the formula, variance ratio $= \hat{\sigma}_v^2 \, / \, \hat{\sigma}_v^2 + \hat{\sigma}_e^2$.

Results

The reliability of ratings by a single rater was estimated to be .381 when the raters used only the typescripts. In contrast, the estimated reliability of a single rater using the typescripts plus sound recordings was .524. The higher reliability of a rater when rating under the latter circumstances and comparison of the two sets of variance estimates given in Table 9.1 indicate that the raters, when using the typescripts alone, were less able to differentiate the verbal samples ($\hat{\sigma}_v^2$ smaller), differed considerably more in their average ratings of the total sample ($\hat{\sigma}_r^2$), and had greater error variance ($\hat{\sigma}_e^2$) than when using typescript plus sound recording. The coefficient of reliability for the sum of the scores of the 16 raters was found to be .908 on the basis of the typescripts alone and .946 on the basis of the typescripts plus sound recordings.

Since the major concern of this study was the comparison of anxiety scores obtained under the two assessment conditions already described, the product-moment correlation between the anxiety scores for the two types of assessment conditions was calculated from the covariance and variance of the sums of the ratings over

TABLE 9.1

Separate Analyses of Variance of Ratings of Verbal Samples Obtained
by Using Typescripts Alone or Typescripts Plus Sound Recordings

Source	SS	df	MS	Expected mean square	Variance estimate
		Typescripts	alone		
Verbal samples	98.042	11	8.913	$16\sigma_v^2 + \sigma_e^2$	$\hat{\sigma}_v^2 = 0.506$
Raters	64.250	15	4.283	$12\sigma_r^2 + \sigma_e^2$	$\hat{\sigma}_r^2 = 0.288$
Residual	135.625	165	0.822	σ_e^2	$\hat{\sigma}_e^2 = 0.822$
Total	297.917	191	.....	....	....
		Typescripts plus sound	recordings		
Verbal samples	119.042	11	10.822	$16\sigma_v^2 + \sigma_e^2$	$\hat{\sigma}_v^2 = 0.640$
Raters	13.667	15	0.911	$12\sigma_r^2 + \sigma_e^2$	$\hat{\sigma}_r^2 = 0.027$
Residual	95.958	165	0.582	σ_e^2	$\hat{\sigma}_e^2 = 0.582$
Total	222.667	191	.....	....	....

the 16 judges. The correlation obtained was .846. This, however, was an underestimate of the degree of agreement existing between the two conditions for assessing anxiety, due to the imperfect reliabilities of the separate ratings under the two conditions. Therefore, the "correction for attenuation" (Gulliksen, 1950, pp. 98–99) was employed in order to obtain an estimate of the correlation between the anxiety scores from typescripts and those from typescripts plus sound recordings of speech if the ratings of the average of the 16 raters for the two separate conditions were perfectly reliable. This correction gave an estimated correlation of .913 between the two sets of anxiety scores; consequently, at least [3] 16.6 percent (i.e., $1-r^2$) of a universe of anxiety scores derived from typescripts plus sound recordings of five-minute speech samples would not be predictable from anxiety scores derived from typescripts of these speech samples alone.

Of possible additional interest was the extent to which the anxiety ratings obtained under the two conditions discussed above —and scaled by means of the Overall-Gorham rating procedure— correlated, separately, with scores derived by means of the Gottschalk-Gleser verbal behavior method. The correlations are given in Table 9.2.

---

[3] The corrected correlation is probably somewhat inflated by the fact that the same raters made both sets of ratings. Thus, the correlation between the two methods contains some specific rater covariance components.

TABLE 9.2

Product-Moment Correlations of Anxiety Scores from Speech Samples

Variables correlated	Correlation
Average Overall-Gorham ratings of anxiety using typescript only with average Overall-Gorham ratings using typescript plus sound recording	.846
Anxiety scores derived by content analysis with average Overall-Gorham ratings using typescript only	.740
Anxiety scores derived by content analysis with average Overall-Gorham ratings using typescript plus sound recording	.837

It may be noted from this table that the product-moment correlation between the anxiety scores of the verbal behavior method and the ratings obtained when only the typescripts were employed (.74) was lower than the correlation between the scores from the verbal behavior method and the ratings obtained by using the typescript plus sound recording (.84).

A *perfectly reliable anxiety rating* of the typescript via the Overall-Gorham scale would correlate .777 with anxiety scores measured by means of the Gottschalk-Gleser method, and a *perfectly reliable anxiety rating* of the typescript plus voice recording would correlate .861 with anxiety scores based on the Gottschalk-Gleser method. If a correction is further made for attenuation due to unreliability in scoring anxiety by the content analysis procedure and .90 is taken as the reliability estimate of such scores for this purpose, the two coefficients become .818 and .905, respectively (see Chapter III).

Discussion

The present study suggests that the reliability of a rater's judgments regarding anxiety made from small verbal samples is somewhat better when he listens to sound tapes of the speech while typescripts are read than when he only reads the typescripts. However, since the research design did not do away with possible sequential effects of having the raters in all instances make their rating from the typescript plus sound recording follow the rating of the typescript alone, the higher reliability obtained when rating under the former circumstances may be in part a result of practice or perhaps marginal familiarity with the verbal sample. Furthermore, the reliability estimates alone do not enable us to conclude that there is necessarily any difference in the average scores that would be obtained by the two methods if enough raters were available to make both methods equally reliable or if the universe scores themselves were available.

The question of construct validity is best answered by the correlation between the two sets of scores corrected for the unreliability in each. From this analysis, we find that 83.4 percent of the variance of either set of measures is shared in common by the other set, while only 16.6 percent of the variance of either one is unique. It is difficult to say to what extent this estimate of common variance was inflated by the fact that the same judges made both ratings.

The correlation (.84) between the anxiety scores derived by the Gottschalk-Gleser content analysis procedure and the average ratings based on soundscript plus typescript yields another piece of evidence regarding the extent of overlap of these sources of information. Since the content scoring was performed completely independently of the ratings, there is no likelihood of a spuriously high correlation between the two measures. Using an estimated reliability of .90 for the content scores (see Chapter III), we obtain a corrected correlation of .905 between content scores and the average ratings using typescript plus sound recording. This value would imply that 81.9 percent of the variance of either score is common variance, and 18.1 percent of the variance is specific— an estimate that is very similar to the previous one. Furthermore, the estimate of specific variance in this case is enhanced slightly by the differences in scaling between the Overall-Gorham scale and that of content analysis.

Clinical observation of psychiatric patients gives corroborative evidence that the lexical and paralanguage aspects of speech do not always go together uniformly. For instance, schizophrenic and severe obsessive-compulsive patients show a dampening of some of the paralanguage components in the expression of their emotions—the characteristic flatness of affect of the schizophrenic or the obsessive-compulsive's psychological defense of isolation. And patients with hysterical character disorder or emotionally unstable personality disorders tend to exaggerate the vocal qualities of their verbal expression of emotions relative to the content of their speech (see also Moses, 1954). Our results, however, indicate that such discrepancies in lexical and paralanguage channels of communication are the exception rather than the rule.

In general, our findings tend to support a theory of the redundancy of lexical and vocal factors in speech rather than an additive theory in the expression and communication of the intensity of affects. Redundancy in different channels of communication could be important for minimizing error in the messages obtained on the receiving end. And the fact that there is considerable duplication of information with respect to the amount of anxiety conveyed in verbal and vocal avenues of communication has probably been of survival value in early man. Other investigators, such as Scheflen (1964, 1966), have emphasized how yet another communication channel, kinesics (which includes posture and gesture), may not necessarily reinforce or be in concordance with the information communicated by other channels of communication, such as the lexical or paralanguage channels, and in fact in some individuals may be contradictory. Such findings do not detract from the predominance of the redundancy aspect in verbal communication. Rather, they indicate the possible ambiguity resulting for the receiver whenever human communication systems do not follow the redundancy principle.

USE OF WRITTEN VERSUS SPOKEN VERBAL SAMPLES

In most of the content analysis we have done, spoken verbal samples have been obtained and used as the source of language behavior to which our scales have been applied.

Because of the relative ease and time-saving aspects of getting written verbal samples into typescript form for scoring, we have thought that there might be advantages in using written verbal samples in certain types of investigations. It has seemed plausible, however, that the writing of language, in response to our standard instructions or for that matter in response to any stimulus, might give the subject time to consider and reconsider what he was going to reveal, so that spontaneity would be lost as compared to what would be uttered in speaking extemporaneously. Hence, we have conjectured that affect scores might be reduced when derived from written as compared to spoken verbal samples. This does not seem to be so, as adjudged from data that we will cite in the studies summarized below. We have also thought that the generalizability of written verbal samples over scores and occasions might be less than that of spoken verbal samples if similar time-units were used for permitting the subject to express himself in language behavior.

This is due to the fact that people speak more than they write per unit of time, and hence a smaller sample of the "stream of consciousness" is available. One can counteract the effect on scoring reliability of the small number of words in the five-minute written sample by increasing the time interval to ten minutes or more; this, however, does not increase the proportion of verbalized affect in an interval. At this point, we are uncertain whether scores from one type of language material can be indiscriminately equated with scores obtained using the other kind of language material. We recommend that all verbal samples in any specific study be either completely spoken or completely written until more detailed answers are obtained to these questions. The studies reported below provide what solid information we have on these issues.

USE OF FIVE-MINUTE WRITTEN VERBAL SAMPLES IN A
PSYCHOPHARMACOLOGIC STUDY

Ross *et al.*, 1963, used two sets of five-minute written verbal samples from 81 medical students to ascertain the differential psychological effects of amobarbital, dextroamphetamine, and a placebo. The average anxiety score was significantly lower in those medical students who received amobarbital than those who were administered the other two agents. The reliability and adequacy of sampling of these written verbal samples, however, was less than is obtainable with spoken samples. For example, the reliability of anxiety scores by a single coder was estimated at .68 as compared to estimates of .73 to .86 for spoken five-minute samples. This reduction in the reliability of anxiety scores was attributed to the paucity of words, since the average number of words obtained in five-minute *spoken* verbal samples in a group of male students (40) was 633.7 ± 180.9; whereas, the average number of words obtained in five-minute verbal samples from this group of medical students was 105.5 ± 35.1. Furthermore, approximately 35 percent of the written records for those on placebo contained no anxiety codings as compared to 14 percent in the spoken samples of employed personnel (see Chapter IV), suggesting an inadequate sampling of anxiety when using the five-minute written sample.

On the basis of this study, it was decided to obtain ten minutes of the written verbal samples in order to increase their reliability and adequacy.

USE OF TEN-MINUTE WRITTEN VERBAL SAMPLES IN A PSYCHOPHARMACOLOGIC STUDY

The affect scores obtained from ten-minute written verbal samples of 103 male college students in a psychopharmacologic study (Gottschalk *et al.*, 1968) did not appear to be appreciably different than comparable affect scores from spoken samples of a group of male college students (see Table 9.3). The standard deviations for both anxiety and hostility, however, were somewhat larger in the written samples than the standard deviation in spoken samples. Furthermore, the number of words written was still only one-third of the number obtained in asking the person to speak. (See Chapter VIII, pp. 225 ff. for a fuller discussion of this study.)

TABLE 9.3

Means and Standard Deviations of Affect Scores Obtained with College Males on Ten-Minute Written Verbal Samples and on Five-Minute Spoken Verbal Samples

Measure	Written ten-minute sample (N = 103)		Spoken five-minute sample (N = 40)	
	Mean	s.d.	Mean	s.d.
Anxiety	1.49	.85	1.45	.64
Hostility outward	1.02	.53	1.12	.46
Hostility inward	.81	.41	.74	.44
Number of words	212.1	44.7	633.7	180.9

USE OF TEN-MINUTE WRITTEN VERBAL SAMPLES AS A PREDICTOR OF OUTCOME WITH PSYCHOTHERAPY

In a recent study (Gottschalk *et al.*, 1967*b*), ten-minute written verbal samples were obtained from acutely disturbed psychiatric outpatients before their admission to a brief psychotherapy outpatient clinic in an investigation designed to predict and evaluate outcome with treatment. The results in an initial group of 20 patients, from whom written and spoken samples were obtained in about equal numbers, generated hypotheses that were tested in a second sample of patients, all of whom gave spoken samples. Written verbal samples were discontinued after the first sample of patients because some of the patients coming to this emergency psychotherapy clinic were too disturbed to write and yet could speak for five minutes. Nevertheless, the predictors of outcome with psychotherapy derived from the written verbal samples of the preliminary study with the first small group of patients proved to be of prognostic value in the second group of patients using spoken verbal samples. The comparable rank-order correlations are indicated in Table 9.4.

TABLE 9.4

Correlations Between Scores before and after Psychotherapy Using Written and Spoken Verbal Samples

	Pretreatment verbal behavior scores					
	Human relations scores		Social alienation-personal disorganization scores		Anxiety scores	
Psychiatric morbidity scores (PMS)	10-min. written v.s.*	5-min. spoken v.s.†	10-min. written v.s.	5-min. spoken v.s.	10-min. written v.s.	5-min. spoken v.s.
Posttreatment (PMS$_2$) ..	—.33	—.32	.54	.39	.54	.14

* N = 10; correlations are Spearman rank order.
† N = 23; correlations are Spearman rank order.

The pretreatment human relations score, the social alienation–personal disorganization score, and the anxiety score—derived from either written or spoken verbal samples—have correlations in the same directions with posttreatment measures.

EFFECT OF PERSONALITY OF INTERVIEWER ON VERBAL BEHAVIOR PATTERNS OF THE INTERVIEWEE

The effects of the personality of the observer on the observed have been dealt with from many points of view. The literature itself is voluminous, and its language varies with the scientific disciplines involved. The reader can explore the range of interest of scientists in this area among physicists (Mulligan and McDonald, 1957; Thewlis, 1962), psychologists (McGuigan, 1963; Rosenthal, 1964), and psychoanalysts (Orr, 1954).

When verbal behavior has been elicited by means of our standard procedure, we have been inclined to assume that the interviewer may have relatively little effect on the content scores obtained, for the standard method of eliciting speech recommends that the interviewer keep his facial expression relatively immobile as he reads the instructions to elicit speech and that he continue doing so as the subject talks (see Gottschalk *et al.*, 1969). However, interviewer differences in sex, general appearance, tone of voice, and pretesting acquaintance with the interviewee cannot be successfully standardized. Hence, some differences in the content of speech of the subject can occur as the result of these factors. Ordinarily, we do not believe that the effects of such factors are significant over such brief time periods as the five or ten minutes necessary to produce a verbal sample. Nevertheless, we have consistently recommended the use of the same interviewer for each research project when it is desirable to minimize interviewer differences.

Recently, we have analyzed data, collected much earlier, for interviewer effects on anxiety and hostility and have also undertaken some studies to explore possible effects of the interviewer on other aspects of content. The studies, indeed, suggest that different patterns of response can be obtained with different interviewers.

EFFECT OF PERSONALITY OF INTERVIEWER ON ANXIETY AND HOSTILITY SCORES

Two male interviewers (Gottschalk and Hambidge, 1956), each obtained two five-minute verbal samples from eight normal, employed subjects. The first sample was elicited by using the so-called "visual" method of induction (see Preface, p. ix; also, Gottschalk and Hambidge, 1955), which involved giving each subject a series of TAT cards (7 GF, 13 MF, 2 BM, 3 BM) and asking the subject to tell stories about the pictures for five minutes. The second sample was elicited by using the standard "verbal" method of induction, in which the subjects were asked to speak for five minutes about any interesting or dramatic life experiences they had ever had.

The order of obtaining verbal samples by each interviewer was balanced; that is, one interviewer elicited verbal samples first from four of the subjects and the other interviewer elicited verbal samples first from the other four subjects. Anxiety and hostility outward scores were determined by a technician unfamiliar with the study. The effects of interviewer, method of induction of speech ("visual" or "verbal"), order, and their interactions on affect scores were computed by analysis of variance. The results of the study are presented in Table 9.5.

Anxiety scores were significantly lower (p < .005) when obtained by interviewer A than by interviewer B. This difference

TABLE 9.5

The Different Effect of Two Interviewers on Anxiety Scores Derived from Speech Samples from Eight Subjects

| Interviewer | Mean anxiety scores | | |
| | Method of eliciting speech samples | | |
	Visual stimulus	Verbal stimulus	Total
A	1.21	.85	1.03
B	1.59	1.42	1.50
Average	1.40	1.13	1.26

| Source | Analysis of variance | | | |
	df	MS	F	p
Investigator	1	1.781	16.95	< .005
Stimulus	1	.554	......	......
Occasion	1	.002	......	......
Subjects	7	1.018	9.68	< .001
Investigator × stimulus	1	.069	......	......
Stimulus × occasion	1	.044	......	......
Stimulus × subjects	7	.479	4.55	< .025
Residual	12	.105	......	......

was consistent over both methods of obtaining verbal samples. No differences in hostility outward scores were noted with respect to which interviewer obtained the verbal samples.

EFFECT OF PERSONALITY OR SEX OF INTERVIEWER ON SEXUAL REFERENCES, SELF REFERENCES, AND AFFECT SCORES [4]

This study was designed to test the hypothesis that the sex of the interviewer, as one aspect of personality, influences the response patterns of the interviewee. It was reasoned that such an effect would manifest itself most clearly in the frequency of references to others of a specified sex and self references made by the interviewee in the presence of an interviewer of the same sex versus one of the opposite sex. We recognized that one difficulty in such a study was that of controlling other personality variables in the interview, such as the interviewer's behavior and verbal comments, tone of voice, or other vocal factors that might differ in reaction to the gender of the subject. We attempted to control, as much as possible, some of these factors, that is, the overall behavior, facial expression, and content of speech of the interviewer,

[4] This study, heretofore unpublished, was carried out by L. A. Gottschalk, E. J. Hanson, J. Niemiller, and G. C. Gleser in 1964d.

and to observe principally the effect of the appearance of the interviewer on the verbal messages evoked from the interviewee.

Method

The interview sessions were scheduled so that each subject would, alternately, speak in the presence of one or another of the interviewers over three occasions. The order of presentation of the interviewer was balanced. Thus with our 19 subjects in this study, for five of the male and five of the female subjects, the sex of the interviewers for the three sessions was male-female-male; for the remainder of the subjects, it was female-male-female. This was done to eliminate the effect that the schedule of interviews, apart from the interviewers, might have upon the subjects' behavior. Sessions for each subject were at least one day apart.

The setting for the interview did not vary, being in the office in which one of the interviewers ordinarily saw patients in psychotherapy. A tape recorder was placed in full view of the subject with a microphone on a desk before him. At the beginning of the first session for each subject, the standard instructions were given to elicit five minutes of verbal communication.

When with the subject, and especially when he was speaking, the interviewers were instructed to give no behavioral or facial cues or encouragement whatsoever, but to sit quietly and silently throughout the session.

Subjects

The group of subjects numbered 19, ten males and nine females, all unpaid volunteers. The age range was 19 to 25 years, and all were students at the University of Cincinnati at the undergraduate or graduate level. They were told that they would be participating in a study of certain aspects of speech.

Interviewers

The interviewers were a male psychiatric resident physician (E. H.) and a female graduate student in psychology (J. N.), and both were identified to the subjects as "Doctor" ————. Both interviewers were aware of the nature of the experiment.

Scoring procedure

Each interview session was transcribed verbatim and the typescripts were scored for masculine and feminine sexual references according to the guidelines in Table 9.6. Also, each verbal sample was scored for anxiety and three types of hostility by our verbal behavior method.

The task of reliably and validly classifying references to others according to sex turned out to be more difficult and intricate than was immediately apparent. Colby (1960), who classified sexual references in his study on speech patterns in the presence and absence of another person, did not make explicit the rules by which he made these classifications. We initially set out to ascertain all the sexually identifiable verbal units that could be found in verbal samples, but we found that interjudge reliability of scoring was unsatisfactory when we included possible abstract and symbolic criteria of sexual designation. Finally, we agreed on a system of scoring (Table 9.6), resigning ourselves to the fact that in assuring ourselves of an interscorer reliability of .85, we probably lost some data.

TABLE 9.6

Principles for Scoring Verbal Samples for Male-Female (Sexual) References

Code symbol	Description and explanation
M	Clearcut, unequivocal masculine references.
MI	References are likely to a male or males, but there is some uncertainty about this decision because the sex is not specifically designated. One may infer that the sexual designation is masculine, e.g., the words "shoemaker" or "coal miner" refer to males. No inferences based on a symbolic or figurative basis are allowable.
MS	References to the self when the speaker is a male.
F	Clearcut, unequivocal female references.
FI	Analogous to MI references, but pertaining to females, e.g., "seamstress" or "beauty parlor operator."
FS	References to the self when the speaker is a female.
G	Impersonal nouns, pronouns or other expressions denoting a person or persons but not specifying the sex.

The counts of sexual references were summated in each category and expressed in terms of frequency of occurrence per 100 words spoken.

After the subjects had completed their participation in the "interviews," they were all asked to take a brief, modified Thematic Apperception Test (TAT), which was scored for heterosexual compatibility and incompatibility. The TAT cards selected for this test were: 2, 4, 6 GF, 10, 13 MF, 6 BM. The subject's TAT stories were tape-recorded and typed .The typescripts were scored by one

of the investigators (E. H.), after preliminary trials of testing
interjudge scoring reliability on eight TAT protocols by two of the
investigators (L. A. G. and E. H.) produced a coefficient of reliability of .85. The principles followed for scoring these TAT
records are summarized in Table 9.7.

TABLE 9.7

Principles for Scoring Brief Thematic Apperception Tests (TAT) for
Heterosexual Compatibility and Incompatibility

Code symbol	Description and explanation
+	All statements which refer to heterosexual interaction in which there is pleasure, satisfaction, affectionate moving toward one another and so on.
−	All statements which refer to heterosexual interaction in which there is displeasure, dissatisfaction, pain, avoidance, hostile moving away from one another, and so forth.
0	Neutral heterosexual references.

Scores for heterosexual compatibility-incompatibility were
expressed in terms of the positive themes minus the negative themes
per 100 words.

When scores were derived from our TAT heterosexual compatibility-incompatibility measure, it was found that scores per
interviewee from the three TAT cards (4, 6 GF, 13 MF)—which
depicted heterosexual settings involving young people similar in
age to the subjects and the two interviewers—yielded more consistent scores [5] than did scores from the other three cards (2, 6 BM,
10) which depict son-mother, father-mother, etc., types of human
relationships. Hence, the kinds of scores derived from our brief
TAT heterosexual compatibility-incompatibility measures were
those based only on the former three cards.

The tentative hypotheses were principally nonspecific with
respect to the anxiety and hostility scores; that is, a difference
would occur in the magnitude of anxiety and of hostility depending
on the sex of the interviewer and the heterosexual compatibility
score of the interviewee. With the sexual references, however, it
was conjectured that the subjects would verbalize, during the five-minute period of free association, a greater percentage of content

---

[5] Reliability (internal consistency) estimate for these three TAT cards (4,
6 GF, 13 MF) was .62 for males and .24 for females. For all six cards, the reliability was .29 for males and .14 for females.

items identified as masculine when in the presence of a male interviewer and a greater percentage of feminine references in the
presence of a female interviewer. An alternate hypothesis was that
the above hypothesis would hold true with respect to female subjects but not with male subjects, who might in such initial encounters shy away from speaking of women when in the presence of a
female interviewer.

Results

The first interview session was regarded as a training and
introductory period for the interviewee, and except where noted,
scores from this session were not used in the analyses of the data.
One reason why this was done was to eliminate any "first-time"
effect (see p. 111).

With regard to sexual references, it was found that scores and
results were not appreciably different when the less certain categorizations involving gender were dropped. Accordingly, only references coded M and F in Table 9.6 are reported here, and those
coded MI and FI are omitted. The references to self (MS and FS)
are treated separately. The averages of male and female references
per 100 words spoken in the presence of both a male and a female
interviewer by all subjects are summarized in Table 9.8.

TABLE 9.8

Average Male and Female References (per 100 words) Spoken in the Presence of a
Male and Female Interviewer (Second and Third Interviews only)

| | Male interviewee | | Female interviewee | |
| | Av. verbal references | | Av. verbal references | |
Interviewer	Male (M)	Female (F)	Male (M)	Female (F)
Male	3.60	1.21	1.66	2.30
Female	1.12	.22	1.05	3.33
Average	2.36	.72	1.35	2.82

Table 9.8 illustrates the following findings:
1. Males, with both interviewers, made more references to
   males than to females (2.36 > .72); females made more
   references to females (2.82 > 1.35).
2. With both interviewers, females made significantly more
   references to females than did males (2.82 > .72, p =
   .025).

3. Males talked more about people (M plus F) with the interviewer of the male sex than with the female interviewer (4.81 > 1.34); females made approximately the same total number of male plus female refrences to the two kinds of interviewers (i.e., 3.96 and 4.38). On the other hand, no difference was found in the average number of references made to people without designating sex (code symbol G, Table 9.6) by subjects of either sex in the presence of interviewers of either sex.

4. Both sexes made more references to males with the male interviewer than with the female interviewer (3.60 + 1.66 > 1.12 + 1.05, p = .05).

5. Males made fewer references to females with the female interviewer than with the male interviewer; whereas, females made more references to females with the female interviewer than with the male interviewer (.22 < 1.22 and 3.33 > 2.30, p < .05).

Although this was not a purpose of this study, it is interesting that females were found to give more self references (FS) than males. This trend was significant (p < .05) when all three interviews were taken into account, but did not reach significance when only the last two interviews were considered (see Table 9.9). The

TABLE 9.9

Differences in References to Self Among Male and Female Interviewees

| Interviewer | Male interviewee | | | | Female interviewee | | | |
| | Interview | | | | Interview | | | |
	1st	2d	3d	Av.	1st	2d	3d	Av.
Male	4.19	4.30	5.33	4.46	5.48	6.05	8.21	6.58
Female	4.48	6.47	3.30	4.56	8.18	9.16	4.48	7.27

tendency of women to show significantly more self-references than do men corroborated an earlier finding (Gottschalk et al., 1957). Table 9.9 also indicates that no differences were found in overall level of self references by male or female subjects due to the sex of the interviewer.

There was a nonsignificant trend for males to have more anxiety (.95 > .66) in interviews with the male interviewer than with the female interviewer when all three interviews were considered. There was a nonsignificant trend for females to have higher hostility outward scores with the male than the female interviewer ($1.24 > 1.06$) when all three interviews were considered.

The following interesting correlations were found, using Spearman's rank difference rho (see Table 9.10).

TABLE 9.10

Correlations (Rank Difference) of TAT Heterosexual Compatibility-Incompatibility Scores with Hostility Outward and Hostility Inward Scores

	Correlations with TAT heterosexual compatibility-incompatibility scores			
	Male interviewees (10)		Female interviewees (9)	
Interviewer	Hostility outward	Hostility inward	Hostility outward	Hostility inward
Male	−.33	.00	+.55	−.57
Female	−.76	+.25	−.12	+.48

The higher the TAT heterosexual compatibility scores of our male interviewees, the more likely they were to have low hostility out scores in the presence of a female interviewer (and also to a lesser extent when with a male interviewer). On the other hand, the higher the TAT heterosexual compatibility score of our female interviewees, the more likely they were to have high hostility out scores and low hostility in scores when in the presence of a male interviewer.

Discussion

The findings from this study tend to support the hypothesis that the sexes behave differently with interviewers of different sexes or personalities, even when the "interviews" are extremely brief, that is, only five minutes in duration, and when the cues and interactions from the interviewer are standardized and minimal.

One explanation for these findings is that courting behavior is involved. Thus males may make fewer references to a female with a female interviewer than with a male interviewer because, at the age range of our interviewees, males may look upon the female interviewer as a possible person with whom to manifest courting behavior and, hence, inhibit a show of interest in women other than the interviewer. Also, an explanation of the differences in correlations between hostility outward and hostility inward scores and the TAT heterosexual compatibility-incompatibility scores when the sexes were interviewed by a member of either sex is, again, that courting behavior is involved. The findings suggest that men do not readily verbalize hostility in the presence of a woman when they are inclined to have predominantly positive feelings toward women in general. Women, however, especially those highly polarized to a receptive and positive attitude toward men in general, are likely to show hostile reactions readily if their wishes to be responded to warmly by a man are frustrated and met with the formalized aloofness our interviewers were instructed to manifest. It is plausible, furthermore, that women with high heterosexual compatibility scores (and by extension and inference good father-daughter relationships) are not likely to have strong attitudes of self-criticism and self-repudiation; and, hence, hostility inward scores of female interviewees, when interviewed by a male, correlate —.60 with their scores of heterosexual compatibility.

The findings in this investigation did not conclusively prove that the differences in verbal content found with male and female interviewers were entirely due to the sex of the interviewer. These differences may, indeed, have occurred in reaction to nonsexual personality differences in the two interviewers. Another study was carried out in order to ascertain those verbal responses which seemed to be related specifically to the sex of the interviewer rather than to nonsexual characteristics.

EFFECT OF SEX AND PERSONALITY OF INTERVIEWER
ON VERBAL SCORES

The opportunity to study further the effect of the sex or personality of the interviewer on the content of verbal samples was afforded us by a study of 170 freshman college students, participating in pre-academic orientation exercises. These subjects, who were paid a dollar each to volunteer their services, all gave five-minute verbal samples on the same day in response to standard instructions to one of four interviewers, two male and two female. The assignment of interviewer was unsystematic. When the verbal samples were sorted, it was found that one interviewer had seen only ten subjects of each sex, so an equal number of each sex was selected randomly from the verbal samples of the other three interviewers. These 80 verbal samples were scored for anxiety, hostility, male and female references, and self references. Differences in the scores attributable to the sex or personality of the interviewer were sought using a mixed model, nested analysis of variance, assuming both interviewer and interviewee effects to be random while sex effects were considered fixed.

Affect scores

The average anxiety scores for male and female subjects classified according to interviewer are shown in Table 9.11. From the analysis of variance of these data,[6] it was determined that the sex of the interviewer per se had no effect on anxiety scores, but that some interviewers, regardless of their sex, obtained higher anxiety scores on the average than did others ($F = 3.60$, $p \leqq .05$). Furthermore, some interviewers consistently obtained higher anx-

TABLE 9.11

Anxiety Scores for Male and Female Subjects Interviewed by Different Interviewers

	Subjects (10 per cell)		
Interviewer	Males	Females	Total
Male A	.98	1.82	1.40
Male B	1.28	1.08	1.18
Female C	1.57	1.43	1.50
Female D	1.15	.99	1.07
Total av.	1.25	1.33	1.29

	Analysis of variance		
Source	df	MS	F
Sex of subject	1	.144	....
Sex of interviewer	1	.000	....
Sex of sub. × sex of int.*	1	1.095	....
Int. given sex (int./sex) †	2	1.171	3.598 p ≦ .05
Sex of sub. × int./sex‡	2	1.337	4.109 p ≦ .025
Within cell	72	.325	....

* Sex of subject by sex of interviewer.
† Interviewer effects for interviewers of the same sex, whether male or female.
‡ Sex of subject by interviewer effects for interviewers of the same sex, whether male or female.

---

[6] A mixed-model analysis of variance nested design was used in this and the subsequent analyses, with interviewer and subject effects considered random.

iety scores from female subjects; for other interviewers, the higher scores were obtained with male interviewees.

The findings on hostility inward were similar to those for anxiety, as indicated in Table 9.12. For this variable, however, the interviewer effect (for a given sex) reached a higher level of significance than for anxiety.

TABLE 9.12

Hostility Inward Scores for Male and Female Subjects Interviewed by Different Interviewers

Interviewer	Subjects (10 per cell)		
	Males	Females	Total
Male A	.45	.76	.61
Male B	.64	.42	.53
Female C	.97	.95	.96
Female D	.60	.59	.59
Total av.	.67	.68	.67

Source	Analysis of variance		
	df	MS	F
Sex of subject	1	.004	....
Sex of interviewer	1	.869	1.23 n.s.
Sex of sub. × sex of int.*	1	.012	....
Int. given sex (int./sex) †	2	.705	5.56 p ≤ .01
Sex of sub. × int./sex‡	2	.716	5.64 p ≤ .01
Within cell	72	.127	....

* Sex of subject by sex of interviewer.
† Interviewer effects for interviewers of the same sex, whether male or female.
‡ Sex of subject by interviewer effects for interviewers of the same sex, whether male or female.

The hostility outward scores, averaged according to interviewer and sex of subject, are shown in Table 9.13. Again, the sex of the interviewer had no significant effect on scores, but certain interviewers, regardless of sex, differed significantly in the amount of hostility outward they elicited from both male and female subjects.

Ambivalent hostility scores, unlike those of the other three affects, showed a definite interaction effect of sex of interviewer with sex of interviewee (p ≤ .001). Female subjects responded with higher ambivalent hostility scores when interviewed by males than when interviewed by females. Male subjects, on the other hand, had higher ambivalent hostility scores when interviewed by females than when interviewed by males (see Table 9.14).

TABLE 9.13

Hostility Outward Scores for Male and Female Subjects Interviewed by
Different Interviewers

Interviewer	Subjects (10 per cell)		
	Males	Females	Total
Male A	.91	1.13	1.02
Male B	.97	.87	.92
Female C	1.01	.90	.96
Female D	.70	.59	.65
Total av.	.90	.87	.88

	Analysis of variance		
Source	df	MS	F
Sex of subject	1	.014	....
Sex of interviewer	1	.558	....
Sex of sub. × sex of int.*	1	.136	....
Int. given sex (int./sex) †	2	.519	3.123 p ≤ .05
Sex of sub. × int./sex‡	2	.133	....
Within cell	72	.168	....

* Sex of subject by sex of interviewer.
† Interviewer effects for interviewers of the same sex, whether male or female.
‡ Sex of subject by interviewer effects for interviewers of the same sex, whether
male or female.

TABLE 9.14

Ambivalent Hostility Scores for Male and Female Subjects Interviewed by
Different Interviewers

Interviewer	Subjects (10 per cell)		
	Males	Females	Total
Male A	.36	.84	.60
Male B	.51	.54	.52
Female C	.81	.53	.67
Female D	.58	.45	.52
Total av.	.57	.59	.58

	Analysis of variance		
Source	df	MS	F
Sex of subject	1	.010	....
Sex of interviewer	1	.022	....
Sex of sub. × sex of int.*	1	1.086	8.94§ p ≤ .001
Int. given sex (int./sex) †	2	.148	....
Sex of sub. × int./sex‡	2	.284	2.43 n.s.
Within cell	72	.117	....

* Sex of subject by sex of interviewer.
† Interviewer effects for interviewers of the same sex, whether male or female.
‡ Sex of subject by interviewer effects for interviewers of the same sex, whether
male or female.
§ Denominator is a pooled error term from within cell and sex of sub. × int./sex.

Male, female, and self-references

In this study, as in the previous one (pp. 265 ff.), male subjects spoke more about males than females; females made more references to females (Table 9.15). In fact, while male and female subjects, averaged over all interviewers, referred to males with about equal frequency, the females referred to females significantly more than did male interviewees ($F = 13.01$, $p \leqq .001$). In the present study, unlike the previous one, there were no significant main effects attributable to the sex of the interviewer. Rather, it was found that the personality of interviewers, regardless of sex, had a differential effect on male references ($F = 7.02$, $p \leqq .005$). Thus, for example, interviewer B elicited far more male references from subjects of both sexes than did interviewer A and also more than did either of the female interviewers. Also, in this study, males made more references to males with a female interviewer; in contrast, females made more references to males with a male interviewer ($F = 7.23$, $p \leqq .01$). The corresponding interaction effect for female references was not significant.

TABLE 9.15

Male and Female References (per Hundred Words) for Male and Female Subjects Seen by Different Interviewers

Interviewer	Male subjects		Female subjects		Total	
	Male ref.	Female ref.	Male ref.	Female ref.	Male ref.	Female ref.
Male A	.50	.26	1.03	1.22	.77	.74
Male B	1.66	.07	2.08	2.30	1.87	1.18
Female C	1.59	.15	.59	1.23	1.09	.69
Female D	.94	.63	.53	.98	.73	.80
Average, male interviewers (A and B)	1.08	.17	1.55	1.76	1.32	.96
Average, female interviewers (C and D)	1.26	.39	.56	1.10	.91	.75
Total average	1.17	.28	1.06	1.43	1.11	.85

Self-references were also examined. These showed no differences attributable to interviewer. There was, however, the usual difference between sexes in the relative frequency of self-references, the females making significantly more such references (4.6 vs. 3.6, $p \leqq .025$) than did the males.

In the light of the findings of this study, it is reasonable to conclude that most, if not all, of the differences attributable to interviewers in the prior study were a result of more subtle factors in their personality than their sex. One notable exception was the effect of sex of interviewer on ambivalent hostility scores, which interacted with the sex of the interviewee. Whether the more subtle influence of personality is conveyed by mannerisms, gestures, or tone of voice, we do not know, but evidently some interviewers elicit more emotional content from subjects than do others. Furthermore, these subtle cues may be such that they arouse relatively more hostility and anxiety in subjects of one sex than in the other.

CAN THE INTERVIEWER DELIBERATELY INFLUENCE THE FREQUENCY OF THE VERBAL RESPONSE OF THE SPEAKER WITHOUT THE SPEAKER'S AWARENESS?

We have raised the question and attempted to investigate to what extent the situational context and the personality of the interviewer are capable of influencing the content of an interview. A further question which might be raised is whether subtle, nonvocal activities of the same interviewer can induce changes in the verbal behavior of an interviewee without the latter's awareness. We have undertaken one such study, which we report here (Gottschalk *et al.*, 1963b). Its importance is that it underlines the fact that in investigations of such interpersonal phenomena as verbal communication, interview process, and psychotherapy, the interviewer may have considerable potential influence in shaping interviewee behavior.

Methods

The basic approach in this study was the application of operant conditioning procedures to the verbal behavior of normal subjects asked to give five-minute verbal samples on three occasions in response to our standard instructions.

The subjects were 20 medically and psychiatrically healthy male paid volunteers, all members of the same college social fraternity. The subjects were divided into two groups, matched, of course, for sex and also for age and educational level. The social class, religious affiliation, and cultural background of these young men were quite similar.

The subjects were all told, in a group, that this was a study of speaking and conversational habits and that we wanted to observe their verbal behavior on three successive sessions, spaced approximately within a period of one week. The sessions spread over more than eight days for only four subjects, two in each group.

The specific procedure on each experimental day was for the interviewer to read to the subject our standard instructions for eliciting speech. The subject's speech was tape recorded and transcribed to a typescript.

With one group of subjects (Group A), the interviewer—instead of presenting an immobile facial expression to the interviewee, the expression we usually recommend for our procedure—slowly nodded his head affirmatively in an inconspicuous manner for about two seconds every time the interviewer used self references in the form of words, such as "I," "we," "me," "mine," and "ours." The interviewer continued this behavior during all three sessions when the members of Group A were producing five-minute verbal samples.

For Group B, the interviewer wagged his head gently from side to side for about two seconds to denote negation whenever the subjects used any of the above designated words of self-reference. Again, the interviewer behaved this way during all three five-minute verbal sessions of Group B.

The average number of self-references per 100 words in the three verbal samples of each member of Groups A and B were calculated. Furthermore, the average number of self-references per 100 words for the first half and second half of each five-minute verbal sample (split on the basis of number of words) was computed. The rationale for obtaining these data was that it was considered probable that the frequency of the conditioned response patterns, that is, increase or decrease of self references, was likely to be more prominent with longer exposure to the experimenter's reinforcing behavior per five-minute session.

Results

Both groups obtained a significant decrease in corrected frequency of self reference from the first to the second half of the five-minute verbal sample averaged over all three sessions ($p < .05$). Likewise, both groups showed a trend toward decreasing self references from the first to the third session, when the first half of the verbal sample was considered alone ($p < .01$ for combined groups, no significant interaction). When the trends for the second half of the sessions were analyzed, however, it was found that while the combined linear decreasing trend was again significant, the differential trend was also significant (p < .025). The group receiving negative reinforcement had a very significant decreasing trend in self-references; whereas, the positively reinforced group made about the same number of self-references in all three sessions (see Fig. 9.1 and Table 9.16).

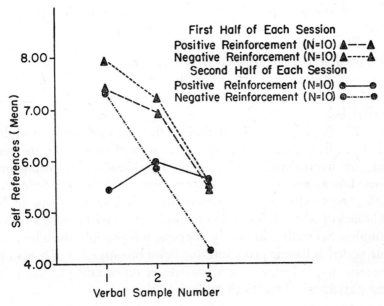

Fig. 9.1. Operant conditioning over three sessions of self-references in five-minute speech samples through affirmative and negative head nodding by the interviewer.

TABLE 9.16

Frequency of Self-References (per 100 words) by Session for Positively (N = 10) and Negatively (N = 10) Reinforced Groups

Segment of speech sample	Positive reinforcement Sessions			Negative reinforcement Sessions			Combined groups Sessions		
	1	2	3	1	2	3	1	2	3
First half	7.36	7.12	5.54	7.93	6.95	5.46	7.64	7.03	5.50
Second half	5.41	5.96	5.61	7.23	5.94	4.10	6.32	5.95	4.86

Linear trend over sessions, first half = 45.92, MS_e = 6.07, F = 7.57, p ≤ .01.
Linear trend over sessions, second half = 21.49, MS_e = 4.71, F = 4.56, p ≤ .05.
Reinforcement × linear trend, second half = 27.39, MS_e = 4.71, F = 5.82, p ≤ .025.

These findings strongly suggest that even minimal kinesic, nonvocal cues, if consistently presented by an interviewer, can influence the content of speech of an interviewee. Furthermore, these changes in speech can occur outside the speaker's awareness. In this study, for instance, not only did the speaker not know that the content of his speech was being influenced, but he did not recognize or recall—on questioning—that the interviewer was moving his head in any specific direction while the interviewee was speaking.

Elsewhere, Krasner (1966) has reviewed the literature and discussed verbal behavior conditioning under the broad title "Behavior modification research and the role of the therapist." There is here cited ample evidence that operant conditioning can change verbal behavior.

The implications of our findings here are primarily twofold. First of all, they underline the importance of controlling the verbal and nonverbal behavior of an interviewer when using our procedure as a means to measure emotions and other psychological states, especially when sequences of verbal samples are to be obtained or when different interviewers are used to collect verbal samples. Secondly, this study suggests the possible usefulness of our verbal behavior procedure for those investigators who plan to examine the influence of the interviewer on certain psychological and physiological reactions of the interviewee.

APPLICATION OF THE CONTENT ANALYSIS SCALES TO VERBAL MATERIAL OTHER THAN THE LANGUAGE BEHAVIOR OBTAINED BY OUR STANDARD INSTRUCTIONS

Some readers may be interested in learning about data we have that concerns the applications of our scales to verbal material that is elicited by other means than the standard instructions. As a convenience to the reader, let us repeat here what the standard instructions are: "This is a study of speaking and conversational habits. Upon a signal from me, I would like you to speak for five minutes about any interesting or dramatic personal life experiences you have had. Once you have started, I will be here listening to you, but I would prefer not to reply to any questions you may feel like asking until the five-minute period is over. Do you have any questions you would like to ask me now before we start? Well, then, you may begin."

It is obvious that the standard instructions lead the speaker to expect a temporary period of nonverbal interaction on the part of the interviewer in which the speaker will be listened to but not spoken to. In addition, with these instructions, a relative lack of gestural and facial signs of encouragement or disapproval are prescribed for the interviewer as he listens to the speaker. The interviewer, in fact, is advised to remain relatively immobile and expressionless while the five-minute speech sample is being uttered.

Many investigators wanting to use our content analysis scales have asked whether samples of verbal behavior obtained under other circumstances can be analyzed according to our scales. We believe that these content scales can be applied to data obtained in different situations than the standard one. But under such circumstances, the distribution of scores we have given (Chapter IV) would, of course, not be relevant. Our content analysis scales have been applied to a variety of different materials, sometimes with interesting results. Let us enumerate and briefly discuss some examples.

DREAMS

Three studies involving the content analysis of dreams (Karacan et al., 1966; Witkin et al., 1969; Gottschalk et al., 1966b) have been reported. Because of the relative shortness of the verbal communications in reporting dreams, some precautions have to be taken toward selecting dream reports above a minimum number of words to insure adequate sampling reliability. We have recommended (Gottschalk et al., 1966b) not including dreams for affect scoring by these scales where there are fewer than 70 words. Even this number of words is somewhat inadequate as a sample of affect, but it was taken as a compromise between inadequate sampling and the complete loss of data.

DIAGNOSTIC OR PSYCHOTHERAPEUTIC INTERVIEWS

Several studies have been reported in which interviews were used as the source of the verbal behavior for scoring content by our scales (Gottschalk and Kaplan, 1958b; Gottschalk et al., 1961b, 1963, 1966a; Witkin et al., 1966, 1968). The procedure has varied from coding successive two- or five-minute sequences of the patient's and/or therapist's speech, the first 500 words of the interview, or successive 500-word sequences of the same. The latter two methods are easier in that they do not require a timing device to mark time-units.

The scores from sequences of time units or word units of interview material are likely, in our opinion, to be influenced not only by the nature of the interpersonal relationship and context in which the speech is elicited, but also by the fact that the sequences of speech are, obviously, not independent and hence are likely to be influenced by the preceding psychologic states and what the speaker anticipates may be the permissible range of psychologic response later and before termination of the interview.

The findings obtained between the dimensions of field dependence and shame anxiety as derived from 500 word units of psychotherapeutic interviews (Witkin et al., 1966, 1968) and single five-minute verbal samples elicited by our standard instructions (de-Groot et al., 1967) give quite different results (see pp. 112 f., 164 f.). Further studies are scheduled to explore the bases for such differences.

Another study compared the concordance between hostility out clinical ratings of five-minute segments in psychoanalytic interviews and verbal anxiety scores derived from the typescripts of these five-minute segments (Gottschalk et al., 1963), and a correlation of .76 was found (see p. 162).

One study explored the correlations between two- and five-minute sequences of two psychotherapeutic interviews and skin temperature as well as pulse rate (Gottschalk et al., 1961b). These data revealed a negative correlation between verbal anxiety and heart rate over each of the two interviews. A significant negative correlation was also found between skin temperature and anxiety in the second interview but not the first. Subsequent analysis, however, of the change in skin temperature from the beginning to the end of each five-minute interval indicated that the change was significantly related to the anxiety occurring in this time interval for both interviews (rank-order correlation = $-.57$ and $-.46$ for the eighth and eighteenth psychotherapeutic interviews, respectively).

Unpublished studies of successive plasma free fatty acid determinations and anxiety scores summated in successive five-minute intervals of a 45-minute affect-eliciting interview on each of five psychiatric patients (Gottschalk et al., 1964c) yielded a positive correlation between free fatty acid and anxiety scores for only three of the patients but corroborated previous findings that patients with higher average free fatty acid levels have higher average anxiety scores. Sequential correlations appeared maximal for the three patients when free fatty acid determinations were lagged by ten minutes.

This would correspond to the notion that the free fatty acids rise relatively slowly in response to psychological stress, reaching a peak in 15 to 25 minutes (Gottschalk et al., 1965b, 1969). However, this model is probably too simple to describe the temporal relationship of free fatty acid and anxiety in successive intervals of time, which may differ slightly from subject to subject and under various experimental conditions; nor does it take into account other factors that may affect the relationship.

It should be noted that sequential units of speech that are arbitrarily unitized and are likely to be contextually and emotionally interrelated may yield different relationships, in phase and magnitude, with continuous physiological variables as compared to what occurs with numerous discrete verbal samples collected over a period of time. With discrete sampling of affects, the inhibition of the expression of emotions imposed by the experimental conditions may influence the magnitude of such emotions when they are elicited. Furthermore, during the period in which the individual is not speaking, his personality dynamics and his perception of the total experimental situation may result in changes in the quality of affects experienced. This does not imply that one type of verbal approach represents a truer picture of the psychophysiological relations than does the other. Rather, information gained from both types of studies can contribute to our knowledge. In other words, the psychoeconomics of emotional expression may be different when the individual is permitted to speak continuously for an hour or more as compared to speaking during separate five-minute intervals.

PROJECTIVE TESTS

Five-minute verbal samples of speech have been elicited, in a standardized manner, by having subjects tell stories in response to a set of four TAT cards, the "visual" method of induction (Gottschalk and Hambidge, 1955; Hambidge and Gottschalk, 1958). Some differences have been noted in certain categories of words per 100 words in verbal samples obtained by such means as compared to using the standard method—the "verbal" method of induction—of asking subjects to talk about any interesting or dramatic personal life experiences. The design of these studies, however, did not involve balancing the order of the "visual" and "verbal" methods of induction of speech, the visual one always being first. Thus, some of these differences may be due to order.

A number of studies, reported elsewhere in this book, have discussed the use of our content analysis scales on TAT material: anxiety (pp. 63, 109), hostility (pp. 66, 163), and human relations (p. 227). These scales do appear to be applicable to TAT protocols, and the results are, in general, in the expected direction. It should be noted here that references to self having various feelings or carrying out various actions are not scorable directly from TAT data.

LETTERS, AUTOBIOGRAPHICAL MATERIALS, AND LITERATURE IN GENERAL

Some interesting content analyses have been done by others on letters, a striking example being the analysis by the electronic computer (Paige, 1964) and by hand (Baldwin, 1942; Anonymous, 1946) of the letters of Jenny.

Our scales have not been applied in any systematic way to letters or literature in general. However, one application to suicide notes (Gottschalk and Gleser, 1960a) turned up some interesting results using our "atomistic" scales.

It seems reasonable to assume that, with properly designed studies, our content scales can be applied to such material. Holsti (1967) has discussed the broader applications of content analysis to language materials from the social sciences (including political science), the behavioral sciences, and literature in general.

CHAPTER X
Applications of Verbal Behavior Analysis Procedure

APPLICATIONS TO PSYCHOPHYSIOLOGY AND PSYCHOSOMATIC MEDICINE

As noted in the Preface, the initial impetus for this verbal behavior analysis procedure came from psychophysiological studies in epilepsy, where it was found that a serious need existed for a method that would provide measures of transient psychological states that might have a cause or effect relationship with paroxysmal electroencephalographic activity or epileptic behavioral manifestations. The content analysis of five-minute verbal samples has now become an important method for measuring labile emotional and other psychological events. The method can be used to investigate such psychophysiological processes as the relationship of anxiety, hostility, or other psychologic states to pulse rate and blood pressure (Gottschalk *et al.*, 1964*b*), galvanic skin response (Fox *et al.*, 1965), oropharyngeal bacterial flora (Gottschalk and Kaplan, 1958*b*; Kaplan *et al.*, 1957, 1958), skin temperature (Gottlieb *et al.*, 1967)[1], phases of the menstrual cycle (Gottschalk *et al.*, 1962; Ivey and Bardwick, 1968), penile erections during dreams (Karacan *et al.*, 1966), plasma hydroxycorticosteroids (Sholiton *et al.*, 1963; Gottschalk *et al.*, 1963), and plasma-free fatty acids in subjects who are awake (Gottschalk *et al.*, 1965*b*, 1969) or those who are asleep and dreaming (Gottschalk *et al.*, 1966*b*). Further, using our content analysis method, the relative levels of various psychological states have been explored in coronary heart disease (Miller, 1965; Gottschalk *et al.*, 1964*c*), essential hypertension (Kaplan *et al.*, 1961; Gottschalk *et al.*, 1964*b*), dermatologic inpatients(Gottschalk *et al.*, 1960*b*), inpatients with

---

[1] See also above, p. 278.

lung cancer as compared to inpatients with nonneoplastic diseases of the chest (Sholiton *et al.*, 1963), inpatients suffering progressive phases of terminal cancer (Kunkel and Gottschalk, 1966; Gottschalk and Kunkel, 1966), general medical inpatients as compared to general psychiatric inpatients or outpatients (Gottschalk and Gleser, 1964*a*), patients with acute or chronic impairment of brain function (Gottschalk *et al.*, 1969), and so forth.

By means of the content analysis method we have developed, many other kinds of investigations can now be pursued involving the relationships of momentary psychological states, as well as more stable and fixed psychologic states, to somatic disease. The possible applications of this verbal behavior content analysis procedure to psychophysiology and psychosomatic medicine have, in our opinion, only begun to be explored.

APPLICATIONS OF CONTENT ANALYSIS METHOD TO PSYCHOPHARMACOLOGY

An independent survey and appraisal of the application of verbal behavior methods to psychopharmacology has been made by Waskow (1967). She has described and discussed not only our content analysis approach, but that of others, and she has emphasized the pioneering aspects of our work.

As has been indicated earlier in this book (pp. 13, 96), psychopharmacological studies have been attractive to us because they provide an avenue for exploring the relationship in humans of neurochemical correlates to feelings, thoughts, and behavior. The biochemical alterations induced by psychoactive pharmacological agents, although in some instances incompletely understood, provide an experimental approach to the psychobiochemistry and psychopharmacology of the mind, now that the use of pharmacological agents in emotional disturbances is a therapeutic procedure which is quite in fashion.

Our own studies in the area of psychopharmacology have, indeed, explored the applications of the content analysis of speech as one means of determining what psychological and behavioral changes are induced by various pharmacological agents. In previous sections of this book dealing with validation studies, we have looked at these psychopharmacologic studies from a somewhat different perspective, namely, how such studies contribute to the construct validation of some of the scales, especially the anxiety and hostility scales. Most of the psychopharmacological studies we have done using our verbal behavior method have not had as an urgent or immediate goal the assessment of the effectiveness of a psychopharmacological agent in any specific type of emotional disorder or mental illness, although there are a few exceptions to this statement. Rather, the focus has been to determine in what way the administration of the psychoactive agent has influenced various key psychological states, drives, or psychopathological symptoms, and quite often these psychopharmacological studies have not involved psychiatric patients (Gottschalk *et al.*, 1968a).

To illustrate some of the kinds of potential applications of these content analysis scales, let us describe briefly some of our own psychopharmacological studies.

Using our content analysis method, a dose of 2–6 mg. pipradrol (Meratran—a psychomotor stimulant), as compared to a placebo, was found to increase significantly not only the number of words spoken in three minutes, but also the number of references to actual or expected accomplishments and strivings for recognition (Gottschalk *et al.*, 1956). Ross *et al.* (1963) along a somewhat similar line asked 80 medical students to *write* five-minute verbal samples in a double-blind, placebo-drug study in which one-third of the students received, by mouth, either a placebo, 10 mg. of dextroamphetamine, or 65 mg. of amobarbital. No significant differences in hostility scores, by the Gottschalk-Gleser content analysis measure, were found with dextroamphetamine. A significantly lower mean anxiety score (p < .05) was found with amobarbital, as compared with dextroamphetamine or the placebo. Also, more words were written, on the average (p < .10), by subjects on amphetamine (108) than on the placebo (95) or amobarbital (86). Gottschalk *et al.* (1968a) explored the influence of the mental set or doctor's attitude on the patient's response to psychoactive medication, using 108 male college students, and having them write ten-minute verbal samples while on either a placebo, secobarbital (90 mg.), or racemic amphetamine sulphate (10 mg). The subjects were exposed to one of three mental sets as to the possible reaction they might expect from the drug. Interesting drug and mental set effects were noted.

Several studies have been reported using these content analysis procedures in psychopharmacological investigations of tranquilizers. In one study (Gleser *et al.*, 1965a), 46 juvenile delinquent boys were administered 20 mg. of chlordiazepoxide (Librium) in a double-blind, placebo-drug study. Adjusting for initial values by covariance analysis, significant decreases were found in anxiety ($p < .01$), ambivalent hostility ($p < .05$), and overt hostility out ($p < .06$) 40 to 120 minutes after ingesting 20 mg. of chlordiazepoxide. No psychological changes were found using the content analysis of five-minute verbal samples 24 hours after ingesting 30 mg. of chlordiazepoxide. In another study (Gottschalk et al., 1960b), 20 dermatologic inpatients (10 men and 10 women, age range 17 to 79) were given 16 to 24 mg. a day of perphenazine (Trilafon) by mouth for one week alternating with a placebo for one week, using a double-blind, cross-over design. Analysis of the content of five-minute verbal samples obtained from these patients showed with perphenazine a reduction of median hostility out scores in 16 of the 20 patients ($p < .01$) and a significant increase in references to feelings of bodily and emotional well being ($p < .02$). With perphenazine, there also occurred a decrease in anxiety scores at the elevated end of the spectrum of anxiety scores derived from the speech samples, but this trend did not quite reach a 0.05 level of confidence. Longitudinal studies of psychopharmacological effects of drugs have also been carried out using the major tranquilizer thioridazine (Mellaril) (Gottschalk et al., 1963–1965, 1968), and the antidepressant imipramine (Tofranil) (Gottschalk et al., 1965a).

Studies of the content analysis of the speech of individuals administered psychotomimetic drugs (LSD-25, Ditran, or Psilocybin) or a placebo showed that people receiving psychotomimetic drugs have significantly higher content analysis scores on our Cognitive and Intellectual Impairment Scale than when they receive a placebo (see Chapter VIII, Cognitive and Intellectual Impairment Scale, pp. 228 f.). Such investigations are useful in supporting the concept that such drugs produce cognitive impairment rather than a schizophrenic psychosis.

APPLICATIONS OF CONTENT ANALYSIS METHOD TO PSYCHOTHERAPY RESEARCH

The applications of our content analysis method to psychotherapy research—both research in the process and outcome of psychotherapy—have just begun to be explored. Our own ventures in this research area may serve to illustrate several of the many approaches. Two of the studies attempted to pursue evaluation of sequential changes in affects or other psychological variables in successive two- or five-minute units of psychotherapeutic interviews.

In one study (Gottschalk *et al.*, 1961*b*), two widely spaced treatment interviews were broken down into successive two- and five-minute units, and these were scored for anxiety, hostility outward, social alienation–personal disorganization (schizophrenia), achievement strivings, and a number of other psychologic states. There was an opportunity in this study to make some preliminary comparisons (specifically, correlations) of the time-unit scores on these psychological variables with either comparable psychological variables focused on by other investigators, for example, the type-token-ratio (Jaffe, 1961) and the speech disturbance ratio (Mahl, 1961), or two physiological variables, for example, pulse rate and skin temperature (DiMascio, 1961).

In another study (Gottschalk *et al.*, 1966*a*), we formulated the assumptions and hypotheses on which we based our method of quantification of affects. Also, we again illustrated the quantification of anxiety and hostility in successive five-minute units of a psychotherapeutic interview, a breakdown of relative amounts of different kinds of anxiety per five-minute units, and the differences in anxiety scores when only the typescript of the interview was used for scoring as compared to the use of both a typescript and tape recording of the interview (see also, Gottschalk and Frank, 1967). Alternate ways of handling the therapist's contribution to the interview process and of the levels of affect were also suggested.

An approach to using our verbal behavior procedure in prediction and outcome research in psychotherapy has recently been completed (Gottschalk *et al.*, 1967). Here was examined and discovered the predictive value of pretreatment five-minute verbal sample scores of human relations, social alienation–personal disorganization (schizophrenia), anxiety, and hostility obtained from acutely disturbed patients coming to an emergency, brief psychotherapy clinic that patients could not attend for more than six treatment sessions. The use of certain scores derived from five-minute verbal samples as outcome measures was also explored; for these kinds of patients, the most promising content analysis scales appeared to be the Human Relations Scale, the Social Alienation–Personal Disorganization (Schizophrenic) Scale, the Anxiety Scale, and the Hostility Inward Scale. An exploration was carried out of the possible use of ten-minute written verbal samples as a substitute for five-minute spoken verbal samples, and some evidence was obtained that ten-minute written verbal samples may provide as adequate predictive and evaluative data. If this finding holds up in further studies, the use of the written verbal samples may be preferential in certain types of investigations, especially where economy and speed is an issue, for transcribing tape recordings of speech is a relatively costly and time-consuming procedure.

In Chapter IX of this book, we have described several studies indicating how our content analysis may be used to investigate the effect of the personality of an interviewer on the verbal behavior patterns of the interviewee (pp. 259 f.). These studies suggest avenues for further research in unplanned effects of the therapist on his patients.

There is no doubt that considerably more complex psychodynamic relationships can be objectively examined using our verbal behavior content analysis method by itself or in combination with other psychological measures or even physiological or biochemical variables. It is only a matter of time before further exploratory scientifically objective and rigorous steps will be taken into the area of psychotherapy, a research area that has been and still is highly impressionistic, inexact, and heavily burdened with heretofore untestable clinical hypotheses.

APPLICATIONS OF CONTENT ANALYSIS PROCEDURE TO PERSONALITY THEORY AND RESEARCH

The range of applications of this content analysis method to personality theory has not been fully explored. We have purposely chosen the broad term "personality theory" here so as to include a wide variety of theories relating to development, psychopathology, personality determinants—psychological, social, cultural, genetic, congenital, traumatic, histogenic—and so forth.

Personality variables may be classified as invariant, stable, labile, transient, behavioral versus psychological, interrelated versus discrete, psychodynamic, conflicted, occurrent, dispositional, conscious, and unconscious and in many other ways. Our content analysis method provides a means of measuring most of these kinds of personality variables. The successful application of these scales is to a large extent determined by the ingenuity of the researcher and the kind of design he is able to originate and develop.

So far, we have not used our procedure to any great extent

for the purpose of measuring unvarying features of personality, such as traits. Rather, we have tended to focus on the more change-able aspects of personality, such as the emotions of anxiety and hostility. We have, however, attempted to develop measures of some more stable traits or characterological makeups, such as the schizoid or the schizophrenic person.

We have also worked on the variables that appear to give a measure of primarily dispositional characteristics, such as the capacity to have constructive and satisfying human relations. Also, there are scales we have developed which appear to measure per-sonality responses that are prominently influenced by the environ-mental context or social field in which the individual is located; one such scale, for example, is the Dependency Strivings Scale.

Witkin *et al.* (1966, 1968) have used our scales, particularly the shame and guilt subscales of our Anxiety Scale, to explore the relationship of these affects to certain cognitive and perceptual styles, namely, the field-dependent and field-independent classifi-cations. Using psychotherapeutic interviews as the conversational material from which shame and guilt have been measured, Witkin has reported preliminary findings of a positive relationship of shame anxiety with field dependence and of guilt anxiety with field independence when the Witkin rod and frame test (1954) is used as the principal criterion of field dependence and field independence. In our laboratory, however, deGroot *et al.* (1967) have found a different relationship between these psychological variables when using five-minute verbal samples as the source of shame and guilt anxiety scores instead of psychotherapeutic inter-view material and the Embedded Figures Test (Witkin, 1950) as a criterion of field dependence and field independence. It is quite possible that interviewer effects or interviewee differences may be responsible for these different correlations; the content analysis procedures and scales lend themselves nicely to the investigation of these subtle interactions.

Sequential analysis of content within psychiatric interviews might provide some means of exploring psychodynamic relation-ships between different psychological variables, such as dependency strivings conflicting with shame. Also, conceivably one could ex-plore one of the psychoanalytic hypotheses that hostility directed outwards, if it increases beyond a certain intensity, can lead to increases in hostility directed inwards and depression. This would require sequential quantitative analysis of these affects per unit time during a psychiatric interview.

Some of our newer scales have promising applications to the exploration of social and cultural determinants of attitudes and behavior. The Human Relations Scale and the Achievement Strivings Scale are good examples of such scales, and the Scale of Cognitive and Intellectual Impairment might be useful in investigating transient, potentially reversible impairment of brain function as well as more chronic brain syndromes.

Actually, the possible applications of such a content analysis method to personality as we have broadly conceived it are so numerous that it would be futile to try to enumerate them. We refer the reader to a recent review of the literature on content analysis which points out some of the possibilities (Holsti *et al.*, 1967).

CHAPTER XI
The Future of Content Analysis Procedures

IMMEDIATE PROSPECTS

In Chapter X we have described some recent applications of this content analysis procedure and have pointed to directions for further applications.

At the present time, there are several choices open to the clinical or basic researcher who wants to explore the use of content analysis of interview material or of written or spoken speech obtained by any other of a myriad of methods.

One general choice of content categories is a classification system which includes largely nonlexical areas, such as uhs, ahs, and ers; expletives; laughs; sighs; aposiopeses, and so forth. Although we briefly explored this approach to content analysis early in our work in this area (Gottschalk and Hambidge, 1955), we gave it up soon thereafter.

A second level of content analysis is one that classifies content according to single word categories, based on such classifications as, grammatical ones or according to persons, things, places, abstractions, thought processes, emotional processes, action processes, states of being, and so forth. In such simple classifications, the researcher—after making counts of such content categories— may subsequently have to decide how he is going to put together such information in order to draw more meaningful conclusions. Our own "atomistic" system (Gottschalk *et al.*, 1955, 1957) is one example, and that of Hall and Van de Castle (1966), which has been applied to the content analysis of dreams, is another.

We discontinued our own efforts in the first and second approaches to content analysis for two principal reasons. First, we felt we could not adequately progress in this area of investigation if we tried to cover all facets of communication and that we had to limit the concentration of our energies to the most immediately promising facet. Second, we felt reasonably certain that very simple approaches to content analysis, as exemplified above, might be capable of providing a reliable tally of the phenomena described but most certainly would tend to lack the specifiable relevance to clinically observable and psychiatrically observable phenomena and to psychodynamically and psychoanalytically oriented personality theory.

The researcher can choose a third type of approach to content analysis system based on larger and more complex units of communications, such as the grammatical clause or sentence. Under such circumstances, the content categories may relate to directly or indirectly stated content. Especially in the case of the latter, more theory is likely to be already built into the categorization and scaling than with word categorization systems. Our own content analysis procedure belongs to this third classification of content analysis approaches.

Although there are conceivably some disadvantages in letting categorization of content be influenced too early by some theoretical vantage point, we contend that all categorizations of content are based on some selective principle and, hence, are ordered according to some hypothesis, even though it is not made explicit or has not been formulated. We are of the opinion that if the content analysis is to be carried out in order to pursue answers to psychologic, social, or psychiatric questions, content categories based on psychodynamic and clinical psychoanalytic hypotheses are likely to provide more meaningful use of the data than categories which have no obvious relevance to psychodynamic personality theory or any specifiable type of personality theory.

At present there is some awareness among researchers working in the area of content analysis that there are different theoretical approaches and, within these, different levels of integration and meaning. Intercommunication between these researchers has been limited, but there are signs of attempts at interdisciplinary and intradisciplinary cross-fertilization as exemplified in the recent U.S. Public Health Service-sponsored Verbal Behavior Conference, the proceedings of which have been published under the editorship of K. Salzinger and S. Salzinger (1967). More such conferences and other means of exchange of information should be sought by investigators in this area to enhance research progress.

COMPUTER APPLICATIONS TO CONTENT ANALYSIS

Content analysis procedures may eventually be capable of adaptation to computer analysis. A tremendous saving of time, an increase in uniformity of scoring, and a broad survey of the qualitative and quantitative interrelationships between many different kinds of psychologic states are all possible results of computer assistance in this area of research.

Preparing a faithful typescript from written or spoken speech is time consuming. A shortcut would be a system whereby speech could be transformed to recognizable and classifiable bits of information which could be directly fed to a computer programmed to analyze the material for any specifiable psychologic dimensions. Investigators (Presti, 1966; Mathews and McMahon, 1966; Denes, 1966) have made considerable progress in transforming speech spoken into a microphone directly into a typescript produced by an automated typewriter. This has been accomplished by studying phonetic patterns on the spectrograph which result from the utterance of certain sounds and words and constructing a machine which decodes (recognizes and identifies) the patterns to activate keys and clusters of keys in an electric typewriter. As far as this system goes, it already provides a saving of time and money. An electronic computer could, conceivably, accomplish even more: the scoring of such typescripts to provide the quantitative indices of psychologic variables we have described. Ideally, in fact, it is conceivable that the computer could handle these separate operations without the necessity of obtaining a typescript of the speech. That is, the content analysis could be done directly from a tape recording and an automated print-out could be obtained giving, for example, running scores every three to five minutes of anxiety or hostility from an ongoing interview. Much more complicated evaluations, in fact, could be obtained based on psychodynamic theories.

One of the biggest stumbling blocks to such an automated system is that, at the present time, a human being has to label each word in a sample of speech with the appropriate syntactical tag indicating how it is used in a sentence so that the computer can put together the words in meaningful sentences approximating the information intended by the speaker. If this step is carried out, it is now possible to write a program encompassing a large variety of contents, so that the computer can count the frequency of occurrence of these categories of content and can perform certain statistical evaluations of these data.

Several interesting and promising attempts have been made to apply computer analysis to content analysis. Philip Stone and his collaborators (Stone et al., 1962, 1963, 1967; Stone, 1963; Paige, 1964) have pioneered a large group of these studies and have set up computer programs capable of classifying content (the General Inquirer System) and of ordering these content categories with one another in meaningful ways, for example, by use of the Concept Learner (Hunt, 1962), a computer program system for building rules for discriminating between two text sources. Briefly, it is a computer program for automatically analyzing themes, and Stone and his associates have used it successfully in combination with his content analysis computer program.

Jaffe (1964) has also worked on using the computer as a tool in content analysis with some interesting results. He has not directed his attention thus far to the more complex meanings in verbal communications, as have Stone et al. Rather, he has focussed on the more atomistic aspects of content, concentrating on grammatical categories and the type-token ratio (TTR),[1] as well as on certain noncontent aspects of speech, such as rate of speech.

Holsti et al. (1967) have recently reviewed the literature on the use of computers in content analysis; they have, moreover, supplied many suggestions concerning uses of content analysis.

Hopefully, application of computer techniques to content analysis will evolve and progress rapidly, so that some of the present tedious and laborious aspects of content analysis will be eliminated.

The computer will not be able to generate hypotheses with regards to meaningful communication aspects of language. These will come from those who read and listen to language and who try to formulate general principles from what they see and hear about how human beings communicate the range of feelings and thoughts they experience. At this stage in our development of the computer, its power appears to be its capacity to help us test the hypotheses which we instruct it to examine, at a speed and efficiency that has never before been possible.

---

[1] The TTR is a measure of verbal diversification (Johnson, 1944). It is defined as the number of different words (types) divided by the number of word units (tokens).

DISTANT GOALS AND PROSPECTS

When automated analysis of the superficial and underlying content of speech becomes a current reality, many scientific wonders will be possible. It may be difficult to overcome some of the current obstacles to such an achievement, not only in the area of automation, but also in the area of defining operationally and conceptually what clusters of content serve as cues of different levels of meaning. These are problems that need to be systematically investigated—carefully, patiently, and rigorously. As such research progresses, the behavioral sciences and clinical psychiatry will obtain a channel for more effective cross-fertilization. Moreover, clinical psychology and psychiatry will obtain a powerful tool for testing many of their working hypotheses, which today, unfortunately, sometimes masquerade as scientific truths only on the basis of archaic tradition, new fashion, or the unfounded endorsement of some persons of prominence.

As content analysis becomes perfected, the prediction of educational, vocational, or marital success from small samples of written or spoken speech will be possible on a probability basis. The assessment, on a moment-to-moment basis, of the emotional and cognitive functioning and intactness of a person anywhere on earth or in outer space will be possible by monitoring an individual's speech and obtaining simultaneous automated analysis of it. Evaluation and prediction of emotional adjustment, cognitive impairment, value orientations, political views, and so forth of political candidates or of industrial and business executives will be made in a brief time. Noxious effects of the environment—air pollution, radiation, heavy metals, even stressful effects of sudden disasters—will be ascertained by a proximal or remote assessment team monitoring the speech of exposed individuals. Psychophysiological, psychobiochemical, and psychopharmacological relationships will be capable of much more adequate and exact measurement than has ever been possible and will provide new methods of medical diagnosis and treatment.

Will psychotherapy ever be possible by a preprogrammed machine, capable of analyzing and appropriately responding to a speaker? Although the idea has been playfully and informally suggested in recent years, it seems too fantastic and mechanical to consider seriously. Our current perspective about such a matter, in fact, would put us in the position that, although a machine could be trained by our best psychotherapists, its effectiveness and congeniality could never equal a human therapist. Perhaps on such an issue we should keep an open mind. Perspectives can change when facts are persuasive.

BIBLIOGRAPHY

Abraham, K. (1916). The First Pregenital Stage of the Libido, in *Selected Papers on Psycho-Analysis*. London: Hogarth Press, 1927*a*.
————. (1924). A Short Study of the Development of the Libido, in *Selected Papers on Psycho-Analysis*. London: Hogarth Press, 1927*b*.
Albrink, M. J. Triglycerides, lipo-proteins, and coronary artery disease, *Arch. Int. Med.*, 109: 345, 1962.
Alexander, F. The influence of psychologic factors upon gastrointestinal disturbances: General principles, objectives, and preliminary results, *Psa. Quart.*, 3: 501, 1934.
————. A case of peptic ulcer and personality disorder, *Psychosom. Med.*, 9: 320–330, 1947.
Amarel, M., and F. E. Cheek. Some effects of LSD-25 on communication, *J. Abnorm. Psychol.*, 70: 453–456, 1965.
Anonymous. Letters from Jenny, *J. Abnorm. Soc. Psychol.*, 41: 315–350, 449–480, 1946.
Arieti, S. Special logic of schizophrenia and other types of autistic thought, *Psychiat.*, 11: 325–338, 1948.
————. Autistic thought: Its formal mechanisms and its relationship to schizophrenia, *J. Nerv. Ment. Dis.*, 111: 288–303, 1950.
————. Some aspects of the psychopathology of schizophrenia, *Am. J. Psychother.*, 8: 396–414, 1954.
Aserinsky, E., and N. Kleitman. Regularly occurring periods of eye motility, and concomitant phenomena, during sleep, *Science*, 118: 273–274, 1953.
————. Two types of ocular motility in sleep, *J. Appl. Physiol.*, 8: 1–10, 1955.
Auld, F., Jr., and J. Dollard. Measurement of Motivational Variables in Psychotherapy, in *Methods of Research in Psychotherapy*, ed. L. A. Gottschalk and A. H. Auerbach. New York: Appleton-Century-Crofts, 1966.
Ax, A. F. The physiological differentiation between fear and anger in humans, *Psychosom. Med.*, 15: 433–442, 1953.
Axelrod, J., and J. Glowinski. Inhibition of uptake of tritiated norepinephrine in the intact rat brain by imipramine and structurally related compounds, *Nature*, 204: 1318, 1964.
Baldwin, A. L. Personal structure analysis: A statistical method for investigating the single personality, *J. Abnorm. Soc. Psychol.*, 37: 163–183, 1942.
Bales, R. L. *Interaction Process Analysis*. Cambridge, Mass.: Addison-Wesley, 1950.
Bass, B. M. Development of a structured disguised personality inventory, *J. Appl. Psychol.*, 40: 393–397, 1956.
Beck, A. T., C. H. Ward, M. Mendelson, J. Mock, and J. Erbaugh. An inventory for measuring depression, *Arch. Gen. Psychiat.*, 4: 561–571, 1961.
Beecher, H. *Measurement of Subjective Responses*. New York: Oxford University Press, 1959.
Bellak, L., and M. B. Smith. An experimental exploration of the psychoanalytic process, *Psa. Quart.*, 25: 385–414, 1956.
Bellak, L., and P. K. Benedict, eds. *Schizophrenia: A Review of the Syndrome*. New York: Logos Press, 1958.
Bellak, L., and L. Small. *Emergency Psychotherapy and Brief Psychotherapy*. New York: Grune and Stratton, 1965.
Berelson, B. *Content Analysis in Communication Research*. Glencoe, Ill.: The Free Press, 1952.

Birdwhistell, R. L. The Kinesic Level in the Investigation of the Emotions, in *Expression of the Emotions in Man*, ed. P. H. Knapp. New York: International Universities Press, 1963.

Bjerstedt, A. Critical Review of the Rosenzweig P-F Study, in *The Sixth Mental Measurements Yearbook*, ed. O. K. Buros. Highland Park, N.J.: The Gryphon Press, 1965.

Bleuler, E. (1911). *Dementia Praecox or the Group of Schizophrenias*. Trans. J. Zinkin. New York: International Universities Press, 1950.

Bogdonoff, M. D., and E. H. Estes, Jr. Energy dynamics and acute states of arousal, *Psychosom. Med.*, 23: 23, 1961.

Boomer, D. C., and D. W. Goodrich. Speech disturbances and judged anxiety, *J. Consult. Psychol.*, 25: 160, 1961.

Bowlby, J. Separation anxiety, *Int. J. Psa.*, 41: 89–113, 1960.

Brady, J. V. Psychophysiology of Emotional Behavior, in *Experimental Foundations of Clinical Psychology*, ed. A. J. Bachrach. New York: Basic Books, 1962.

Brodie, B. B., S. Spector, and P. A. Shore. Interaction of drugs with norepinephrine in the brain, *Pharmacol. Rev.*, 11: 548, 1959.

Bruce, R. A., L. A. Cobb, and R. H. Williams. Effects of exercise and isoproterenol on free fatty acids and carbohydrates in cardiac patients, *Am. J. Med. Sci.*, 241: 59, 1961.

Buss, A. H. *The Psychology of Aggression*. New York: John Wiley and Sons, Inc., 1961.

Buss, A. H., A. Durkee, and M. Baer. The measurement of hostility in clinical situations, *J. Abnorm. Soc. Psychol.*, 52: 84–86, 1956.

Cameron, J. L., T. Freeman, and A. McGhie. Clinical observations on chronic schizophrenia, *Psychiat.*, 19: 271–281, 1956.

Cannon, W. B. *Bodily Changes in Pain, Hunger, Fear, and Rage*. 2d ed.; New York: Appleton-Century-Crofts, 1936.

Carlson, L. A. Determination of serum glycerides, *Acta Soc. Med. Upsal.*, 64: 208, 1959.

Carroll, J. B. *The Study of Language*. Cambridge, Mass.: Harvard University Press, 1955.

Carroll, J. B., F. B. Agard, D. E. Dulany, S. S. Newman, L. Newmark, C. E. Osgood, T. A. Sebeok, and R. L. Solomon. Report and Recommendation of the Interdisciplinary Summer Seminar in Psychology and Linguistics, pp. 27–29. Ithaca, N.Y., 1951.

Cattell, R. B. *Handbook for the IPAT Anxiety Scale*. Champaign, Ill.: Institute for Personality and Ability Testing, 1957.

Cattell, R. B., and H. W. Eber. *Handbook for the Sixteen Personality Factor Questionnaire*. Champaign, Ill.: Institute for Personality and Ability Testing, 1957 (1964 Supplementation).

Cattell, R. B., and I. H. Scheier. *The Meaning and Measurement of Neuroticism and Anxiety*. New York: Ronald Press, 1961.

Chance, E. Content Analysis of Verbalizations about Interpersonal Experience, in *Methods of Research in Psychotherapy*, ed. L. A. Gottschalk and A. H. Auerbach. New York: Appleton-Century-Crofts, 1966.

Clements, W. H. Marital Adjustment and Marital Interaction. Unpublished Ph.D. dissertation, University of Cincinnati, 1968.

Clyde, D. J. *Clyde Mood Scale*. Washington, D.C.: George Washington University, 1961.

Colby, K. M. Experiment on the effects of an observer's presence on the imago system during psychoanalytic free-association, *Behav. Sci.*, 5: 216–232, 1960.

Cook, W. W., and D. M. Medley. Proposed hostility and pharisaic-virtue scales for the MMPI, *J. Appl. Psychol.*, 38: 414–418, 1954.

Corboz, R. J. Proprietes et indications therapeutiques du chlordiazepoxyde (Librium) chez l'enfant et l'adolescent, *Med. Hyg.*, 20: 190–191, 1962.

Cronbach, L. J., N. Rajaratnam, and G. C. Gleser. Theory of generalizability: A liberalization of reliability theory, *Brit. J. Statist. Psychol.*, 16: 137–163, 1963.

Darrow, C. W. Differences in the physiological reactions to sensory and ideational stimuli, *Psychol. Bull.*, 26: 185–201, 1929.

Darwin, C. (1872). *The Expression of the Emotions in Man and Animals.* New York: Philosophical Library, 1955.

Davis, H. L. Role of ionic fatty acids in stress and their determination, *Circulation*, 26: 650, 1962.

deGroot, J. C., G. C. Gleser, and L. A. Gottschalk. The relationship between field dependence-independence, a psychometric measure of response tendency, and certain affect dimensions. Unpublished study, 1967.

Denes, P. B. Real-Time Speech Research, in *The Human Use of Computing Machines. Proceedings of a Symposium Concerned with Diverse Ways of Enhancing Perception and Intuition.* Murray Hill, N.J.: Bell Telephone Laboratories, 1966.

Dengler, H. J., I. A. Michaelson, H. E. Spiegel, and E. O. Titus. The uptake of labeled norepinephrine by isolated brain and other tissues of the cat, *Int. J. Neuropharmacol.*, 1: 23, 1962.

DeVos, G. A. A quantitative approach to affective symbolism in Rorschach responses, *J. Proj. Techn.*, 16: 133–150, 1952.

DiMascio, A. Some Physiologic Correlates of the Psycholinguistic Patterns of Two Psychiatric Interviews, in *Comparative Psycholinguistic Analysis of Two Psychotherapeutic Interviews*, pp. 139–150, ed. L. A. Gottschalk. New York: International Universities Press, 1961.

Dinwiddie, F. W. An application of the principle of response generalization to the prediction of aggressive responses. Unpublished doctor's dissertation, Catholic University of America, 1954.

Dittmann, A. T., and L. C. Wynne. Linguistic techniques and the analysis of emotionality in interviews, *J. Abnorm. Soc. Psychol.*, 63: 201–204, 1961.

Dole, V. P. Relation between non-esterified fatty acids in plasma and metabolism of glucose, *J. Clin. Invest.*, 35: 150, 1956.

Dollard, J., and F. Auld, Jr. *Scoring Human Motives: A Manual.* New Haven: Yale University Press, 1959.

Dollard, J., and O. H. Mowrer. A method of measuring tension in written documents, *J. Abnorm. Soc. Psychol.*, 42: 3–32, 1947.

Dykman, R. A., P. T. Ackerman, C. R. Galbrecht, and W. G. Reese. Physiological reactivity to different stressors and methods of evaluation, *Psychosom. Med.*, 25: 37–59, 1963.

Edwards, A. L. *Edwards Personal Preference Schedule Manual.* New York: The Psychological Corp., 1954.

Eldred, S., and D. B. Price. A linguistic evaluation of feeling states in psychotherapy, *Psychiat.*, 21: 115–121, 1958.

Elizur, A. Content analysis of the Rorschach with regard to anxiety and hostility, *J. Proj. Techn.*, 13: 247–284, 1949.

Endler, N. S., J. McV. Hunt, and A. J. Rosenstein. An S-R inventory of anxiousness, *Psychol. Monogr.*, 76: 1–33, 1962.

Fenichel, O. *The Psychoanalytic Theory of Neurosis.* New York: W. W. Norton and Co., 1945.

Fillenbaum, S., and L. V. Jones. An application of "Cloze" technique to the study of aphasic speech, *J. Abnorm. Soc. Psychol.*, 65: 183–189, 1962.

Finney, B. C. Rorschach test correlates of assaultive behavior, *J. Proj. Techn.*, 19: 6–17, 1955.

Firth, J. R. Linguistic Analysis and Translation, in *For Roman Jakobson: Essays on the Occasion of His Sixtieth Birthday.* The Hague: Mouton, 1956.

Fischer, M. G. The prediction of assaultiveness in hospitalized mental patients. Unpublished doctor's dissertation, Pennsylvania State University, 1956.

Fisher, C. Psychoanalytic implications of recent research on sleep and dreaming, Part I, Empirical findings, *J. Amer. Psa. Assn.*, 13: 197–262, 1965.

Fishman, J. R., P. S. Mueller, and V. Stoeffler. Changes in emotional state and in plasma free fatty acids induced by hypnotic suggestion (Abstract), *Psychosom. Med.*, 24: 522, 1962.

Flegel, H. Erassung schizophrener Morbiditatsverlaufe mit Gottschalks verbaler Stich-probe, verglichen mit Wittenborns Rating Scales und der BPRS, *Zeitschrift für Psychotherapie und medizinische Psychologie*, 5: 186–194, 1967 (Stuttgart).

Fox, R., L. A. Gottschalk, and G. C. Gleser. Relation of anxiety levels to GSR variables. Unpublished studies, 1965.

Freud, S. (1917). Mourning and Melancholia, in *Collected Papers*, Vol. IV. London: Hogarth Press, 1925.

———. *The Problem of Anxiety*. New York: W. W. Norton and Co., 1936.

———. (1915–1916). *Introductory Lectures on Psychoanalysis* (Standard Edition, 15–16). London: Hogarth Press, 1963.

Friedman, M., and R. H. Rosenman. Association of specific overt behavior patterns with blood cholesterol levels, blood clotting time, incidence of arcus senilis, and coronary artery disease, *J.A.M.A.*, 169: 1286, 1959.

———. Overt behavior patterns in coronary disease: Detection of overt behavior pat-terns in patients with coronary disease by a new psychophysiologic procedure, *J.A.M.A.*, 173: 1320, 1960.

Funkenstein, D. H. Norepinephrine-like and epinephrine-like substances in relation to human behavior, *J. Nerv. Ment. Dis.*, 124: 58–67, 1956.

Funkenstein, D. H., M. Greenblatt, and H. C. Solomon. Norepinephrine-like and epinephrine-like substances in psychotic and psychoneurotic patients, *Am. J. Psychiat.*, 108: 652–662, 1952.

Gellhorn, E., and G. N. Loofbourrow. *Emotions and Emotional Disorders. A Neuro-physiological Disorder*. New York: Hoeber-Harper, 1963.

Gershon, E. S., M. Cromer, and G. L. Klerman. Hostility and depression, *Psychiatry*, 31: 224–235, 1968.

Gey, K. F., and A. Pletscher. Activity of monoamine oxidase in relation to the 5-hydroxytryptamine and norepinephrine content of the rat brain, *J. Neurochem.*, 6 (3) : 239–243, 1961.

Gleser, G. C. An adjective checklist for measuring affect. Unpublished study, 1960.

Gleser, G. C., L. A. Gottschalk, and W. John. The relationship of sex and intelligence to choice of words: A normative study of verbal behavior, *J. Clin. Psychol.*, 15: 182–191, 1959.

Gleser, G. C., L. A. Gottschalk, and K. J. Springer. An anxiety scale applicable to verbal samples, *Arch. Gen. Psychiat.*, 5: 593–605, 1961.

Gleser, G. C., L. A. Gottschalk, R. Fox, and W. Lippert. Immediate changes in affect with Chlordiazepoxide in juvenile delinquent boys, *Arch. Gen. Psychiat.*, 13: 291–295, 1965a.

Gleser, G. C., L. J. Cronbach, and N. Rajaratnam. Generalizability of scores influ-enced by multiple sources of variance, *Psychometrika*, 30: 395–418, 1965b.

Gleser, G. C., L. A. Gottschalk, W. N. Stone, and J. A. Cleghorn. Changes in the severity of social alienation–personal disorganization in chronic schizophrenic pa-tients; psychometric and psychopharmacological factors. Presented at the *Sym-posium on Schizophrenia* at the Waldorf-Astoria, New York City, Nov. 12–14, 1968.

Gluck, M. R. The relationship between hostility in the TAT and behavioral hostility, *J. Proj. Techn.*, 19: 21–26, 1955a.

———. Rorschach content and hostile behavior, *J. Consult. Psychol.*, 19: 475–479, 1955b.

Goodstein, L. D. The language of schizophrenia, *J. Genet. Psychol.*, 45: 95–104, 1951.

Gordon, R. S., Jr., and A. Cherkes. Unesterified fatty acid in human blood plasma, *J. Clin. Invest.*, 35: 206, 1956.

Gottlieb, A., G. C. Gleser, and L. A. Gottschalk. Verbal and physiological responses to hypnotic suggestion of attitudes, *Psychosom. Med.*, 24: 172–183, 1967.

Gottschalk, L. A. Effects of intensive psychotherapy on epileptic children. *Arch. Neurol. Psychiat.*, 70: 361–384, 1953.

———. Psychologic conflict and electroencephalographic patterns. Some notes on the problem of correlating changes in paroxysmal electroencephalographic patterns with psychologic conflicts, *Arch. Neurol. Psychiat.*, 73: 656–662, 1955.

————. The Relationship of Psychologic State and Epileptic Activity. Psychoanalytic Observations on an Epileptic Child, in *Psychoanalytic Study of the Child*, Vol. XI. New York: International Universities Press, Inc., 1956.

————. Introspection and Free Association as Experimental Approaches to Assessing Subjective and Behavioral Effects of Psychoactive Drugs, ch. 48, in *Drugs and Behavior*, ed. L. M. Uhr and J. G. Miller. New York: John Wiley & Sons, 1960.

————. Depressions—Psychodynamic Considerations, ch. 11, in *Pharmacotherapy of Depressions*, pp. 30–46, ed. J. O. Cole and J. R. Wittenborn. Springfield, Ill.: Charles C Thomas, 1966.

————. Some applications of the psychoanalytic concept of object-relatedness: Preliminary studies on a human relations scale applicable to verbal samples. Presented at the Topeka Psychoanalytic Society, April 20, 1967. *Compr. Psychiat.*, 9: 608–620, 1968.

Gottschalk, L. A., and A. H. Auerbach, eds. *Methods of Research in Psychotherapy.* New York: Appleton-Century-Crofts, 1966.

Gottschalk, L. A., and R. L. Kunkel. Changes in Emotional and Intellectual Functioning after Total Body Radiation, in *Metabolic Changes in Humans Following Total Body Radiation*, ed. E. L. Saenger, B. J. Friedman, J. G. Keriakes, and H. Perry. Report period February, 1960, through April, 1966, to Defense Atomic Support Agency, Washington, D.C., on Research Grant DA-49-146-XZ-315. Prepared by the University of Cincinnati College of Medicine, Cincinnati General Hospital, Cincinnati, Ohio.

Gottschalk, L. A., R. L. Kunkel, T. H. Wohl, E. L. Saenger, C. N. Winget. Total and half body irradiation: Effect on cognitive and emotional processes. *Arch. Gen. Psychiat.* (in press), 1969.

Gottschalk, L. A., and G. Hambidge, Jr. Verbal behavior analysis: A systematic approach to the problem of quantifying psychologic processes, *J. Proj. Techn.*, 19: 387–409, 1955.

Gottschalk, L. A., and G. Hambidge, Jr. Effect of interviewer on anxiety and hostility of interviewee. Unpublished study, 1956.

Gottschalk, L. A., F. T. Kapp, W. D. Ross, S. M. Kaplan, H. Silver, J. A. MacLeod, J. B. Kahn, Jr., E. F. Van Maanen, and G. H. Acheson. Explorations in testing drugs affecting physical and mental activity. Studies with a new drug of potential value in psychiatric illness, *J.A.M.A.*, 161: 1054–1058, 1956.

Gottschalk, L. A., G. C. Gleser, and G. Hambidge, Jr. Verbal behavior analysis: Some content and form variables in speech relevant to personality adjustment, *Arch. Neurol. Psychiat.*, 77: 300–311, 1957.

Gottschalk, L. A., G. C. Gleser, R. S. Daniels, and S. L. Block. The speech patterns of schizophrenic patients: A method of assessing relative degree of personal disorganization and social alienation, *J. Nerv. Ment. Dis.*, 127: 153–166, 1958a.

Gottschalk, L. A., and S. M. Kaplan. A quantitative method of estimating variations in intensity of a psychologic conflict or state, *Arch. Neurol. Psychiat.*, 79: 688–696, 1958b.

Gottschalk, L. A., and G. C. Gleser. An analysis of the verbal content of suicide notes, *Brit. J. Med. Psychol.*, 33: 195–204, 1960a.

Gottschalk, L. A., G. C. Gleser, K. J. Springer, S. M. Kaplan, J. Shanon, and W. D. Ross. Effects of Perphenazine on verbal behavior patterns, *Arch. Gen. Psychiat.*, 2: 632–639, 1960b.

Gottschalk, L. A., G. C. Gleser, E. B. Magliocco, and T. L. D'Zmura. Further studies on the speech patterns of schizophrenic patients. Measuring inter-individual differences in relative degree of personal disorganization and social alienation, *J. Nerv. Ment. Dis.*, 132: 101–113, 1961a.

Gottschalk, L. A., K. J. Springer, and G. C. Gleser. Experiments with a Method of Assessing the Variations in Intensity of Certain Psychological States Occurring During Two Psychotherapeutic Interviews, ch. 7, in *Comparative Psycholinguistic Analysis of Two Psychotherapeutic Interviews*, ed. L. A. Gottschalk. New York: International Universities Press, 1961b.

Gottschalk, L. A., S. M. Kaplan, G. C. Gleser, and C. M. Winget. Variations in magnitude of emotion: A method applied to anxiety and hostility during phases of the menstrual cycle, *Psychosom. Med.*, 24: 300–311, 1962.

Gottschalk, L. A., G. C. Gleser, and K. J. Springer. Three hostility scales applicable to verbal samples, *Arch. Gen. Psychiat.*, 9: 254–279, 1963.

Gottschalk, L. A., G. C. Gleser, W. N. Stone, J. M. Cleghorn, and C. M. Winget. Drugs, Personality, and Verbal Behavior. U.S.P.H.S. Research Project Grant MH-08282. Unpublished studies, 1963–1965.

Gottschalk, L. A., G. C. Gleser, and E. J. Hanson. Positive and negative conditioning of self-references. Unpublished study, 1963b.

Gottschalk, L. A., and G. C. Gleser. Distinguishing Characteristics of the Verbal Communications of Schizophrenic Patients, in *Disorders of Communication A.R.-N.M.D.*, 42: 400–413. Baltimore: William and Wilkins, 1964a.

Gottschalk, L. A., G. C. Gleser, T. L. D'Zmura, and I. B. Hanenson. Some psychophysiological relationships in hypertensive women. The effect of Hydrochlorothiazide on the relation of affect to blood pressure, *Psychosom. Med.*, 26: 610–617, 1964b.

Gottschalk, L. A., J. M. Cleghorn, and G. C. Gleser. Studies of inpatients with acute myocardial infarction and coronary insufficiency. Foundations Fund for Research in Psychiatry–Fluid Research Grant. Unpublished studies, 1964c.

Gottschalk, L. A., E. J. Hanson, J. Niemiller, and G. C. Gleser. Effect of personality or sex of interviewer on sexual references, self-references, and affect scores. Foundations Fund for Research in Psychiatry–Fluid Research Grant. Unpublished study, 1964d.

Gottschalk, L. A., G. C. Gleser, H. W. Wylie, Jr., and S. M. Kaplan. Effects of Imipramine on anxiety and hostility levels, *Psychopharmacologia*, 7: 303–310, 1965a.

Gottschalk, L. A., J. M. Cleghorn, G. C. Gleser, and J. M. Iacono. Studies of relationships of emotions to plasma lipids, *Psychosom. Med.*, 27: 102–111, 1965b.

Gottschalk, L. A., C. M. Winget, G. C. Gleser, and K. J. Springer. The Measurement of Emotional Changes During a Psychiatric Interview: A Working Model Toward Quantifying the Psychoanalytic Concept of Affect, in *Methods of Research in Psychotherapy*, ed. L. A. Gottschalk and A. H. Auerbach, New York: Appleton-Century-Crofts, 1966a.

Gottschalk, L. A., W. N. Stone, G. C. Gleser, and J. M. Iacono. Anxiety levels in dreams: Relation to changes in plasma free fatty acids, *Science*, 153: 654–657, 1966b.

Gottschalk, L. A., W. N. Stone, G. C. Gleser, and J. M. Iacono. Anxiety and plasma free fatty acids (FFA), *Life Sciences*, 8: 61–69, 1969.

Gottschalk, L. A., and E. C. Frank. Estimating the magnitude of anxiety from speech, *Behav. Sci.*, 12: 289–295, 1967.

Gottschalk, L. A., P. Mayerson, and A. Gottlieb. The prediction and evaluation of outcome in an emergency brief psychotherapy clinic, *J. Nerv. Ment. Dis.*, 144: 77–96, 1967.

Gottschalk, L. A., G. C. Gleser, W. N. Stone, and R. L. Kunkel. Studies of Psychoactive Drug Effects on Non-Psychiatric Patients. Measurement of Affective and Cognitive Changes by Content Analysis of Speech, in *Psychopharmacology of Drugs of Abuse*, ed. J. Wittenborn, W. Evans, N. Kline, and J. Cole. Springfield, Ill.: Charles C Thomas, 1968.

Gottschalk, L. A., G. C. Gleser, and W. A. Stone. Language as a measure of change in schizophrenia: Effect of a tranquilizer (phenothiazine derivative) on anxiety, hostility, and social alienation–personal disorganization in chronic schizophrenic patients. Presented at the *Symposium on Language and Thought in Schizophrenia, 1968*, Newport Beach, California, Nov. 21–24, 1968.

Gottschalk, L. A., C. N. Winget, and G. C. Gleser. *Manual of Instructions for Using the Gottschalk-Gleser Content Analysis Scales.* Berkeley and Los Angeles: University of California Press, 1969.

Greenacre, P., ed. *Affective Disorders: Psychoanalytic Contributions to Their Study.* New York: International Universities Press, Inc., 1953.

Grinker, R. R., Sr., J. Miller, M. Sabshin, R. Nunn, and J. C. Nunnally. *The Phenomena of Depressions.* New York: Paul B. Hoeber, Inc., 1961.

Guilford, J. P. *Personality.* New York: McGraw-Hill Co., 1959.

Gulliksen, H. *Theory of Mental Tests.* New York: John Wiley & Sons, 1950.

Hafner, A. J., and A. M. Kaplan. Hostility content analysis of the Rorschach and TAT, *J. Proj. Techn.*, 24: 137–143, 1960.

Hall, C. S., and R. L. Van de Castle. *The Content Analysis of Dreams.* New York: Appleton-Century-Crofts, 1966.

Halstead, W. C. *Brain and Intelligence*, pp. 206 f. Chicago: University of Chicago Press, 1947.

Hambidge, G., Jr., and L. A. Gottschalk. Verbal Behavior Analysis—Psychodynamic, Structural, and Temporal Correlates of Specific Variables, in *Psychopathology of Communication*, ed. P. H. Hoch and J. Zubin. New York: Grune and Stratton, Inc., 1958.

Hamburg, D. A. Plasma and Urinary Corticosteroid Levels in Naturally Occurring Psychological Stresses, in *Ultra Structure and Metabolism of the Nervous System*, pp. 406–413, ed. S. Korey. Baltimore: William and Wilkins, 1962.

Havel, R. J., and A. Goldfien. Role of the sympathetic nervous system in the metabolism of the free fatty acids, *J. Lipid Res.*, 1: 102, 1960.

Hoijer, H., ed. *Language in Culture.* Chicago: University of Chicago Press, 1954.

Holsti, O. R., J. K. Loomba, and R. C. North. Content Analysis, in *The Handbook of Social Psychology*, ed. G. Lindzey and E. Aronson. Cambridge, Mass.: Addison-Wesley, 1967.

Horney, K. *Our Inner Conflicts. A Constructive Theory of Neurosis.* New York: W. W. Norton and Co., Inc., 1945.

Hunt, E. B. *Concept Learning: An Information Processing Problem.* New York: John Wiley & Sons, 1962.

Hurley, J. R. The Iowa picture interpretation test: A multiple choice version of the TAT, *J. Consult. Psychol.*, 19: 372–376, 1955.

Iversen, L. L. Inhibition of norepinephrine uptake by drugs, *J. Pharm. Pharmacol.*, 17: 62, 1965.

Ivey, M. E., and J. M. Bardwick. Patterns of affective fluctuation in the menstrual cycle, *Psychosom. Med.*, 30: 336–345, 1968.

Jacobson, E. Contribution to the Metapsychology of Cyclothymic Depression, in *Affective Disorders: Psychoanalytic Contributions to Their Study*, ed. P. Greenacre. New York: International Universities Press, 1953.

Jaffe, J. Language of the dyad: A method of interaction analysis in psychiatric interviews, *Psychiat.*, 21: 249–258, 1958.

———. Dyadic Analysis of Two Psychotherapeutic Interviews, in *Comparative Psycholinguistic Analysis of Two Psychotherapeutic Interviews*, pp. 73–90, ed. L. A. Gottschalk. New York: International Universities Press, 1961.

———. Verbal Behavior Analysis in Psychiatric Interviews with the Aid of Digital Computers, in *Disorders of Communication A.R.N.M.D.*, vol. 42. Baltimore: William and Wilkins Co., 1964.

Jenkins, R. L. The schizophrenic sequence: Withdrawal, disorganization, psychotic reorganization, *Am. J. Orthopsychiat.*, 22: 738–748, 1952.

Johnson, L. C. Some attributes of spontaneous autonomic activity, *J. Compr. Physiol. Psychol.*, 56: 415–422, 1963.

Johnson, W. Studies in language behavior, I, A program of research, *Psychol. Monogr.*, 56: 1–15, 1944.

Kamano, O. K., and D. J. Arp. Effects of chlordiazepoxide (Librium) on the acquisition and extinction of avoidance responses, *Psychopharmacologia*, 6: 112–119, 1964.

Kaplan, S. M., L. A. Gottschalk, and D. E. Fleming. Modifications of oropharyngeal bacteria with changes in the psychodynamic state. A preliminary study, *Arch. Neurol. Psychiat.*, 78: 656–664, 1957.

Kaplan, S. M., and L. A. Gottschalk. Modifications of the oropharyngeal bacteria with changes in the psychodynamic state, II, A validation study, *Psychosom. Med.*, 20: 314–320, 1958.

Kaplan, S. M., L. A. Gottschalk, E. B. Magliocco, D. D. Rohovit, and W. D. Ross. Hostility in verbal productions and hypnotic dreams of hypertensive patients: Studies of groups and individuals, *Psychosom. Med.*, 23: 311–322, 1961.

Kapp, F. T., M. Rosenbaum, and J. Romano. Psychological factors in men with peptic ulcers, *Am. J. Psychiat.*, 103: 700–704, 1947.

Kapp, F. T., and L. A. Gottschalk. Drug Therapy, ch. 32, in *Progress in Neurology and Psychiatry*, 17: 536–538. New York: Grune and Stratton, Inc., 1962.

Karacan, I., D. R. Goodenough, A. Shapiro, and S. Starker. Erection cycle during sleep in relation to dream anxiety, *Arch. Gen. Psychiat.*, 15: 183–189, 1966.

Kasanin, J. S., ed. *Language and Thought in Schizophrenia.* Berkeley: University of California Press, 1946.

Katkin, E. S. Relationship between manifest anxiety and two indices of autonomic response to stress, *J. Personal. Soc. Psychol.*, 2: 324–333, 1965.

Kelley, J. Q., and D. I. Gisvold. The use of MMPI in the evaluation of Librium, *Colorado GP*, 2: 3–8, 1960.

Kierkegaard, S. *The Concept of Dread.* Trans. W. Lowrie. Originally published in Danish, 1844. Princeton: Princeton University Press, 1944.

Klages, W. Produktive hyponoische Sprachenthemmung (Ein Beitrag zur Sprach-psychopathologie Schizophrener), *Arch. Psychiat.*, 192: 383–392, 1954.

Knapp, P. H., ed. *Expression of the Emotions in Man.* New York: International Universities Press, 1963.

Knapp, P. H., C. Mushatt, and S. J. Nemetz. Collection and Utilization of Data in a Psychoanalytic Psychosomatic Study, in *Methods of Research in Psychotherapy*, ed. L. A. Gottschalk and A. H. Auerbach. New York: Appleton-Century-Crofts, 1966.

Kraeplin, E. *Lectures on Clinical Psychiatry.* New York: William Wood and Co., 1904.

Krakowski, A. J. Chlordiazepoxide in treatment of children with emotional disturbances, *New York J. Med.*, 63: 3388–3392, 1963.

Kramer, E. Judgment of personal characteristics and emotions from nonverbal properties of speech, *Psychol. Bull.*, 60: 408–420, 1963.

Krasner, L. Behavior Modification Research and the Role of the Therapist, in *Methods of Research in Psychotherapy*, ed. L. A. Gottschalk and A. H. Auerbach. New York: Appleton-Century-Crofts, 1966.

Krause, M. S. The measurement of transitory anxiety, *Psychol. Rev.*, 68: 178–189, 1961.

Krayer, O., ed. *Symposium on Catecholamines.* Held at the National Institutes of Health, U.S. Department of Health, Education, and Welfare, Bethesda, Md., October 16–18, 1958. Baltimore: William and Wilkins Co., 1959.

Kunkel, R. L., and L. A. Gottschalk. Hope and denial in metastatic carcinoma—a preliminary report. Presented at the 11th Annual Conference V.A. Cooperative Studies in Psychiatry, New Orleans, La., March, 1966. *U.S. Medicine*, 2: 31, 1966.

Lacey, J. T. Psychophysiological Approaches to the Evaluation of Psychotherapeutic Process and Outcome, in *Research in Psychotherapy*, ed. E. A. Rubinstein and M. B. Parloff. Washington, D.C.: National Publishing Co., 1959.

Lauterbach, C. G. The Taylor A Scale and clinical measures of anxiety, *J. Consult. Psychol.*, 22: 314, 1958.

Leary, T. *Interpersonal Diagnosis of Personality: A Functional Theory and Methodology for Personality Evaluation.* New York: The Ronald Press Co., 1957.

Leary, T., and M. Gill. The Dimensions and a Measure of the Process of Psychotherapy: A System for the Analysis of the Content of Clinical Evaluations and Patient-Therapist Verbalizations, in *Research in Psychotherapy*, ed. E. A. Rubinstein and M. B. Parloff. Washington, D.C.: National Publishing Co., 1959.

Leconte, S., and J. Orval. Analyse de l'action du Librium sur le comportement d'enfants inadapte's, *Ann. Med. Psychol.*, 1: 139, 1963.

Levitt, E. E., H. Persky, and J. P. Brady. *Hypnotic Induction: A Psychoendocrine Investigation.* Springfield, Ill.: Charles C Thomas, 1964.

Lorenz, M. Language as expressive behavior, *Arch. Neurol. Psychiat.*, 70: 277–285, 1953.

———. Expressive behavior and language patterns, *Psychiat.*, 18: 353–366, 1955.

Lorenz, M., and S. Cobb. Language patterns in psychotic and psychoneurotic subjects, *Arch. Neurol. Psychiat.*, 72: 665–673, 1954.

Lorr, M., D. M. McNair, W. W. Michaux, and A. Raskin. Frequency of treatment and change in psychotherapy, *J. Abnorm. Soc. Psychol.*, 64: 281–292, 1961.

Lorr, M., D. M. McNair, and G. J. Weinstein. Early effects of chlordiazepoxide (Librium) used with psychotherapy, *J. Psychiat. Res.*, 1: 257–270, 1962.

Lorr, M., C. J. Klett, D. M. McNair, and J. J. Lasky. *Inpatient Multidimensional Psychiatric Scale: Manual.* Palo Alto, Calif.: Consulting Psychological Press, 1963.

Lorr, M., and D. M. McNair. Methods Relating to Evaluation of Therapeutic Outcome, in *Methods of Research in Psychotherapy*, ed. L. A. Gottschalk and A. H. Auerbach. New York: Appleton-Century-Crofts, 1966.

Lubin, B. Fourteen brief depression adjective check lists, *Arch. Gen. Psychiat.*, 15: 205–208, 1966.

MacLean, P. D. The limbic system (visceral brain) in relation to central gray and reticulum of the brain stem. Evidence of interdependence in emotional processes, *Psychosom. Med.*, 17: 355–366, 1955.

MacLeod, J. A., and L. W. Tinnin. Special service project: A solution to problems of early access, brief psychotherapy, *Arch. Gen. Psychiat.*, 15: 190–197, 1966.

Mahl, G. F. Disturbance and silences in the patient's speech in psychotherapy, *J. Abnorm. Soc. Psychol.*, 53: 1–15, 1956.

———. Exploring Emotional States by Content Analysis, in *Trends in Content Analysis*, ed. I. D. Pool. Urbana: University of Illinois Press, 1959.

———. Measures of Two Expressive Aspects of a Patient's Speech in Two Psychotherapeutic Interviews, in *Comparative Psycholinguistic Analysis of Two Psychotherapeutic Interviews*, pp. 91–114, ed. L. A. Gottschalk. New York: International Universities Press, 1961.

McGuigan, F. J. The experimenter: A neglected stimulus object, *Psychol. Bull.*, 4: 421–428, 1963.

McQuown, N. A. Linguistic transcription and specification of psychiatric interview material, *Psychiat.*, 20: 79–86, 1957.

Mandler, G., and S. B. Sarason. A study of anxiety and learning, *J. Abnorm. Soc. Psychol.*, 47: 166–173, 1952.

Marsden, G. Content-analysis studies of therapeutic interviews: 1954 to 1964, *Psychol. Bull.*, 68: 298–321, 1965.

Mason, J. W., F. E. Wherry, J. V. Brady, G. A. Tolliver, A. C. Goodman, and B. Beer. Psychological influences on plasma insulin levels in monkeys. Presented at the Annual Meeting of the American Psychosomatic Society, Chicago, Ill., 1966.

Masserman, J. H. *Behavior and Neurosis.* Chicago: Chicago University Press, 1943.

Mathews, M. V., and L. E. McMahon. Computers and English Text, in *The Human Use of Computing Machines: Proceedings of a Symposium Concerned with Diverse Ways of Enhancing Perception and Intuition.* Murray Hill, N.J.: Bell Telephone Laboratories, 1966.

May, R. *The Meaning of Anxiety.* New York: The Ronald Press Co., 1950.

Mednick, M. T., and O. W. Lindsley. Some clinical correlates of operant behavior, *J. Abnorm. Soc. Psychol.*, 57: 13–16, 1958.

Miller, C. K. Psychological correlates of coronary artery disease, *Psychosom. Med.*, 27: 257–265, 1965.

Mirin, B. The formal aspects of schizophrenic verbal communication, *Genet. Psychol. Monogr.*, 52: 149–190, 1955.

Mirsky, I. A., R. E. Miller, and J. V. Murphy. The communication of affect in Rhesus monkeys, I, An experimental method, *J. Amer. Psa. Assn.*, 6: 433–441, 1958.

Mittenecker, E. New quantitative method of speech analysis. Application to schizophrenics, *Monatsschr. Psychiat. Neurol.*, 121: 364–375, 1951.

Moldawski, P. A study of personality variables in patients with skin disorders. Unpublished doctor's dissertation, Iowa State University, 1953.

Moses, P. *The Voice of Neurosis.* New York: Grune and Stratton, Inc., 1954.

Mueller, P. S., and D. Horwitz. Plasma free fatty acid and blood glucose responses to analogues of norepinephrine in man, *J. Lipid Res.,* 3: 251, 1962.

Mulligan, J. F., and D. F. McDonald. Some recent determinations of the velocity of light, II, *Am. J. Physics.,* 25: 180–192, 1957.

Murray, H. A. *Thematic Apperception Test: Manual.* Cambridge, Mass.: Harvard University Press, 1943.

Murray, J. A content analysis method for studying psychotherapy, *Psychol. Monogr.,* 70: #13, 1956.

Murstein, B. I. The projection of hostility on the Rorschach and as a result of ego-threat, *J. Proj. Techn.,* 20: 418–428, 1956.

Muscholl, E. The action of nialamide on the concentration of catecholamines in heart and brain stem, *Medicina Experimentalis,* 1: 363–367, 1959.

Nowlin, J. B., W. G. Troyer, W. S. Collins, G. Silverman, C. R. Nichols, H. D. McIntosh, E. H. Estes, Jr., and M. D. Bogdonoff. The association of nocturnal angina pectoris with dreaming, *Ann. Int. Med.,* 63: 1040–1046, 1965.

Nowlis, V., and H. H. Nowlis. The description and analysis of mood, *Ann. New York Acad. Sci.,* 65: 345–355, 1956.

Oken, D. An experimental study of suppressed anger and blood pressure, *Arch. Gen. Psychiat.,* 2: 441–456, 1960.

Orr, Douglas W. Transference and countertransference: A historical survey, *J. Amer. Psa. Assn.,* 2: 621–670, 1954.

Ostwald, P. F. *Soundmaking. The Acoustic Communication of Emotion.* Springfield, Ill.: Charles C Thomas, 1963.

Overall, J. E., and D. P. Gorham. The brief psychiatric rating scale, *Psychol. Rpts.,* 10: 799–812, 1962.

Paige, J. M. Automated content analysis of "Letters From Jenny." A study in individual personality. Unpublished paper, Department of Social Relations, Harvard University, 1964.

Persky, H., D. A. Hamburg, H. Bosowitz, R. R. Grinker, M. Sabshin, S. J. Korchin, M. Herz, F. A. Board, and H. A. Heath. Relation of emotional responses and changes in plasma hydrocortisone level after stressful interview, *Arch. Neurol. Psychiat.,* 79: 434–447, 1958.

Persky, H., M. Zuckerman, G. K. Basu, and D. Thornton. Psychoendocrine effects of perceptual and social isolation, *Arch. Gen. Psychiat.,* 15: 499–505, 1966.

Piers, G., and M. D. Singer. *Shame and Guilt.* Springfield, Ill.: Charles C Thomas, 1953.

Pittenger, R. E., and H. L. Smith, Jr. A basis for some contributions of linguistics to psychiatry, *Psychiat.,* 20: 61–78, 1957.

Pittenger, R. E., C. F. Hockett, and J. J. Danehy. *The First Five Minutes.* Ithaca, N.Y.: Paul Martineau, 1960.

Pool, I. D. Trends in Content Analysis Today: A Summary, in *Trends in Content Analysis,* ed. I. D. Pool. Urbana: University of Illinois Press, 1959.

Presti, A. J. High-speed sound spectrograph, *J. Acoustical Society of America,* 40: 628–634, 1966.

Randall, L. O. Pharmacology of chlordiazepoxide (Librium), *Dis. Nerv. Syst.,* 22 (Suppl.): 7–15, 1961.

Randall, L. O., W. Schallek, G. A. Heise, E. F. Keith, and R. E. Bagdon. The psychosedative properties of methaminodiazepoxide, *J. Pharmacol. Exp. Therap.,* 129: 163–171, 1960.

Rechtschaffen, A., and P. Verdone. Amount of dreaming: Effect of incentive, adaptation to laboratory and individual differences. Presented at the Fourth Annual Meeting of the Association for Psychophysiological Sleep, Palo Alto, Calif., 1964.

Reitan, R. M. Validity of the trail-making test as an indicator of organic brain damage, *Percept. Mot. Skills,* 8: 271–276, 1958.

Rosen, I. M. Defense and communication in the language of schizophrenia, *Dis. Nerv. Syst.,* 16: 315–317, 1955.

Rosenthal, R. The Effect of the Experimenter on the Results of Psychological Research, in *Progress in Experimental Personality Research*, vol. 1, ed. B. A. Maher. New York: Academic Press, Inc., 1964.

Rosenzweig, S. Revised norms for the adult form of the Rosenzweig Picture-Frustration Study, *J. Person.*, 3: 344–346, 1950.

———. Validity of the Rosenzweig Picture-Frustration Study with felons and delinquents, *J. Consult. Psychol.*, 27: 535–536, 1963.

Rosenzweig, S., E. E. Fleming, and H. J. Clarke. Revised scoring manual for the Rosenzweig Picture-Frustration Study, *J. Psychol.*, 24: 165–208, 1947.

Ross, W. D., N. Adsett, G. C. Gleser, C. R. B. Joyce, S. M. Kaplan, and M. E. Tieger. A trial of psychopharmacologic measurement with projective techniques, *J. Proj. Techn.*, 27: 223–225, 1963.

Sachar, E. J., J. W. Mason, H. S. Kolmer, Jr., and K. L. Artiss. Psychoendocrine aspects of acute schizophrenic reactions, *Psychosom. Med.*, 25: 510–537, 1963.

Salzinger, K., and S. Salzinger, eds. *Research in Verbal Behavior and Some Neurophysiological Implications.* New York: Academic Press, 1967.

Saporta, S. Preface, in *Psycholinguistics*, ed. S. Saporta. New York: Holt, Rinehart and Winston, 1961.

Saporta, S., and T. A. Sebeok. Linguistics and Content Analysis, Ch. 4, in *Trends in Content Analysis*, ed. I. D. Pool. Urbana: University of Illinois Press, 1959.

Sarason, I. G. Empirical findings and theoretical problems in the use of anxiety scales, *Psychol. Bull.*, 57: 403–415, 1960.

Sargent, H. D. Intrapsychic change: Methodological problems in psychotherapy research, *Psychiat.*, 24: 93–108, 1961.

Saul, L. J., E. Sheppard, D. Selby, W. Lhamon, B. Sachs, and R. Master. The quantification of hostility in dreams with reference to essential hypertension, *Science*, 119: 382–383, 1954.

Schachter, J. Pain, fear, and anger in hypertensives and normotensives, *Psychosom. Med.*, 19: 17–29, 1957.

Scheflen, A. E. On the significance of posture in communication systems, *Psychiat.*, 27: 316–331, 1964.

———. Natural History Method in Psychotherapy: Communicational Research, in *Methods of Research in Psychotherapy*, pp. 263–289, ed. L. A. Gottschalk and A. H. Auerbach. New York: Appleton-Century-Crofts, 1966.

Schultz, S. D. A differentiation of several forms of hostility by scales empirically constructed from significant items on the Minnesota Multiphasic Personality Inventory. Unpublished doctor's dissertation, Pennsylvania State College, 1954.

Scott, J. Blood plasma free fatty acids and sleep. Presented at the Fifth Annual Meeting of the Association for the Psychophysiological Study of Sleep, Washington, D.C., 1965.

Seitz, P. F. D. The effects of infantile experiences upon adult behavior in animal subjects, I, Effects of litter size during infancy upon adult behavior in the rat, *Am. J. Psychiat.*, 110: 916–927, 1954.

———. Infantile experience and adult behavior in animal subjects. II. Age of separation from the mother and adult behavior in the cat. *Psychosom. Med.*, 21: 353–378, 1959.

———. The Consensus Problem in Psychoanalytic Research, in *Methods of Research in Psychotherapy*, ed. L. A. Gottschalk and A. H. Auerbach. New York: Appleton-Century-Crofts, 1966.

Shneidman, E. S., and N. L. Farberow. *Clues to Suicide*. New York: McGraw-Hill, 1957.

Sholiton, L., T. Wohl, and E. Werk. The correlation of two psychological variables, anxiety and hostility, with adrenal cortical function in patients with lung cancer, *Cancer*, 16: 223–230, 1963.

Shore, P. A. Recent biochemical developments with monoamine oxidase inhibitors, *Dis. Nerv. Syst.*, 21 (Suppl.) : 62–63, 1960.

———. Release of serotonin and catecholamines by drugs, *Pharmacol. Rev.*, 14: 531–550, 1962.

Siegel, S. M. The relationship of hostility to authoritarianism, *J. Abnorm. Soc. Psychol.*, 52: 368–373, 1956.

Silverman, J. Scanning control mechanism and "cognitive filtering" in paranoid and non-paranoid schizophrenia, *J. Consult. Psychol.*, 28: 385–395, 1964.

Silverman, J., P. S. D. Berg, and R. Kantor. Some perceptual correlates of institutionalization, *J. Nerv. Ment. Dis.*, 141: 651–657, 1965.

Sjoerdoma, A., and S. Undenfriend. Pharmacology and biochemistry of a-methyl-DOPA in man and experimental animals (Abstract), *Biochem. Pharmacol.*, 8: 164, 1961.

Sloane, R. B., J. Inglis, and R. W. Payne. Personal traits and maternal attitudes in relation to blood lipid levels, *Psychosom. Med.*, 24: 278, 1962.

Smith, J. G. Influence of failure, expressed hostility, and stimulus characteristics on verbal learning and recognition, *J. Person.*, 22: 475–493, 1954.

Snyder, F. Progress in the new biology of dreaming, *Am. J. Psychiat.*, 122: 377–391, 1965.

Sperry, W. M., and M. Webb. A revision of the Schoenheimer-Sperry method for cholesterol determination, *J. Biol. Chem.*, 187: 97, 1950.

Spitzer, R. L. Immediate available record of mental status exam, *Arch. Gen. Psychiat.*, 13: 76–78, 1965.

————. The mental status schedule: Potential use as a criterion measure of change in psychotherapy research, *Am. J. Psychol.*, 20: 156, 1966.

Spitzer, R. L., J. L. Fleiss, E. I. Burdock, and A. S. Hardesty. The mental status schedule: Rationale, reliability, and validity, *Comp. Psychiat.*, 5: 384–395, 1964.

Spitzer, R. L., J. L. Fleiss, W. Kernohan, J. C. Lee, and I. T. Baldwin. Mental Status Schedule, *Arch. Gen. Psychiat.*, 13: 448–455, 1965.

Spitzer, R. L., J. L. Fleiss, J. Endicott, and J. Cohen. Mental status schedule: Properties of factor analytically derived scales, *Arch. Gen. Psychiat.*, 16: 479–493, 1967.

Starkweather, J. A. The communication value of content-free speech, *Am. J. Psychol.*, 69: 121–123, 1956a.

————. Content-free speech as a source of information about the speaker, *J. Abnorm. Soc. Psychol.*, 52: 394–402, 1956b.

Stone, H. The TAT aggressive content scale, *J. Proj. Techn.*, 20: 445–452, 1956.

Stone, P. J. Letters to a psychiatrist: An analysis of the writings of Eve White, Eve Black, and Jane. Unpublished paper, Department of Social Relations, Harvard University. Presented at the American College of Neuropsychopharmacology, Washington, D.C., January, 1963.

Stone, P. J., R. F. Bales, J. Z. Namewirth, and D. M. Ogilvie. The general inquirer: A computer system for content analysis and retrieval based on the sentence as a unit of information, *Behav. Sci.*, 7: 484–498, 1962.

Stone, P. J., and E. B. Hunt. A Computer Approach to Content Analysis: Studies Using the General Inquirer System, in *Proceedings of the Western Management Science Institute—Spring Joint Computer Conference*, Reprint #7, 241–256. Graduate School of Business Administration, University of California, Los Angeles, 1963.

Stone, P. J., D. C. Dunphy, M. S. Smith, and D. M. Ogilvie. *The General Inquirer: A Computer Approach to Content Analysis.* Cambridge, Mass.: The M.I.T. Press, 1967.

Strupp, H. H., J. B. Chassan, and J. A. Ewing. Toward the Longitudinal Study of the Psychotherapeutic Process, in *Methods of Research in Psychotherapy*, pp. 361–400, ed. L. A. Gottschalk and A. H. Auerbach. New York: Appleton-Century-Crofts, 1966.

Sullivan, H. S. *Schizophrenia as a Human Process.* New York: W. W. Norton and Co., Inc., 1962.

Taylor, J. A. A personality scale of manifest anxiety, *J. Abnorm. Soc. Psychol.*, 48: 285–290, 1953.

Taylor, W. L. Cloze procedure: A new procedure for measuring readability, *Journalism Quart.*, 30: 415–433, 1956.

Thewlis, J., ed. *Encyclopedic Dictionary of Physics*, 5: 345. Oxford: Pergamon Press Ltd., 1962.

Tillich, P. Existential philosophy, *J. Hist. Ideas*, 5: 44–70, 1944.

Trager, G. L. Paralanguage: A first approximation, *Studies in Linguistics*, 13: 1–12, 1958.

――――. Language and Psychotherapy, in *Methods of Research in Psychotherapy*, ed. L. A. Gottschalk and A. H. Auerbach. New York: Appleton-Century-Crofts, 1966.

Trout, D. L., E. H. Estes, Jr., and S. J. Friedberg. Titration of FFA of plasma: A study of current methods and a new modification, *J. Lipid. Res.*, 1: 199, 1960.

Von Euler, U. S., and F. Lishajko. Effect of some drugs on noradrenaline release from nerve granules (Abstract), *Biochem. Pharmacol.*, 8: 62, 1961.

Walker, R. G. A comparison of clinical manifestations of hostility with Rorschach and MAPS test performance, *J. Proj. Techn.*, 15: 444–460, 1951.

Waskow, I. The Effects of Drugs on Speech: A Review, in *Research in Verbal Behavior and Some Neurophysiological Implications*, ed. K. Salzinger and S. Salzinger. New York: Academic Press, 1967.

Weiner, H., M. F. Reiser, M. Thaler, and I. A. Mirsky. Etiology of duodenal ulcer, I, Relation of specific psychological characteristics to rate of gastric secretion (serum pepsinogen), *Psychosom. Med.*, 19: 1–10, 1957.

Welsh, G. S. Factor Dimensions A and B, in *Basic Readings on the M.M.P.I. in Psychology and Medicine*, ed. G. S. Welsh and G. W. Dahlstrom. Minneapolis: University of Minnesota Press, 1956.

Welsh, G. S., and W. G. Dahlstrom, eds. *Basic Readings on the M.M.P.I. in Psychology and Medicine*. Minneapolis: University of Minnesota Press, 1956.

White, M. A. A study of schizophrenic language, *J. Abnorm. Soc. Psychol.*, 44: 61–74, 1949.

Wilensky, H., and L. Solomon. Characteristics of untestable chronic schizophrenics, *J. Abnorm. Soc. Psychol.*, 61: 155–158, 1960.

Winget, C. N., G. C. Gleser, and W. H. Clements. A method for quantifying human relations, hostility, and anxiety applied to TAT productions, *J. Proj. Techn. & Pers. Assess.* (in press), 1969.

Wirt, R. D. Ideational expression of hostile impulses, *J. Consult. Psychol.*, 20: 185–189, 1956.

Witkin, H. A. Individual differences in use of perception of embedded figures, *J. Person.*, 19: 1–15, 1950.

――――. Experimental manipulation of the cognitive and emotional content of dreams, in *Dream Psychology and the New Biology of Dreaming*, ed. M. Kramer and R. Whitman. New York: Grune and Stratton, 1969.

Witkin, H. A., H. B. Lewis, M. Hertzman, K. Machover, P. B. Messner, and S. Wapner. *Personality Through Perception*. New York: Harper, 1954.

Witkin, H. A., H. F. Faterson, D. R. Goodenough, and S. A. Karp. *Psychological Differentiation*. New York: John Wiley & Sons, 1962.

Witkin, H. A., and H. B. Lewis. The relation of experimentally induced presleep experiences to dreams: A report on method and preliminary findings, *J. Amer. Psa. Assn.*, 13: 819–849, 1965.

Witkin, H. A., H. B. Lewis, and E. Weil. Shame and guilt reactions of more differentiated and less differentiated patients early in therapy. Presented at the Annual Meeting of the American Psychological Association, New York, 1966.

Witkin, H. A., H. B. Lewis, and E. Weil. Affective reactions and patient-therapist interactions among more differentiated and less differentiated patients early in therapy, *J. Nerv. Ment. Dis.*, 146: 193–208, 1968.

Wittenborn, J. R. *Wittenborn Psychiatric Rating Scales*. New York: The Psychological Corp., 1955.

Wolff, C. T., S. B. Friedman, M. A. Hafer, and J. W. Mason. Relationship between psychological defenses and mean urinary 17-hydroxycorticosteroid excretion rates, Part I, A predictive study of parents of fatally ill children, *Psychosom. Med.*, 26: 576–591, 1964.

Wonderlic, E. F. *Wonderlic Personnel Test Manual.* Norfield, Ill.: 1945.

Wynne, L. C., and M. T. Singer. Thought disorder and family relations of schizophrenics. 1. A research strategy, *Arch. Gen. Psychiat.,* 9: 191–198, 1963a.

———. Thought disorder and family relations of schizophrenics. 2. A classification of forms of thinking, *Arch. Gen. Psychiat.,* 9: 199–206, 1963b.

———. Thought disorder and family relations of schizophrenics. 3. Methodology using projective techniques. 4. Results and implications, *Arch. Gen. Psychiat.,* 12: 187–212, 1965.

Zbinder, G., L. O. Randall, and R. A. Moe. Clinical and pharmacological considerations on mode of action of monoamine oxidase inhibitors, *Dis. Nerv. Syst.,* 21 (Suppl.) : 89–100, 1960.

Zegans, L., J. C. Pollard, and D. Brown. The effects of LSD-25 on creativity and tolerance to regression, *Arch. Gen. Psychiat.,* 16: 740–749, 1967.

Zubin, J., C. Windle, and V. Hamwi. Retrospective psychologic tests as prognostic instruments in mental disorders, *J. Person.,* 21: 342–355, 1953.

Zuckerman, M. The development of an affect adjective check list for the measurement of anxiety, *J. Consult. Psychol.,* 24: 457–462, 1960.

INDEX OF AUTHORS

INDEX OF SUBJECTS